Clinical Atlas in Endocrinology and Diabetes
A Case-Based Compendium

Clinical Atlas in Endocrinology and Diabetes
A Case-Based Compendium

Editors

Nihal Thomas MBBS MD (Gen Med) MNAMS DNB (Endo) FRACP (Endo) FRCP (Edin) FRCP (Glas)
Professor and Head
Department of Endocrinology, Diabetes and Metabolism
Vice-Principal (Research)
Christian Medical College, Vellore, Tamil Nadu, India

Felix Jebasingh K MBBS MD (Gen Med)
Senior Resident
Department of Endocrinology, Diabetes and Metabolism
Christian Medical College, Vellore, Tamil Nadu, India

Associate Editors

Simon Rajaratnam MBBS MD (Gen Med) DNB (Endo) MNAMS FRACP (Endo) Phd (Endo) FRCP (EDIN)
Professor
Department of Endocrinology, Diabetes and Metabolism
Christian Medical College, Vellore, Tamil Nadu, India

Thomas V Paul MBBS MD (Gen Med) DNB (Endo) PhD (Endo)
Professor
Department of Endocrinology, Diabetes and Metabolism
Christian Medical College, Vellore, Tamil Nadu, India

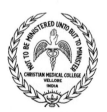

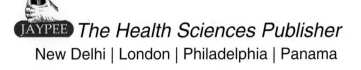

JAYPEE *The Health Sciences Publisher*
New Delhi | London | Philadelphia | Panama

Jaypee Brothers Medical Publishers (P) Ltd

Headquarters
Jaypee Brothers Medical Publishers (P) Ltd.
4838/24, Ansari Road, Daryaganj
New Delhi 110 002, India
Phone: +91-11-43574357
Fax: +91-11-43574314
E-mail: jaypee@jaypeebrothers.com

Overseas Offices
J.P. Medical Ltd.
83, Victoria Street, London
SW1H 0HW (UK)
Phone: +44-20 3170 8910
Fax: +44(0)20 3008 6180
E-mail: info@jpmedpub.com

Jaypee Medical Inc.
325 Chestnut Street
Suite 412
Philadelphia, PA 19106, USA
Phone: +1 267-519-9789
E-mail: support@jpmedus.com

Jaypee-Highlights Medical Publishers Inc.
City of Knowledge, Bld. 237, Clayton
Panama City, Panama
Phone: +1 507-301-0496
Fax: +1 507-301-0499
E-mail: cservice@jphmedical.com

Jaypee Brothers Medical Publishers (P) Ltd.
17/1-B, Babar Road, Block-B, Shaymali
Mohammadpur, Dhaka-1207
Bangladesh
Mobile: +08801912003485
E-mail: jaypeedhaka@gmail.com

Jaypee Brothers Medical Publishers (P) Ltd.
Bhotahity, Kathmandu, Nepal
Phone: +977-9741283608
E-mail: kathmandu@jaypeebrothers.com

Website: www.jaypeebrothers.com
Website: www.jaypeedigital.com

Inquiries for bulk sales may be solicited at: jaypee@jaypeebrothers.com

Clinical Atlas in Endocrinology and Diabetes: A Case-Based Compendium

First Edition: **2016**

ISBN: 978-93-5152-857-9

Printed at Ajanta Offset & Packagings Ltd., New Delhi

Dedication

This compendium is dedicated to all those doctors and colleagues whom we have worked with in the last 20 years in the history of the endocrinology department at Christian Medical College, Vellore, Tamil Nadu, India (CMC). We have partnered with many individuals over this period of time. There have many struggles and many peaks and valleys over the years. The patients we have treated have been beneficiaries of the care at Christian Medical College, Vellore, Tamil Nadu, India. In turn, the knowledge that they have imparted to us in many ways, has lead to the evolution of this book. We would like to thank our teachers, whom we have had the privilege of rubbing shoulders with: Prof MS Seshadri, Prof Aravindan Nair and many others, who have laid the foundations of a rich endocrine legacy in our institution.

Chapter 1: The Terrific Thyroid

Felix Jebasingh K
MBBS MD (Gen Med)
Senior Resident
Department of Endocrinology
Diabetes and Metabolism
Christian Medical College
Vellore, Tamil Nadu, India

Nihal Thomas
MBBS MD (Gen Med) MNAMS DNB (Endo)
FRACP (Endo) FRCP (Edin) FRCP (Glas)
Professor and Head
Department of Endocrinology
Diabetes and Metabolism
Vice Principal (Research)
Christian Medical College
Vellore, Tamil Nadu, India

Anuradha Chandramohan
MBBS MD (Radiology)
DNB (Radiology), FRCR
Department of Radiology
Christian Medical College
Vellore, Tamil Nadu, India

Deepak Abraham
MBBS MS (Gen Sur)
PhD (Endocrine Surgery)
Professor
Department of Endocrine Surgery
Christian Medical College
Vellore, Tamil Nadu, India

Isaac Frank MBBS
Research Officer
Department of Endocrinology
Diabetes and Metabolism
Christian Medical College
Vellore, Tamil Nadu, India

Dukhabhandu Naik
MBBS MD (Gen Med) DM (Endo)
Associate Professor
Department of Endocrinology
Diabetes and Metabolism
Christian Medical College
Vellore, Tamil Nadu, India

Regi Oommen
MBBS DMRT MD (Radiotherapy)
DRM (Nuclear Medicine)
Professor
Department of Nuclear Medicine
Christian Medical College
Vellore, Tamil Nadu, India

Nylla Shanthly
MBBS DRM (Nuclear Medicine)
Professor
Department of Nuclear Medicine
Christian Medical College
Vellore, Tamil Nadu, India

Jasmine John Ponvelil MBBS
Research Officer
Department of Endocrinology
Diabetes and Metabolism
Christian Medical College
Vellore, Tamil Nadu, India

Chapter 2: Diabolical Diabetes

Shilpa Mulky
MBBS MD (Gen Med) F.Diab (MGR Univ)
Tutor
Department of Endocrinology
Diabetes and Metabolism
Christian Medical College
Vellore, Tamil Nadu, India

Isaac Frank MBBS
Research Officer
Department of Endocrinology
Diabetes and Metabolism
Christian Medical College
Vellore, Tamil Nadu, India

Nihal Thomas
MBBS MD (Gen Med) MNAMS DNB (Endo)
FRACP (Endo) FRCP (Edin) FRCP (Glas)
Professor and Head
Department of Endocrinology
Diabetes and Metabolism
Vice Principal (Research)
Christian Medical College
Vellore, Tamil Nadu, India

Felix Jebasingh K
MBBS MD (Gen Med)
Senior Resident
Department of Endocrinology
Diabetes and Metabolism
Christian Medical College
Vellore, Tamil Nadu, India

DM Mahesh
MBBS MD (Gen Med) DM (Endo)
Assistant Professor
Department of Endocrinology
Diabetes and Metabolism
Christian Medical College
Vellore, Tamil Nadu, India

Chaitanya Murthy MBBS
Fellow in Diabetes
Department of Endocrinology
Diabetes and Metabolism
Christian Medical College
Vellore, Tamil Nadu, India

Jubbin Jagan Jacob
MBBS MD (Gen Med) DNB (Endo)
Associate Professor
Department of Endocrinology
Christian Medical College
Ludhiana, Punjab, India

Edwin Stephen
MBBS MS (Gen Surg)
FEVS (Vascular Surgery)
Professor and Head
Department of Vascular Surgery
Christian Medical College
Vellore, Tamil Nadu, India

Judy Ann John
MBBS MD (PMR) DNB (PMR)
Professor, Department of Physical
Medicine and Rehabilitation
Christian Medical College
Vellore, Tamil Nadu, India

Bobeena Rachel Chandy
MBBS MD (PMR) DNB (PMR)
Professor, Department of Physical
Medicine and Rehabilitation
Christian Medical College
Vellore, Tamil Nadu, India

Aaron Chapla MSc (Biochemistry)
Research Associate
Department of Endocrinology
Diabetes and Metabolism
Christian Medical College
Vellore, Tamil Nadu, India

Mercy Jesudoss MSC (N)
Reader in Nursing and
Nurse Manager
Department of Nursing services
Christian Medical College
Vellore, Tamil Nadu, India

Ruth Ruby Murray BSC (N)
Charge Nurse and Diabetes Educator
Department of Endocrinology
Diabetes and Metabolism
Christian Medical College
Vellore, Tamil Nadu, India

Mercy Inbakumari BSC (N)
Charge Nurse and Diabetes Educator
Department of Endocrinology
Diabetes and Metabolism
Christian Medical College
Vellore, Tamil Nadu, India

Bharathi S BSC (N)
Charge Nurse and Diabetes Educator
Department of Endocrinology
Diabetes and Metabolism
Christian Medical College
Vellore, Tamil Nadu, India

Sunitha RN
Diabetes Educator
Department of Endocrinology
Diabetes and Metabolism
Christian Medical College
Vellore, Tamil Nadu, India

Rajan P BOT
Department of Occupational Therapy
Christian Medical College
Vellore, Tamil Nadu, India

Prem Kumar R PHD
Department of Physiotherapy
Christian Medical College
Vellore, Tamil Nadu, India

Chapter 3: Aggressive Adrenal

Felix Jebasingh K
       MBBS MD (Gen Med)
Senior Resident
Department of Endocrinology
Diabetes and Metabolism
Christian Medical College
Vellore, Tamil Nadu, India

Nihal Thomas
MBBS MD (Gen Med) MNAMS DNB (Endo)
   FRACP (Endo) FRCP (Edin) FRCP (Glas)
Professor and Head
Department of Endocrinology
Diabetes and Metabolism
Vice Principal (Research)
Christian Medical College
Vellore, Tamil Nadu, India

MJ Paul
     MBBS MS (Gen Surg) DNB (Gen Surg)
Professor and Head
Department of Endocrine Surgery
Christian Medical College
Vellore, Tamil Nadu, India

Julie Hepzhibah
       MBBS MD (Radiotherapy) DNB
   (Radiotherapy) DNB (Nuclear Medicine)
Associate Professor
Department of Nuclear Medicine
Christian Medical College
Vellore, Tamil Nadu, India

Jambugulam Mohan MBBS
Junior Resident
Department of Medicine
Department of Nuclear Medicine
Christian Medical College
Vellore, Tamil Nadu, India

Chapter 4: Pituitary Passions

Nihal Thomas
MBBS MD (Gen Med) MNAMS DNB (Endo)
   FRACP (Endo) FRCP (Edin) FRCP (Glas)
Professor and Head
Department of Endocrinology
Diabetes and Metabolism
Vice Principal (Research)
Christian Medical College
Vellore, Tamil Nadu, India

Felix Jebasingh K
       MBBS MD (Gen Med)
Senior Resident, Department
of Endocrinology Diabetes
and Metabolism
Christian Medical College
Vellore, Tamil Nadu, India

Simon Rajaratnam
MBBS MD (Gen Med) DNB (Endo) MNAMS
   FRACP (Endo) Phd (Endo) FRCP (Edin)
Professor
Department of Endocrinology
Diabetes and Metabolism
Christian Medical College
Vellore, Tamil Nadu, India

Nitin Kapoor
   MBBS MD (Gen Med) DM (Endo) ABBM
     (USA) Post Doc Fellowship (Endo)
Assistant Professor
Department of Endocrinology
Diabetes and Metabolism
Christian Medical College
Vellore, Tamil Nadu, India

HS Asha
     MBBS DNB (Gen Med) DNB (Endo)
Associate Professor
Department of Endocrinology
Diabetes and Metabolism
Christian Medical College
Vellore, Tamil Nadu, India

Ari G Chacko
       MBBS MCH (Neurosurgery)
Professor and Head
Department of Neurosurgery
Christian Medical College
Vellore, Tamil Nadu, India

Sunithi Elizabeth Mani
   MBBS DMRD (Radiology) MD (Radiology)
Associate Professor
Department of Radiodiagnosis
Christian Medical College
Vellore, Tamil Nadu, India

Sniya Valsa Sudhakar
       MBBS DNB (Radiology)
Associate Professor
Department of Radiodiagnosis
Christian Medical College
Vellore, Tamil Nadu, India

Chapter 5: Bountiful Bone

Thomas V Paul

MBBS MD (Gen Med)
DNB (Endo) PhD (Endo)

Professor
Department of Endocrinology
Diabetes and Metabolism
Christian Medical College
Vellore, Tamil Nadu, India

Felix Jebasingh K

MBBS MD (Gen Med)

Senior Resident
Department of Endocrinology
Diabetes and Metabolism
Christian Medical College
Vellore, Tamil Nadu, India

Nihal Thomas

MBBS MD (Gen Med) MNAMS DNB (Endo)
FRACP (Endo) FRCP (Edin) FRCP (Glas)

Professor and Head
Department of Endocrinology
Diabetes and Metabolism
Vice Principal (Research)
Christian Medical College
Vellore, Tamil Nadu, India

Nitin Kapoor

MBBS MD (Gen Med) DM (Endo)
ABBM (USA) Post Doc
Fellowship (Endo)

Assistant Professor
Department of Endocrinology
Diabetes and Metabolism
Christian Medical College
Vellore, Tamil Nadu, India

Sahana Shetty

MBBS MD (Gen Med) DM (Endo)

Assistant Professor
Department of Endocrinology
Diabetes and Metabolism
Christian Medical College
Vellore, Tamil Nadu, India

Kripa Elizabeth Cherian

MBBS MD (Gen Med)

Senior Resident
Department of Endocrinology
Diabetes and Metabolism
Christian Medical College
Vellore, Tamil Nadu, India

Meera S MBBS MD (Gen Med)

Research Officer
Department of Endocrinology
Diabetes and Metabolism
Christian Medical College
Vellore, Tamil Nadu, India

Chapter 6: Endocrine Miscellany

Nihal Thomas

MBBS MD (Gen Med) MNAMS
DNB (Endo) FRACP (Endo)
FRCP (Edin) FRCP (Glas)

Professor and Head
Department of Endocrinology
Diabetes and Metabolism
Vice Principal (Research)
Christian Medical College
Vellore, Tamil Nadu, India

Felix Jebasingh K

MBBS MD (Gen Med)

Senior Resident
Department of Endocrinology
Diabetes and Metabolism
Christian Medical College
Vellore, Tamil Nadu, India

Samantha S MBBS MD (Gen Med)

Senior Resident
Department of Endocrinology
Diabetes and Metabolism
Christian Medical College
Vellore, Tamil Nadu, India

Rahul Thampi MBBS

Research Officer
Department of Endocrinology
Diabetes and Metabolism
Christian Medical College
Vellore, Tamil Nadu, India

Foreword

Endocrinology is a very visual speciality. While as always, a good and detailed history is essential, probably in no other specialization other than perhaps dermatology is the physical appearance of patients more vital in coming to a correct diagnosis. Patients with Cushing's syndrome and acromegaly, in particular, have languished for years before the diagnosis was suspected and treatment instituted, and in many other areas recognition of clear clinical features are either ignored, missed, or misattributed. In diabetes, many of the changes over time, particularly those due to a variety of complications, require careful clinical inspection and recognition in order to initiate prompt and often life-saving interventions. Furthermore, both diabetes and endocrinology are increasingly dependent on accurate interpretation of radiological imaging, be it with ultrasound, CT scanning, MRI or radionuclide scanning. It is therefore of great importance, that this new volume is focussed on the visualization of all aspects of endocrinology and diabetes, and their complications.

Furthermore, it is now well accepted in medical education circles, that case-based approaches are an ideal form of learning and revision, aiding the trainee doctor and helping educate even experienced clinicians in sharpening their clinical skills, and so assisting in patient management.

It is especially fitting that this dual approach of teaching endocrinology and diabetes by highly visual techniques and case-based studies comes from the Christian Medical College in Vellore, as one of the most highly praised and accomplished medical centres in Tamil Nadu, India. With both a stellar national and indeed international reputation, the Departments of Endocrinology, Diabetes and Metabolism have put together a beautifully illustrated and highly instructive Color Atlas, assisted by extensive collaboration with many other clinical departments. The illustrations are outstanding, the text is clear and informative, and I suspect many practising physicians will read it as much as for pleasure as for knowledge. I am delighted to introduce this volume to the medical public, and know that it is set to become a standard reference in Endocrinology and Diabetes.

Prof Ashley Grossman FMed Sci
Professor of Endocrinology
Oxford Centre for Diabetes
Endocrinology and Metabolism
Radcliffe Dept. of Medicine
University of Oxford, Churchill Hospital
Headington, Oxford, OX3 7LE, UK

Endocrinology is a specialty which encompasses a wide spectrum of disorders. Disorders of thyroid, diabetes, obesity, and osteoporosis involve nearly 30% of the population at a random time point in life. This book focuses on the need of the practicing clinician—whether primary care, physician, surgeon or Endocrine specialist- to handle and identify endocrine problems.

I would like to thank and acknowledge the hard work and dedication that Dr Felix Jebasingh K has put into developing several areas of the book. I would like to also appreciate the multidisciplinary impact of several medical specialties across the board in supporting this endeavor.

Just as much this expedition is meant to aid in improving patient care, and support the academician in their learning endeavors, the case discussions and evaluations provided may have a long term impact on learning processes.

Bonne Lecture!

Nihal Thomas

Acknowledgments

Endocrinology is a specialty which involves teamwork.

The multidisciplinary overlap between several clinical and non-clinical units is a strong feature of the subject. This book would not have been possible but for the strong academic links that the Department of Endocrinology shares with several other departments in the hospital. The care for patients is foundational for such a lucid output.

We would also like to thank Mr Jitendar P Vij (Group Chairman), Mr Ankit Vij (Group President), Ms Chetna Malhotra Vohra (Associate Director), Ms Sheetal Arora Kapoor (Development Editor) and Production team of Jaypee Brothers Medical Publishers (P) Ltd., New Delhi, India.

Nihal Thomas
Felix Jebasingh K

Contents

Contents

Image 1

Mr L is a 36-year-old gentleman, who presented with new onset diabetes, hypertension and proximal muscle weakness. He had cushingoid habitus with purplish striae in the anterior abdominal wall (shown in Fig. 1). His biochemistry investigations were showing features suggestive of ACTH Dependent Cushing's Syndrome. The radiological investigations localized the lesion to the left side of the pituitary gland, which is shown with an arrow in Figure 2. He underwent trans-nasal trans-spenoidal excision of the pituitary microadenoma. On the second postoperative day, he had vomiting and tiredness with a simultaneous serum cortisol level suppressed (0.1 mcg/dL), suggesting a remission. For the hypocortisolemic status, he was started on parenteral hydrocortisone followed by oral prednisolone. He was discharged with the plan to taper the steroid during the subsequent 3 months.

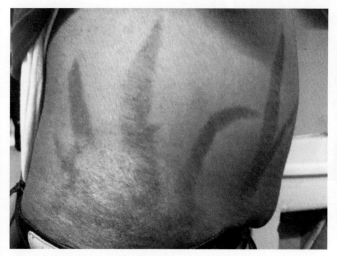

Fig. 1: Clinical image of the patient.

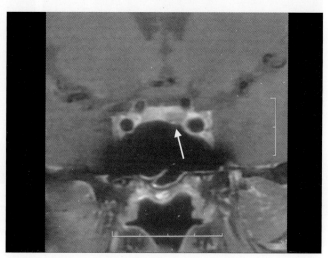

Fig. 2: MRI of the pituitary gland.

Image 2

A 24-year-old Mr C presented to our Endocrine clinic with the complaints of recurrent fractures of the both femurs and left humerus. All the fractures were following a trivial trauma. His biochemical features were normal except for a raised serum alkaline phosphatase level. His radiographs showed osteosclerosis of all the bones. X-ray of the skull showed an opened fontanelles and wormian bones. His X-ray of the hands showed acro-osteolysis of the terminal phalanges (Figs. 1A to C). This radio graphical picture was highly suggestive of Pynknodysostosis also known as osteopetrosis acro-osteolytica or Toulouse-Lautrec syndrome. He was advised to follow fall preventive measures.

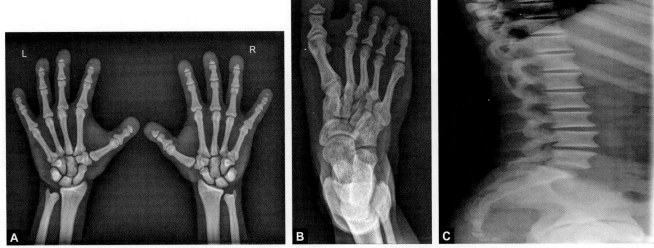

Figs. 1A to C: Patient's radiography.

Image 3

Mrs F was a 50-year-old lady, who presented to our thyroid clinic with history of rapidly increasing neck swelling with associated dysphagia since 20 days prior to the visit (Fig. 1). Clinically she had a hard swelling in the neck which moved with deglutition. Her ultrasonography of the thyroid gland showed multiple thyroid gland nodules with TIRADS 5, suggestive of malignancy. With the clinical and radiological findings, she was diagnosed to have Anaplastic carcinoma, which was confirmed by a Tru-cut biopsy from the dominant nodule. She was then referred to the department of Radiotherapy for further management.

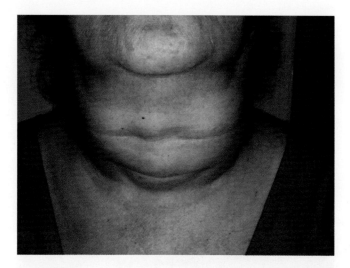

Fig. 1: Patient's clinical image.

Image 4

Mr J a 58-year-old gentleman presented with the history of headache for six months with associated vomiting and giddiness. He also had imbalance while walking for four months. An MRI Brain revealed a posterior third ventricular mass with hydrocephalus (Fig. 1, *Shown with an arrow*). He initially underwent a ventriculo-peritoneal shunt, followed by a midline suboccipital craniectomy with subtotal excision of the mass. The biopsy of the specimen was reported as pineal parenchymal tumor with intermediate differentiation, which falls in the category between pineocytoma and pineoblastoma (based on the prognosis of Pineal gland tumors). He was subjected to radiotherapy for the residual disease. He is at present on follow up with us.

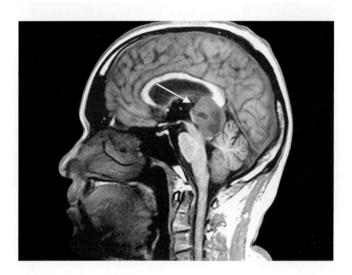

Fig. 1: MRI of the Brain.

Image 5

Mr U, a 44-year-old gentleman, was evaluated for the complaints of breathlessness and productive cough with fever in 2012 and was found to have a mass lesion in the right bronchus. Subsequently, he underwent a right middle and lower lobectomy with Bronchoplasy, and the biopsy of the lesion was reported as atypical neuroendocrine tumor of the bronchus. In the later part of 2014, he presented with history of episodes of flushing (Fig. 1). He was re-evaluated and found to have recurrence of the bronchial carcinoid with metastasis to the liver and bones. He also had a whole body Gallium-68 tagged DOTATATE PET CT scan, which confirmed the distant metastases (Figs. 2 and 3). He was given Lutetium-177 DOTATATE therapy along with an once a month long acting octreotide injection for the metastatic lesions. He is on follow-up since then.

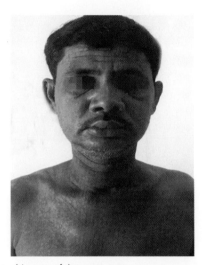

Fig. 1: Clinical Image of the patient.

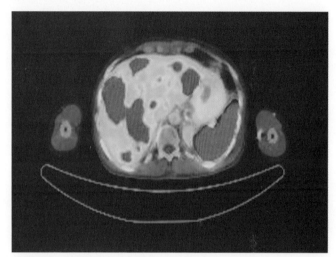

Fig. 2: DOTATATE –PET showing multiple liver metastases (red colour uptakes in the liver).

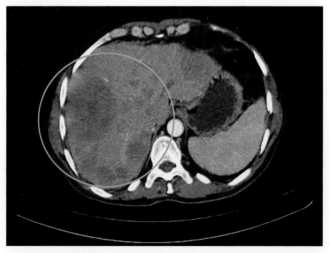

Fig. 3: CT abdomen with multiple liver metastases (shown with a circle).

CHAPTER 1

The Terrific Thyroid
(Thyroid Gland and Related Disease)

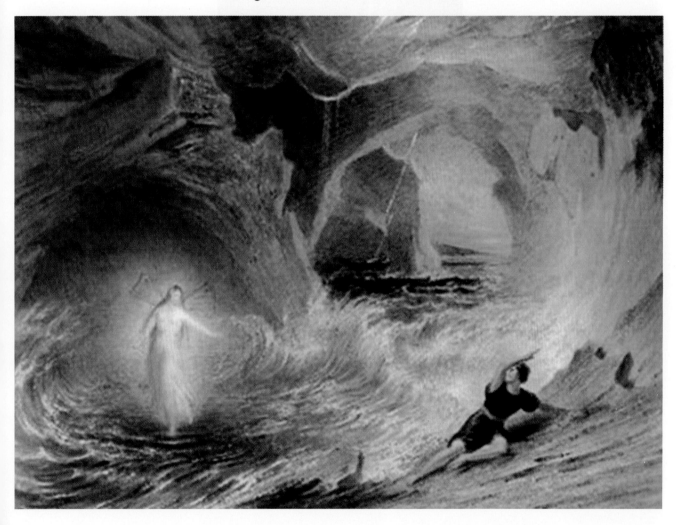

..Who would believe that there were mountaineers dewlapped like bulls,
whose throats had hanging at 'em, wallets of flesh..
—*Shakespeare, The Tempest (Act 3).*

(This is an authentic description of the inhabitants of the Italian Alps,
who had large iodine related goitres in the 16th century)

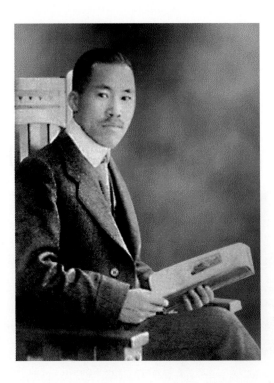

Dr Hakaru Hashimoto was born on May 5, 1881, in the village of Midau, Nishi-tsuge in the Mie prefecture, Iga-Ueno, Japan. He was born in a family that had been practicing medicine for generations whose inspiration was his grandfather, Gen'I Hashimoto who was practicing Dutch medicine.

Dr Hashimoto was one of the first graduates from the Kyusyu Imperial University in Fukuoka in 1907. Between 1908 and 1912, while working in a surgical department, Dr Hashimoto took an interest in thyroid tissue. It was during this time that he extracted thyroid tissue samples from four patients and discovered new pathological characteristics.

In 1912, at the age of 31, Hashimoto published his findings as an independent new disease in Archiv Fur Klinishe Chirurgie, the German journal of clinical surgery. He published a 30 pages monograph with five figures, titled Notes of lymphomatous disease in the thyroid gland (struma lymphomatosa).

At age 52, Dr Hashimoto died on January 9, 1934 due to enteric fever, before receiving wide recognition for the discovery of goitrous lymphocyctic thyroiditis, or Hashimoto's disease.

However the eponym Hashimotos thyroiditis would not be reintroduced to Japan until the 1950s!

As an honor, Kyushu University named a road on its campus "Hashimoto Street". Also The Japan Thyroid Association uses Hakaru Hashimoto's picture in its logo as a tribute to his great discovery.

CASE 1

A 2-year-old girl presented with swelling under her chin from the age of 6 months. The swelling was insidious in onset, painless and gradually progressive in size. It was not associated with any discharge or skin changes. The child did not have any intraoral complaints. A 2 cm by 1 cm firm, non-tender and mobile swelling was detected in the left submental region at level 1A. The skin over the swelling was normal and the swelling was not bi-digitally palpable. The thyroid gland was not palpable. Ultrasound of the neck was done and images are displayed below.

WHAT IS THE DIAGNOSIS?

Laboratory test showed a normal thyroid functions. An Ultrasound scan of the neck showed an absent left lobe of the thyroid with multiple enlarged lymph nodes in level 2, 3 and 4 (Fig. 1).

Subsequently, a thyroid uptake study was done which showed a normal right thyroid lobe, with agenesis of the left lobe (Fig. 2). There was no evidence of functioning thyroid tissue in the submandibular swelling.

The patient has been on regular follow-up with regular thyroid function tests.

DISCUSSION

Thyroid hemiagenesis is a rare embryological condition resulting from the developmental failure of one thyroid lobe. It is seen predominantly in females in a ratio of 3:1.[1] Most patients diagnosed with this disorder have an associated pathology in the remaining thyroid lobe, including benign adenoma, multinodular goiter, hyperthyroidism, chronic thyroiditis, and rarely carcinoma. The most common pathology involved in thyroid hemiagenesis is hyperthyroidism.[2] The molecular mechanism behind hemiagenesis of thyroid has not yet been described in detail. But, a mouse model with $Shh^{-/-}$ mutation showed hemiagenesis of the thyroid or a of non-lobulated gland. Hemiagenesis was also seen in mouse model with a double heterogenous mutation of $Pax8^{+/-}$ and $Tif^{+/+}$.[3] The presence of carcinoma in a patient with hemiagenesis is quite rare and only a few cases have been reported in the world literature.

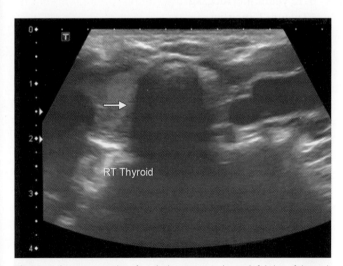

Fig. 1: Ultrasonography of neck showing an absent left lobe of thyroid.

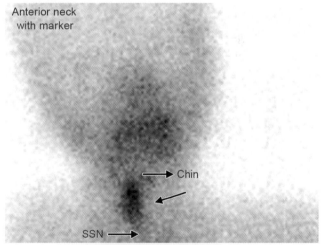

Fig. 2: Radioiodine uptake study showing an absent left lobe of thyroid (shown with arrow). (SSN: Supra Sternal Notch).

REFERENCES

1. Shaha AR, Gujarati R. Thyroid hemiagenesis. J. Surg. Oncol. 65;137–140 (1997).

2. Macchia PE, Fenzi G. Genetic defects in Thyroid Hormone synthesis and action. In Jameson, J. L. & Groot, L. J. D. Endocrinology: Adult and Pediatric. (Saunders, 2010). Vol 2; Page 1723

CASE 2

A young girl, 15 years of age, at present studying in 6th grade was brought by her mother for the evaluation of short stature. On clinical examination, she had a puffy face with a depressed nasal bridge. She also had dry, yellowish discolouration of skin. She was short statured and was mentally challenged (Fig. 1). Her height was less than the third centile for her age.

Radiographic evaluation revealed a bone age that was markedly delayed (presence of only two carpal bones), of 3 years (Fig. 2).

WHAT IS YOUR DIAGNOSIS?

Thyroid scintigraphy was done (Fig. 3) and showed no tracer uptake in the neck in the region of thyroid but abnormal tracer accumulation was seen in the suprahyoid region.

This patient has congenital hypothyroidism associated with an ectopic lingual thyroid gland. The other hormonal axes in this patient were normal. The patient was started on oral thyroxine and has been kept on regular follow-up ever since.

DISCUSSION

Congenital hypothyroidism (CH) is one of the most common treatable causes of intellectual disability (mental retardation). Screening programs have been established in most developed and developing countries to detect and treat this disorder. Primary CH screening has been shown to be effective for the testing of cord blood or heel prick blood collected during the delivery, although the best "window" for testing is 3–5 days of age. Blood is spotted onto special filter paper (known as Guthrie cards), allowed to dry, and eluted into a buffer for TSH analysis. Normally serum TSH levels rises after birth (upto 60 μU/mL with the previous TSH assays) and falls less than 10 μU/mL after 48–72 hours. So a TSH level of upto 8–10 μU/mL can be considered as normal upto 12 week of infancy. With the newer assays TSH values are considered significant for the diagnosis of congenital hypothyroidism when it is around 20–25 μU/mL. The dose of thyroxine is as follows depending upon the age of the patient.

- 0–3 months: 10–15 mcg/kg orally once per day
- 3–6 months: 8–10 mcg/kg
- 6–12 months: 6–8 mcg/kg
- 1–5 years: 5–6 mcg/kg
- 6–12 years: 4–5 mcg/kg
- 12 years: 2–mcg/kg
- Patients in which growth and puberty are complete: 1.6 mcg/kg orally once per day.

The Academy of Pediatrics and the European Society for Paediatric Endocrinology recommend measurement

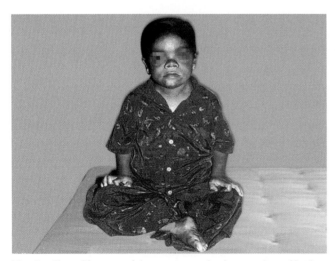

Fig. 1: Clinical features of short stature and a depressed nasal bridge.

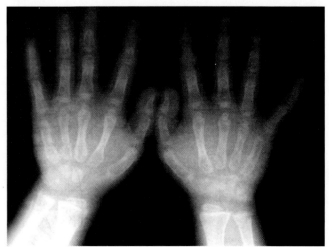

Fig. 2: X-ray of the hands showing bone age of 3 years.

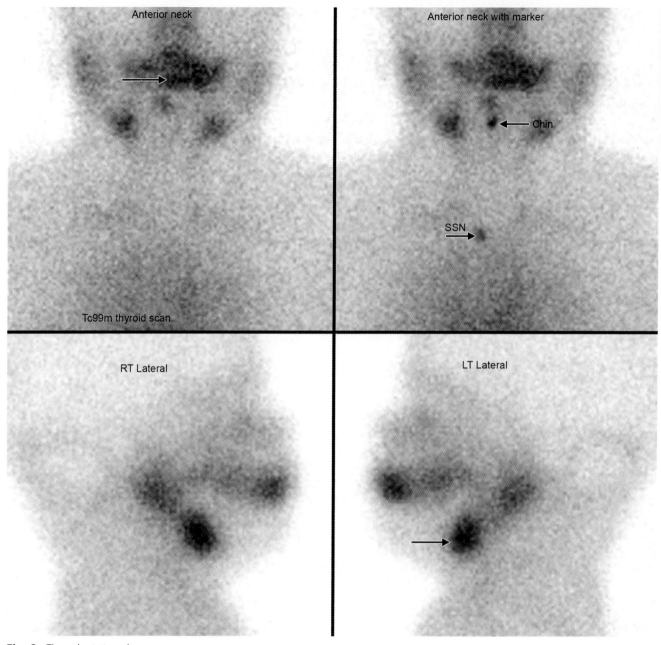

Fig. 3: Thyroid scintigraphy.

of serum T4 or fT4 and TSH at 2 weeks after the initiation of L-T4 treatment, and every 2 weeks until serum TSH level is normalized. Subsequently every 1–3 months during the first 12 months of life, followed by every 2–4 months between 1 and 3 years of age. A follow up once in 6–12 months thereafter until growth is complete is necessary. If a dose of thyroxine is changed with a visit a review visit should be done in a 2 weeks time.[1,2]

REFERENCES

1. Léger J, Olivieri A, Donaldson M, et al. European Society for Paediatric Endocrinology Consensus Guidelines on Screening, Diagnosis, and Management of Congenital Hypothyroidism. J Clin Endocrinol Metab. 2014 Jan 21;99 (2):363–84.
2. Desai MP, Upadhye P, Colaco MP, et al. Neonatal screening for congenital hypothyroidism using the filter paper thyroxine technique. Indian J Med Res. 1994;100:36–42.

CASE 3

A 16-year-old boy, studying in 10th grade, presented with short stature as the boy was concerned about the same was born to nonconsanguinous parents, at term, by caesarean section, with a birth weight of 2.35 kg. He had neonatal jaundice for 5 days which eventually subsided. His mother gave a history of delayed milestones and had noticed that he was lagging behind his peers in height from the age of 10 years. There was no history of headache, visual disturbance or glucocorticoid usage. His academic performance was below average.

On physical examination he was found to be of short stature with a height of 124.5 cm (less than the 3rd centile) with an expected height of 153 + 6.5 cms. Clinically, there was no goitre. He did not have prepubertal testes and his pubic hair was of Tanner stage 4.

WHAT IS THE DIAGNOSIS?

He had a thyroid stimulating hormone (TSH) level of 750 mIU/L with low free thyroxine and total thyroxine levels. He subsequently underwent a thyroid uptake study and images are displayed above. Tc99m thyroid scan shows tracer 2 areas of uptake: at base of tongue and in the midline of the neck above the thyroid bed. It is suggestive of congenital hypothyroidism with ectopic thyroid in lingual and suprahyoid regions (*see* Fig. 1).

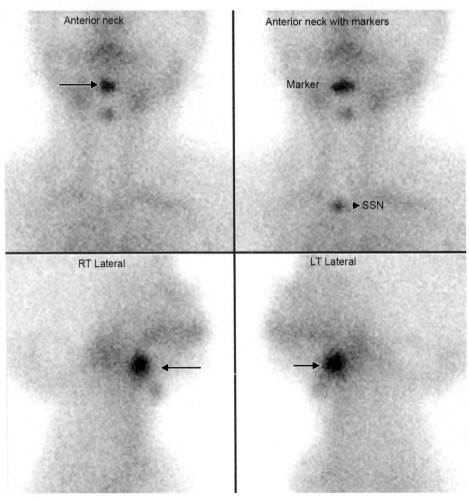

Fig. 1: Thyroid scintigraphy.

DISCUSSION

Ectopic thyroid is a rare developmental anomaly of the thyroid gland which is defined as the presence of thyroid tissue at a site other than the pretracheal area. In most cases, ectopic thyroid is located along the embryologic descent path of migration as either as a lingual thyroid or a thyroglossal duct cyst.[1] A lingual thyroid is the most common presentation of ectopic thyroid. In 70% of cases of ectopic thyroid, the normal thyroid gland is absent and this ectopic gland is the only functional thyroid tissue.[2] Nearly 1–3% of all ectopic thyroids are located in the lateral neck.

REFERENCES

1. Desai MP, Upadhye P, Colaco MP, et al. Neonatal screening for congenital hypothyroidism using the filter paper thyroxine technique. Indian J Med Res. 1994;00:36-42.
2. Boyages S, Halpern JP, Maberly GF, et al. Effects of protracted hypothyroidism on pituitary function and structure in endemic cretinism. Clin Endocrinol (Oxf). 1989;30(1):1-12.

CASE 4

A 69-year-old lady, who was known to have 2 diabetes mellitus, hypertension and coronary artery disease presented with neck swelling for a duration of 9 years (Fig. 1). The swelling was cystic in nature and was pulsatile. There was no history suggestive of either hypothyroidism or hyperthyroidism. There was no history of associated pressure related symptoms. On examination, the thyroid gland was normal in size. There was no tracheal tug and the swelling did not move up with deglutition or protrusion of the tongue. Thyroid function tests were normal.

WHAT IS THE PROBABLE DIAGNOSIS?

A color Doppler of the swelling revealed dilatation of the right innominate artery, which was suggestive of an aneurysm. This swelling was mimicking a thyroid swelling (Fig. 2).

This is a unique patient wherein the aneurysm of the innominate artery (AIA) presented as a thyroid swelling. Since she was clinically, and biochemically euthyroid, she was referred to vascular surgery department for further management.

DISCUSSION

Here are some differential diagnosis for a neck mass:
Congenital Neck Mass:[1,2]

- Branchial cleft cyst
- Thyroglossal duct cyst
- Vascular anomalies
- Laryngocele
- Ranula
- Teratoma
- Dermoid cyst
- Thymic cyst

Inflammatory Neck Mass:
- Infectious inflammatory disorders
  - Reactive viral lymphadenopathy
  - Bacterial lymphadenopathy
  - Parasitic lymphadenopathy
- Noninfectious inflammatory disorders

Neoplastic Disorders:
- Metastatic head and neck carcinoma
- Thyroid masses
- Salivary gland neoplasm
- Paragangliomas
- Schwannoma
- Lymphoma
- Lipoma and benign skin cysts

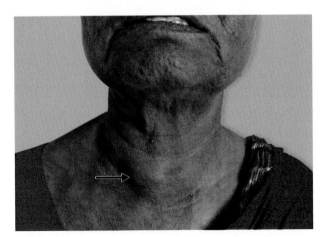

Fig. 1: Cystic neck swelling (shown with arrow).

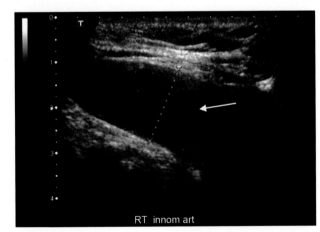

Fig. 2: Color Doppler showing a right innominate artery dilatation (shown with arrow).

REFERENCES

1. Kraus R, Han BK, Babcock DS, et al. Sonography of neck masses in children. AJR Am J Roentgenol. 1986;146(3): 609-13.

2. Josephson GD, Spencer WR, Josephson JS. Thyroglossal duct cyst: the New York Eye and Ear Infirmary experience and a literature review. Ear Nose Throat J. 1998;77(8):642–4, 646–7,651.

CASE 5

A 38-year-old lady presented with the history of a painless swelling in front of the neck for the past 2 years. She had history of weight gain and cold intolerance for which she approached her family physician and was started on oral replacement of thyroxine, after preliminary thyroid function tests. She also had complaints of pain in the proximal interphalangeal joints of both her hand over the past 5 years for which she had taken analgesics off and on, for pain relief.

Clinical examination of the neck showed a diffuse thyroid swelling, rubbery in consistency, with an approximate weight of 40 gm with pyramidal lobe enlargement (Fig. 1). She also had deformity of the fingers (Fig. 2). The rest of systemic examination was unremarkable.

WHAT IS THE DIAGNOSIS?

The biochemical evaluation showed a high thyroid stimulating hormone (TSH) titre of 56 mIU/L and the thyroid peroxidase antibody titres (TPOAb) (normal- less than 35 IU/mL) were 1000 IU/mL. She also was Rheumatoid Factor (RF) positive (100 u/mL). A biopsy of the thyroid swelling showed heterogeneous clusters of lymphocytes (Fig. 3).

With the above mentioned clinical features and investigations this patient was diagnosed to have Hashimoto's thyroiditis with rheumatoid arthritis.

She was started on methotrexate, hydroxychloroquine and on replacement doses of thyroxine. She has been on follow-up ever since.

DISCUSSION

Hashimoto's thyroiditis is considered as an autoimmune disease whose detection was originally based on the tissue biopsy but which now can be reliably detected by the presence of high titre anti-microsomal antibodies. Its relationship to rheumatic diseases seems more frequent than might be expected, but this has not been definitely proved. Hashimoto's thyroiditis frequently leads to hypothyroidism, which in turn progresses to myxoedema. Rheumatic syndromes associated with hypothyroidism include fibrositis, myositis, myalgias, carpal tunnel syndrome, Sjögren's syndrome, joint stiffness and joint effusion.[1,2] Thyroid dysfunction is seen at least three times more often in women with RA than in women with similar demographic features with non-inflammatory rheumatic diseases such as osteoarthritis and fibromyalgia. Most of these manifestations are said to resolve with thyroid replacement.

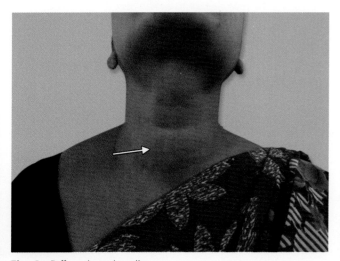

Fig. 1: Diffuse thyroid swelling.

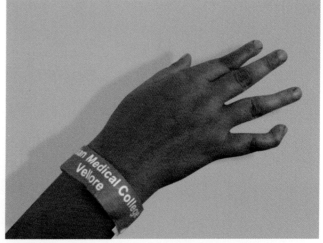

Fig. 2: Deformities in the interphalangeal joints of right hand.

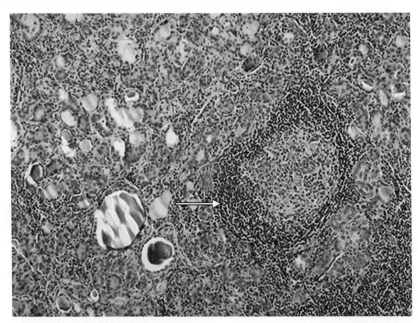

Fig. 3: Dense clusters of lymphocytes (shown with arrow) with loss of normal thyroid architecture on biopsy.

REFERENCES

1. Buchanan WW, Crooks J, Alexander WD, et al. Association of Hashimoto's thyroiditis and rheumatoid arthritis. Lancet 1961;i:245-8.

2. Buchanan WW. The relationship of Hashimoto's thyroiditis to rheumatoid arthritis. Geriatrics. 1965;20:941-8.

CASE 6

A 32-year-old lady presented with intolerance to heat, significant weight loss for over a month. Over the past one week she had also developed pain over the neck, fever and tremors.

On examination, she had a palpable, painful diffuse thyroid swelling. There were no significant findings.

Laboratory investigations showed an erythrocyte sedimentation rate (ESR) of 110 mm and a thyroid stimulating hormone (TSH) of 0.009 mIU/mL. Thyroid uptake study was done and showed very poor uptake of 99 mTc in the thyroid bed (1.7% after 24 hrs) (Fig. 1).

WHAT IS THE DIAGNOSIS?

A biopsy of the thyroid gland was done which showed neutrophils and epithelioid giant cells (Fig. 2).

The clinical and investigative evidence led to the diagnosis of de Quervain's thyroiditis. The patient was given pain relief medicines and sent home.

DISCUSSION

Inflammatory disorders of the thyroid gland are divided into three groups according to their duration: acute, subacute and chronic. De Quervain's thyroiditis (also termed giant cell or granulomatous thyroiditis) is a subacute inflammation of the thyroid, which accounts for 5% of the thyroid inflammatory disorders. The etiology is unknown, but it generally appears two weeks after an upper viral respiratory infection.

The natural history of granulomatous thyroiditis involves four phases: the destructive inflammation results temporarily in hyperthyroidism followed by euthyroidism. After transient hypothyroidism the disease becomes inactive and thyroid function is normalized.[1] Ultrasonography usually shows unilateral or bilateral hypoechoic, poorly defined, non-ovoid, hypovascular, focal lesions and may mimic malignant thyroid nodule. Few may be diffuse and heterogeneously hypoechoic in appearance.[2] The disease often remains unrecognised, or the first phase of the disease is diagnosed and treated as hyperthyroidism. The diagnosis can be confirmed by the presence of thyroid autoantibodies, cold gland (poor uptake) on scintigraphy and fine needle aspiration cytology. There is no definitive treatment. Non-steroidal anti-inflammatory drugs (NSAIDs) or glucocorticoids should be given to relieve the pain.

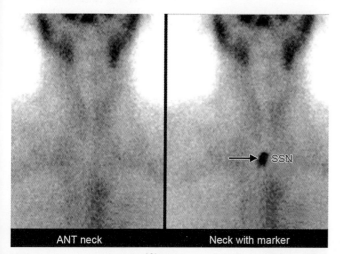

Fig. 1: Thyroid uptake study (I[131]) showing no uptake in the thyroid bed. (SSN: Supra Sternal Notch).

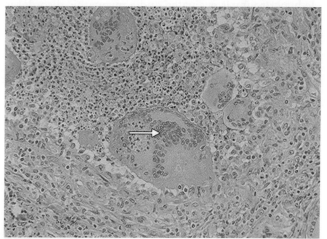

Fig. 2: Biopsy showing Epithelioid Giant Cells (shown with arrow) and Neutrophils.

REFERENCES

1. Thomas N. Thyroiditis in India—profile and management. In: The Association of Physicians of India—Medicine Update, Volume 13. Ed: S Das. 2003;469-74.

2. Frates MC1, Marqusee E, Benson CB, et al. Subacute granulomatous (de Quervain) thyroiditis: grayscale and color Doppler sonographic characteristics. J Ultrasound Med. 2013;32(3):505-11.

CASE 7

A 21-year-old gentleman was referred to our thyroid clinic with a history of progressive proximal muscle weakness, muscle pain and fatigue after minimal exercise. He complained of swelling of the calf muscles over the past few years and constipation.

On general examination he had puffiness of the face, slowness of speech and hypertrophy of the calf muscles bilaterally (Fig. 1). Gower's sign was negative. He had a positive hung up ankle reflex. He had no palpable swelling in the neck and his oral cavity was normal. He did not have any other stigmata of polyglandular autoimmune syndrome type II (PGA-II) (Figs. 1A and B).

WHAT IS THE DIAGNOSIS?

Laboratory tests including muscle biopsy showed features of rhabdomyolysis (Fig. 2), creatinine phosphokinase (CPK) 1500 U/L (25-90 U/L).

This gentleman was diagnosed as having primary hypothyroidism with Hoffmann's syndrome. Hoffmann's syndrome should be considered with other differential diagnoses (Becker's, Duchenne's muscular dystrophy, amyloidosis and focal myositis) when a patient with calf muscle hypertrophy is evaluated and a myopathic disorder is suspected, since it is treatable and mostly reversible.

The patient was put on replacement therapy with levothyroxine, started from 25 µg/d and increased to 100 µg/d. After this, the patient noticed improvement of his symptoms within four weeks.

DISCUSSION

Myopathic changes are seen in 30–80% of patients with hypothyroidism. There are four variants of hypothyroid myopathy which are Hoffmann's syndrome, Kocher-Debre-Semelaigne syndrome, an atrophic form and a myasthenic syndrome. Hoffmann's syndrome was first described by Johann Hoffmann in 1897.

Hoffman's syndrome is an uncommon form of hypothyroid myopathy seen in adults with long standing untreated hypothyroidism. It is characterized by proximal limb muscle weakness and muscle pseudohypertrophy (Fig. 1B). Patients present with muscle cramps, muscle stiffness, weakness, hyporeflexia and delayed deep tendon reflexes. Muscle pseudohypertrophy is a very rare presentation and its etiology remains controversial.[1] The gastrocnemius muscle is almost always involved. Postulated mechanisms for muscle pseudohypertrophy include an increased deposition of glycosaminoglycans, with increased muscle fibre size and number. Elevation of the serum

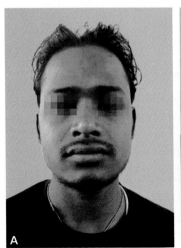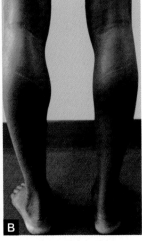

Figs. 1A and B: (A) Clinical features suggestive of hypothyroidism, (B) Pseudohypertrophy of calf muscles.

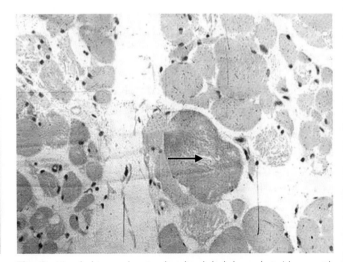

Fig. 2: Muscle biopsy showing localized rhabdomyolysis (shown with arrow).

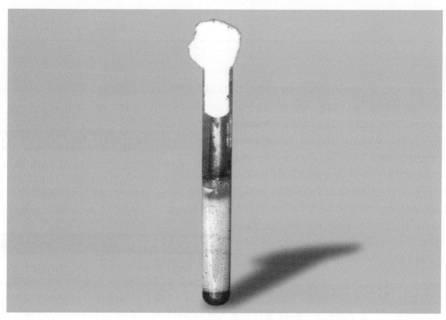

Fig. 3: Lipaemic serum.

CPK level is seen in 70–90% of patients with hypothyroidism indicative of muscle involvement but does not correlate with the severity of weakness. Electrophysiological studies may show myogenic, neurogenic or mixed patterns in hypothyroid myopathy. Biopsy of the affected muscles may show muscle fibre necrosis, atrophy, hypertrophy with increased number of nuclei and increased connective tissue (Fig. 2).

Muscle hypertrophy with weakness and slowness of movement in cretin children is called as Kocher Debre Semelaigne syndrome. The absence of painful spasms and pseudomyotonia differentiates this syndrome from Hoffmann syndrome.[2]

The blood sample of the patient mentioned above was centrifuged. The serum turned milky white as shown above (Fig. 3).

WHY DID THIS HAPPEN?

The milky white serum was seen due to elevated serum triglyceride levels (1800 mg/dL). In primary hypothyroidism there is a reduction in activity of lipoprotein lipase which then in turn causes hypertriglyceridemia. The mechanism of hypercholesterolemia is explained by a reduction in LDL-cholesterol hepatic receptor activity due to hypothyroidism.

REFERENCES

1. Udayakumar N, Rameshkumar AC, Sirinivasan AV: Hoffmann syndrome: presentation in hypothyroidism. J Postgrad Med. 2005:51(4):332-3.
2. Vasconcellos LFR, Peixoto MC, Oliveira TND, et al. Hoffmann syndrome: pseudohypertrophic myopathy as initial manifestation of hypothyroidism. Arq Neuropsiquiatr 2003: 61(3-B):851-4.

CASE 8

A 30-year-old lady presented to the outpatient department with a swelling in front of the neck, hoarseness of voice, fatigue and progressive worsening muscle weakness. She had a significant weight loss of 5 kg over 6 months. She also complained of difficulty in chewing wheat pancakes, but no such symptoms with soft solids. She also gave a history of 2 episodes of sudden onset breathing difficulty in the past requiring invasive ventilation and subsequent tracheotomies. At presentation sequential photographs were taken and show the following clinical findings (Fig. 1).

WHAT IS THE DIAGNOSIS?

Her blood investigations showed TSH of 0.007, FTC of 2.2 and a T4 of 21.2. Anti-acetylcholine receptor antibody was 0.56 (normal <2.1), anti-thyroglobulin antibodies: 22 (<100 IU/mL), anti-microsomal (thyroid peroxidise) 400 (<50 IU/mL). A CT scan of the neck was done and had shown an enlarged thyroid gland with a bulky thymus inconsistent for her age (Fig. 2).

WHAT IS THE DIAGNOSIS NOW?

This patient has a classical history suggestive of autoimmune hyperthyroidism with myasthenia gravis.

She was started on betablockers and was referred to the thoracic surgeons for a thymectomy.

DISCUSSION

It is well known that autoimmune thyroid disorders are known to be present only in 5–7.5% of the myasthenia gravis (MG) patients. However Myasthenia is seen in only 0.2% of the patients with thyroid disease.[1] The higher frequency of ocular myasthenia in autoimmune thyroid disease could well be attributed to the genetic linkage. Certain Human leukocyte antigen (HLA) specificity (B8, DR3, and BW46) between MG and thyroid disease has been reported to be associated with thyrotoxicosis.[2]

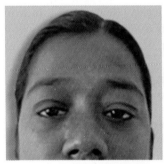 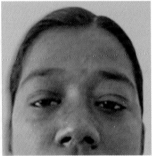 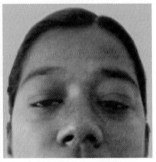

Fig. 1: Sequential photographs at 0 seconds, 30 seconds and 60 seconds of attempted upward gaze.

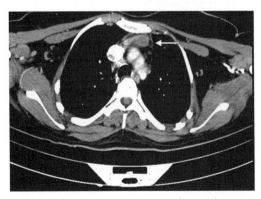

Fig. 2: CT Thorax showing a homogeneous soft tissue density mass in the anterior mediastinum in keeping with enlarged thymus (shown with arrow).

REFERENCES

1. Chhabra S, Pruthvi BC. Ocular myasthenia gravis in a setting of thyrotoxicosis. Indian J Endocrinol Metab. 2013;17(2):341–3.
2. Weetman AP, McGregor AM. Autoimmune thyroid disease: further developments in our understanding. Endocr Rev. 1994;15(6):788–830.

CASE 9

A 19-year-old girl had early satiety towards the evening, tremors and weight loss and underwent radioactive I^{131} ablation two years ago. She presented now with weight gain, yellowish tinged skin and hoarseness of voice (Fig. 1). On examination she was found to have bilateral ptosis with easy fatigability after talking for 2 minutes.

WHAT IS THE DIAGNOSIS?

Her thyroid stimulating hormone (TSH) before ablative treatment was <0.01 mIU/mL and FTC was 10 ng/dL. Pre-ablation iodine uptake studies (I_{131}) showed enlarged thyroid gland (both lobes) with uniform tracer uptake (Fig. 2).

She initially had Graves' disease associated with myasthenia gravis. Following ablation with I_{131} she went into hypothyroidism but ptosis persisted because of the Myasthenia gravis.

DISCUSSION

Graves' disease and myasthenia gravis are both autoimmune diseases and the coexistence of these two diseases is rare but well recognized. Epidemiological studies have shown that autoimmune thyroid disease (AITD) occurs in approximately 5–10% of patients with myasthenia gravis (MG), whereas MG is reported in a fairly low frequency (0.2%) of patients with AITD.[1] The association is thought to be uncommon, and it is generally believed that hyperthyroidism is far more commonly associated with MG than is hypothyroidism. However, no explanation has been offered to account for this difference.

The clinical presentation of MG associated with AITD is frequently restricted to the eye muscles. The reason for this association of AITD with ocular MG is unknown, but several hypotheses can be considered. First, ocular MG and generalized MG might actually represent separate diseases with different spectra of associated conditions. Second, an immunological cross-reactivity against epitopes or auto-antigens shared by the thyroid and the eye muscles might be the basis of this association. In three-quarters of patients with both conditions, thyrotoxic symptoms occur before or concurrently with those of myasthenia.

PAS I, also known as APECED (autoimmune polyendocrinopathy, candidiasis and ectodermal dystrophy) or MEDAC (multiple endocrine deficiency autoimmune candidiasis syndrome), usually appears in childhood in the age of 3–5 years or in early adolescence and, therefore, is also called juvenile autoimmune polyendocrinopathy. It is defined by a spectrum of persistent fungal infection (chronic mucocutaneous candidiasis), the presence of acquired hypoparathyroidism, and adrenal failure (Addison's disease).

PAS II is more common and occurs in adulthood, mainly in the third or fourth decade. It is characterized

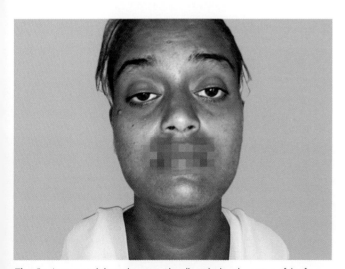

Fig. 1: Assymetric bilateral ptosis with yellowish discolouration of the face.

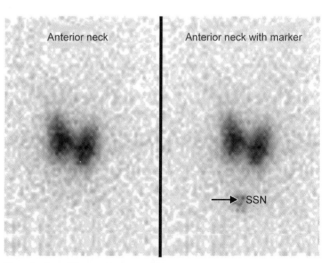

Fig. 2: Pre-ablative uptake studies.

by primary adrenal failure with autoimmune thyroid disease (Schmidt's syndrome) and/or type 1 diabetes (Carpenter's syndrome). Adrenal failure may precede other endocrinopathies. Vitiligo and gonadal failure are occasionally associated with PAS type II than with type I. The other disorders like immunogastritis, pernicious anemia, and alopecia areata may occur in PAS type II. Immunogastritis, eventually leading to pernicious anemia, is an organ-specific autoimmune disease. PAS type II is believed to be polygenic, characterized by an autosomal dominant inheritance.[2]

REFERENCES

1. Drachman DB. Myasthenia gravis and the thyroid gland. N Engl J Med. 1962;15:330-3.
2. Christensen PB, Jensen TS, Tsiropoulos I, et al. Associated autoimmune diseases in myasthenia gravis. A population based study. Acta Neurologica Scandinavica.1995;91:192-5.

CASE **10**

A 12-year-old boy presented with hair loss, a small thyroid swelling, lethargy and drooping of eyelids as shown in Figures 1A and B. His thyroid stimulating hormone (TSH) was 12.0 mIU/L.

WHAT IS THE DIAGNOSIS?

This patient was diagnosed to have autoimmune thyroid disease- Hashimotos thyroiditis with Myasthenia gravis and alopecia, suggestive of Type 2 Autoimmune Polyglandular Endocrinopathy syndrome.

DISCUSSION

Graves' disease and myasthenia gravis are both auto-immune diseases and the coexistence of these two diseases is rare but well recognized. Epidemiological studies have shown that autoimmune thyroid disease (AITD) occurs in approximately 5–10% of patients with myasthenia gravis (MG), whereas MG is reported in a fairly low frequency (0.2%) of patients with AITD.[1] The association is thought to be uncommon, and it is generally believed that hyperthyroidism is far more commonly associated with MG than is hypothyroidism. However, no explanation has been offered to account for this difference.

The clinical presentation of MG associated with AITD is frequently restricted to the eye muscles. The reason for the association of AITD with ocular MG is unknown, but several hypotheses can be considered. First, ocular MG and generalized MG might actually represent separate diseases with different spectra of associated conditions. Second, an immunological cross-reactivity against epitopes or auto-antigens shared by the thyroid and the eye muscles might be the basis of this association. In three-quarters of patients with both conditions, thyrotoxic symptoms occur before or concurrently with those of myasthenia.

PAS I, also known as APECED (autoimmune polyendocrinopathy, candidiasis and ectodermal dystrophy) or MEDAC (multiple endocrine deficiency autoimmune candidiasis syndrome), usually appears in childhood in the age of 3–5 years or in early adolescence and, therefore, is

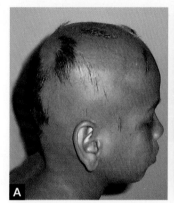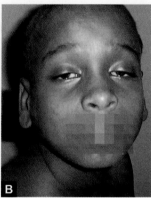

Figs. 1A and B: Hair loss and bilateral ptosis.

also called juvenile autoimmune polyendocrinopathy. It is defined by a spectrum of persistent fungal infection (chronic mucocutaneous candidiasis), the presence of acquired hypoparathyroidism, and adrenal failure (Addison's disease).

PAS II is more common and occurs in adulthood, mainly in the third or fourth decade. It is characterized by primary adrenal failure with autoimmune thyroid disease (Schmidt's syndrome) and/or type 1 diabetes (Carpenter's syndrome). Adrenal failure may precede other endocrinopathies. Vitiligo and gonadal failure are occasionally associated with PAS II than with type I. The, other disorders like immunogastritis, pernicious anemia, and alopecia areata may occur in type II. Immunogastritis, eventually leading to pernicious anemia, is an organ-specific autoimmune disease. PAS II is believed to be polygenic, characterized by an autosomal dominant inheritance.[2]

REFERENCES

1. Drachman DB. Myasthenia gravis and the thyroid gland. N Engl J Med. 1962;15:330–3.
2. Christensen PB, Jensen TS, Tsiropoulos I, et al. Associated autoimmune diseases in myasthenia gravis. A population based study. Acta Neurologica Scandinavica.1995;91:192–5.

CASE 11

A 65-year-old lady who is a known patient of Graves' disease presented to the Thyroid specialty clinic with a history of redness of eyes.

WHAT IS THE CLINICAL ACTIVITY SCORE? WHAT POSSIBLE TREATMENT OPTIONS ARE AVAILABLE?

This patient had an active eye disease due to Graves' ophthalmopathy (GO) with a clinical activity score (CAS) of 4/7 (Figs. 1A and B).

This patient received intravenous glucocorticoid pulse therapy, once a week and intravenous methylprednisolone (1 g weekly for 3 weeks, then 0.5 g, weekly for six weeks each with a total cumulative dose of 4.5 gram).

A CT scan was performed (Fig. 2).

DISCUSSION

For initial clinical activity score (CAS), only items 1–7 are scored.

1. Spontaneous orbital pain
2. Gaze evoked orbital pain
3. Eyelid swelling that is considered to be due to active (inflammatory phase) GO
4. Eyelid erythema
5. Conjunctival redness that is considered to be due to active (inflammatory phase) GO
6. Chemosis
7. Inflammation of caruncle OR plica

Patients assessed during follow-up (after 3 months) can be scored out of 10 by including items 8–10

8. Increase of > 2 mm in proptosis
9. Decrease in uniocular ocular excursion in any one direction of > 5°
10. Decrease of acuity equivalent to 1 Snellen line using a pin hole.[1]

The other treatment modalities for patients who are refractory to steroid therapy include intravenous rituximab or external beam radiation to the affected eyes. The usual dose for treatment of the retro-orbital area is 2000rads (20Gy), administered in 10 doses of 200 rads (2 Gy) over two weeks. Surgical decompression of the affected eye can be attempted in certain patients with sight threatening eye disease. Transantral decompression is a surgical procedure where the floor and medial wall of the orbit is removed to allow decompression of the orbital cavity.[2]

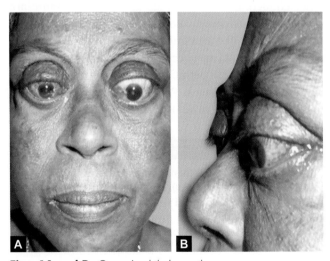

Figs. 1A and B: Graves' ophthalmopathy.

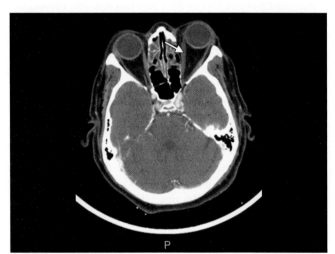

Fig. 2: CT scan showing bilateral proptosis with thickening of the extra ocular muscles (shown with arrow) and retro-orbital fat stranding.

MRI IMAGE OF A PATIENT WITH GRAVES' OPHTHALMOPATHY (FIGS. 3A AND B)

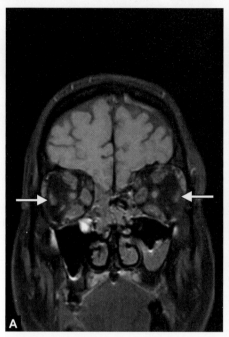 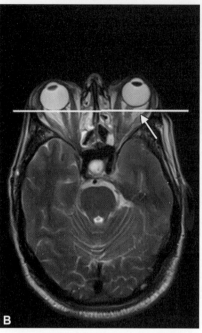

Figs. 3A and B: (A) MRI T1 fat suppressed coronal image showing retro-orbital fat stranding and severe thickening of extraocular muscles. Note the relative sparing of the lateral rectus muscle on both the sides (shown with white arrow). (B) T2 axial MRI showing bilateral proptosis (both globes are entirely anterior to the inter-temporal line) with coke bottle shaped extra-ocular muscles (shown with arrow) (note that the central portion of the muscle is most severely enlarged and tendinous insertions are spared).

OTHER PATIENTS WITH EYE DISEASE (FIGS. 4 TO 7)

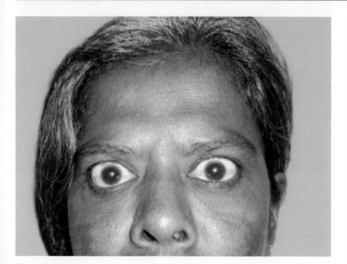 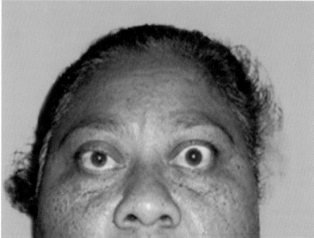

Fig. 4: Mrs K, a patient with known Graves' disease has Graves' ophthalmopathy with a clinical activity score (CAS) of 3/10. The scoring is out of 10 since the patient is a follow-up patient.

Fig. 5: Mrs S, a 50-year-old follow-up patient of Graves' disease with Graves' ophthalmopathy with a clinical activity score (CAS) of 2/7 on initial assessment now has a CAS of 3/10 due to an increase in proptosis.

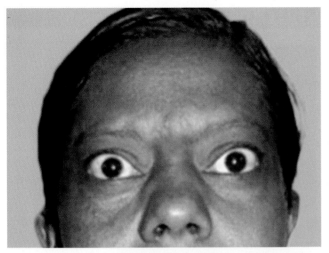

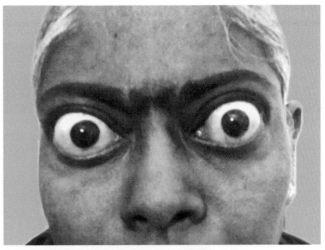

Fig. 6: Mrs A, a new patient was diagnosed to have Graves' disease presented with hyperthyroid/ toxic symptoms of overactiveness, weight loss and diarrhea. She also complained of a bilateral diffuse neck swelling. She was found to have a firm thyroid swelling and also proptosis which was graded with the clinical activity scoring (CAS) system, and she was found to have a score of 3/7. A case of Graves' ophthalmopathy.

Fig. 7: Another patient with Graves' ophthalmopathy on review was found to have worsening ophthalmopathy with a clinical activity score (CAS) of 4/7.

DIFFERENTIAL DIAGNOSIS FOR GRAVES' OPHTHALMOPATHY (FIGS. 8 AND 9)

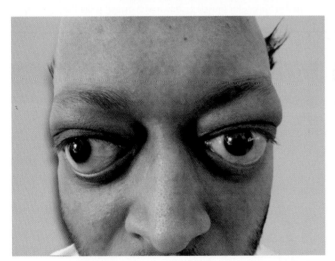

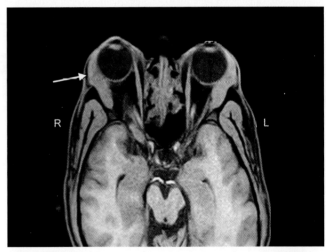

Fig. 8: This patient a 26-year-old presented to the thyroid clinic with bilateral propotosis and was treated elsewhere as dysthyroid (hypothyroid) ophthalmopathy. On further evaluation he was found to have enlarged neck lymph nodes, swollen lacrimal and parotid glands for which MR imaging was done (Fig. 9).

Fig. 9: MRI of the head and neck showing bilateral homogeneous enlargement of the lacrimal glands. Other sections of the MRI showed enlarged parotid and cervical lymph nodes which was suggestive of a lympho-proliferative disorder.

VARIOUS SIGNS AND PRESENTATIONS IN THYROID ILLNESS

A 29-year-old lady presented with history of menorrhagia and progressive weight gain and tiredness. The patient was looking dull and on examination was found to have dry and scaly skin (Figs. 10A and B and Fig. 12). The clinical pictures of the upper limb are shown below.

The patient was evaluated and was found to have high levels of TSH and was started on thyroxine, following which the symptoms of dry skin resolved completely.

A 50-year-old, Mr T, a known patient of hypothyroidism, presented with history of swelling in front of the lower limbs for the past 5 months. The swelling was slowly progressive and not painful. The clinical picture of the patient is shown below (Fig. 11).

He had a slow ankle reflex and also his TSH was more 150 Miu/mL. He was started on thyroxine with which the swelling completely subsided.

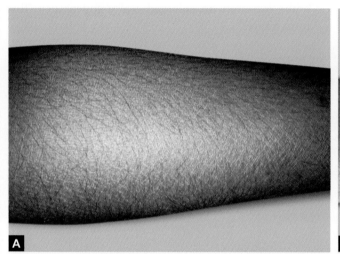 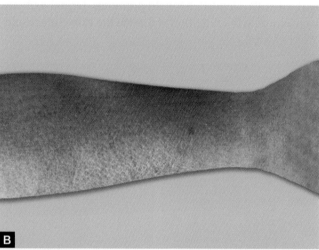

Figs. 10A and B: (A) Ichthyosis in hypothyroidism; (B) Dry skin in hypothyroidism.

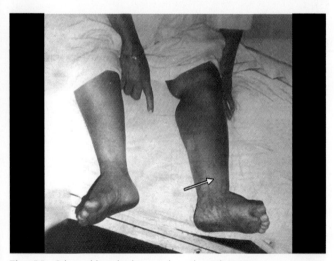

Fig. 11: Bilateral lymphedema in hypothyroidism.

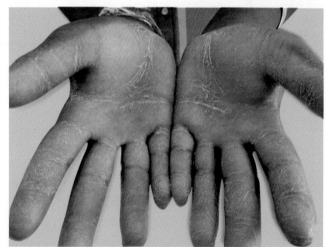

Fig. 12: Dry skin in a patient with hypothyroidism which subsided after treatment with thyroxine.

A 58-year-old man, presented with complaints of neck swelling, protrusion of the eyes and 'bumpy' swelling in the legs. He was evaluated and was found to have a thyroid swelling and deranged thyroid function parameters [TSH <0.001 Miu/mL and T4 >30 (mcg/dL) and free T4 > 10 (ng/dL)] (Figs. 13 to 15).

DISCUSSION

Histopathologically, pretibial myxedema shows deposition of mucin (glycosaminoglycans) throughout the dermis and subcutis. Deposited mucin promotes dermal oedema by promoting the retention of fluid in the skin. This results in compression/occlusion of small peripheral lymphatics and lymphoedema. There are 4 typical types seen:

- Diffuse, non-pitting edema (swelling)—the most common form
- Plaque form—raised plaques on a background of non-pitting edema
- Nodular form—sharply circumscribed tubular or nodular lesions
- Elephantiasic form—nodular lesions with pronounced lymphoedema (swelling due to accumulation of lymphatic tissue fluid). Lesions may coalesce to give the entire extremity an enlarged, warty appearance. This form is rare.

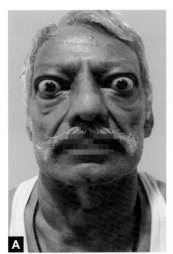 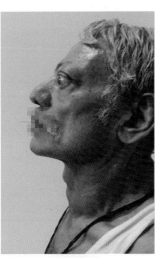 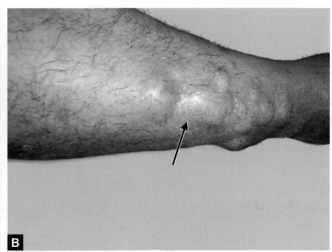

Figs. 13A and B: (A) Graves' ophthalmopathy with a clinical activity score (CAS) of 4/7 with a diffuse bilateral firm thyroid swelling; (B) Pretibial myxedema (shown with arrow) in hyperthyroidism (nodular type).

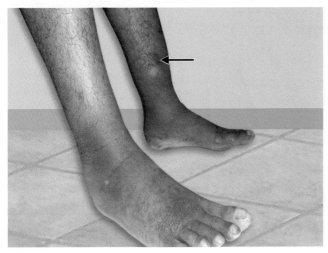 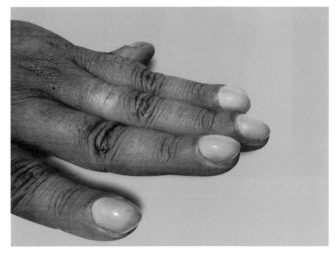

Fig. 14: Thyroid dermopathy, or infiltrative dermopathy (diffuse type of pretibial myxedema).

Fig. 15: Thyroid acropachy.

This affects 0.5–4.3% of patients with Grave's disease; it is seen in up to 13% in those with severe eye disease.

Dermopathy almost always is associated with ophthalmopathy and with acropachy in severe cases. A common antigen with thyroid, in tissues of the skin and the eyes, most likely TSH receptor, is involved in pathogenesis of extra thyroidal manifestations. Presence of dermopathy and acropachy are the predictors of severity of an autoimmune process. Local corticosteroid application is the standard therapy for dermopathy.[2]

REFERENCES

1. Subekti I, Boedisantoso A, Moeloek ND, et al. Association of TSH receptor antibody, thyroid stimulating antibody, and thyroid blocking antibody with clinical activity score and degree of severity of Graves ophthalmopathy. Acta Med Indones. 2012;44(2):114-21.
2. Tortora F, Cirillo M, Ferrara M, et al. Disease activity in Graves' ophthalmopathy: diagnosis with orbital MR imaging and correlation with clinical score. Neuroradiol J. 2013; 26(5):555-64.

CASE 12

A 43-year-old lady presented to the Endocrinology clinic with complaints of swelling in the right side of the neck, which was slowly increasing in size over the past 3 years.

The ultrasound of the swelling showed features as given in Figure 1. After fine needle aspiration (FNA) the swelling subsided markedly.

WHAT IS THE DIAGNOSIS?
WHAT DIFFERENTIAL DIAGNOSES
WILL YOU CONSIDER IN THIS PATIENT?

This patient has a cystic nodule in the right lobe of thyroid which explains the regression of the thyroid nodule after the FNAC. The differential diagnosis in this patient is a cystic parathyroid adenoma. Thyroid scintigraphy showed a hypofunctioning "cold" nodule, as these cystic nodules do not concentrate radioiodine or technetium. Aspiration cytology in this patient showed only colloid (Figs. 2 and 3).

DISCUSSION

The majority of cystic thyroid nodules are benign degenerating thyroid adenomas. Autonomously functioning thyroid adenomas are more likely to undergo cystic degeneration than nonfunctioning adenomas. Purely cystic

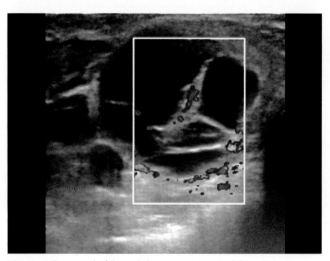

Fig. 1: Ultrasound of thyroid showing a cystic nodule with thin septae.

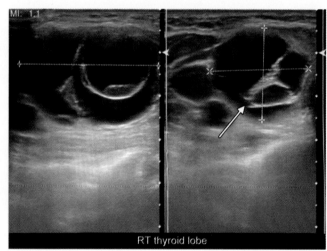

Fig. 2: Ultrasound of thyroid showing an anechoic (cystic) nodule with thin internal septae (shown with arrow).

lesions rarely contain cancer.[1] Size (>4 cm) of the cystic nodule may also be used as a criterion for surgery, although we do not use size as an absolute criteria for surgery.[2]

REFERENCES

1. Tan GH, Gharib H. Thyroid incidentalomas: management approaches to nonpalpable nodules discovered incidentally on thyroid imaging. Ann Intern Med. 1997;126:226.
2. Massoll N, Nizam MS, Mazzagerri EL. Cystic thyroid nodules: Diagnostic and therapeutic dilemmas. The Endocrinologist. 2002;12:185.

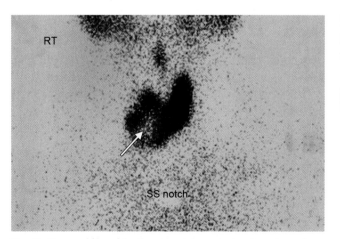

Fig. 3: Scanned film of the thyroid uptake scan showing a hypo-functioning right side nodule (shown with arrow).

CASE 13

A 43-year-old gentleman presented with headache of 3 years duration, failure to gain height from the age of 8 years, underdeveloped secondary sexual characteristics and mental retardation.

On examination he was disproportionately short statured with a height of 132 cms (<3rd centile) with an upper segment and lower segment ratio of 1.2:1 suggestive of shortened limbs. He looked dysmorphic, with prominent temporal bones and hypertelorism. He did not have a palpable thyroid gland (Fig. 1A).

On biochemical evaluation, his thyroid stimulating hormone (TSH) level was 775 uIU/mL with a T4 of 1.7 ng/dL. Other hormonal studies were normal. Radiology of the left hand revealed a bone age of 12 years (Fig. 1B).

Computed tomography (CT) scan of the head was done, which revealed a sellar mass of the size 7.1 × 5.9 × 4.2 cm with supra sellar extension into the third ventricle causing obstructive hydrocephalus (Fig. 2, shown with arrow).

WHAT IS THE DIAGNOSIS?

The presence of short stature, with a mentally challenged state, led to the clinical suspicion of congenital hypothyroidism. His I^{131} uptake study was 0.3% which was grossly reduced, thereby suggestive of thyroid hypoplasia and confirmed the diagnosis.

The differential diagnosis considered raised the possibilities of non-functioning pituitary macroadenoma or a craniopharyngioma or a pituitary pseudotumor which could have been caused by long-standing untreated primary hypothyroidism.

He was started on thyroxine (100 microgram/day). Following thyroid hormone replacement, he gained a height of 4.5 cm over a subsequent period of 3 years. An magnetic resonance imaging (MRI) done after 3 years showed significant reduction in the size of the pituitary mass with resolution of hydrocephalus favouring thyrotroph hyperplasia causing a pituitary pseudotumor.

Pituitary hyperplasia secondary to unrecognised and untreated primary hypothyroidism has been reported in both adults and children. The radiological diminution of the pituitary mass and the mass effects such as visual field improvement after thyroid replacement therapy confirms the possibility of pituitary hyperplasia, rather than a pituitary adenoma. There was a significant reduction in the sellar mass on treatment with thyroxine with

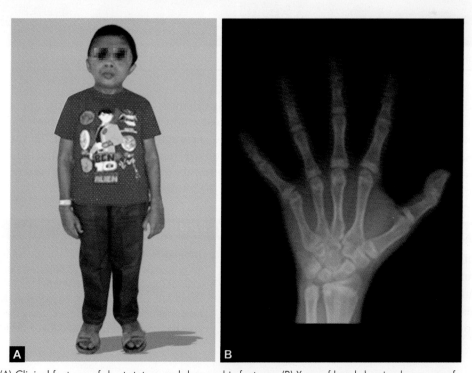

Figs. 1A and B: (A) Clinical features of short stature and dysmorphic features, (B) X-ray of hand showing bone age of around 10-12 years.

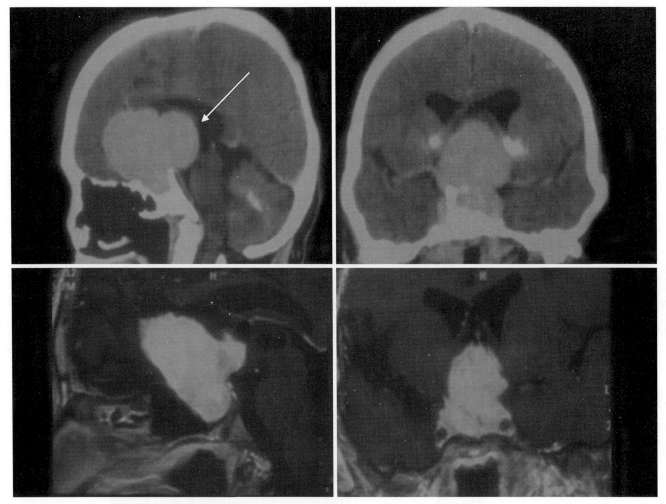

Fig. 2: CT scan of the head done before treatment.

normalization of TSH favouring a pituitary pseudotumour. The incomplete resolution may suggest the co-existence of a non-functioning adenoma or occurrence of a thyrotroph adenoma. Such thyrotroph adenomas are presumed to occur as the result of protracted pituitary stimulation secondary to long-standing thyroid deficiency.

Disturbances of growth, puberty, and sexual function in those with CH as seen in our subject can be explained by the secondary effects of thyroid hormone deficiency on pituitary function.[2] Severe protracted thyroid hormone deficiency may therefore result in thyrotrophin adenomas of the pituitary gland.

DISCUSSION

Congenital hypothyroidism (CH) is a common preventable cause of a mentally challenged state. The estimated incidence in India is 1:2500–2800 live births with a varied age of onset and clinical features.[1] Much of the etiology is due to thyroid ectopia, aplasia or hypoplasia.

REFERENCES

1. Thomas N. Thyroid disorders in the transitional age group—an Indian perspective. In: Promoting Childhood Wellbeing-Vellore Experiences. 2002:38-46
2. Desai MP, Upadhye P, Colaco MP, et al. Neonatal screening for congenital hypothyroidism using the filter paper thyroxine technique. Indian J Med Res. 1994;00:36-42.

CASE 14

A 36-year-old gentleman presented with holocranial headache for over 2 months and weight gain of 10 kg in 5 months. He had a dull look with slow relaxation of the ankle joint reflexes. He did not have vomiting or postural hypotension (Fig. 1).

The thyroid stimulating hormone (TSH) levels were 320 mIU/mL (normal: 0.3–4.5 mIU/mL). The creatine phosphokinase (CPK) levels were markedly elevated. A CT scan brain showed a sellar mass with suprasellar extension (Fig. 2).

WHAT IS THE DIAGNOSIS?

With the above clinical and investigative findings he was diagnosed to have primary hypothyroidism with pituitary pseudotumor.

The patient was started with oral levothyroxine following which he had a relief towards his headache.

DISCUSSION

Pituitary pseudotumor (pituitary thyrotroph hyperplasia) caused by unrecognized and untreated hypothyroidism has been described mostly in adults. Treatment with levothyroxine results in normalization of the size of the pituitary gland.[1] The myolysis in hypothyroid patients are caused by the change of fast twitching type 2 muscle fibre to slow twitching type 1 muscle fibre, deposition of glycosaminoglycan, poor contractility of the actin-myosin filaments, low myosin ATPase activity and low ATP turn-over. This is associated with elevated CPK levels which usually subside after levothyroxine treatment.[2]

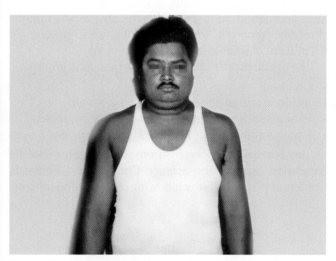

Fig. 1: Clinical features of the patient with dull face and a lethargic look.

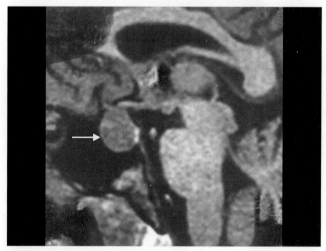

Fig. 2: CT Scan of the brain showing a sellar mass (shown with arrow).

REFERENCES

1. Larson NS, Pinsker JE. Primary hypothyroidism with growth failure and pituitary pseudotumor in a 13-year-old female: a case report. J Med Case Rep. 2013,31;7(1):149. doi: 10.1186/1752-1947-7-149.

2. Al-Shraim M, Syro LV, Kovacs K, et al. Inflammatory pseudotumor of the pituitary: case report. Surg Neurol. 2004; 62(3):264-7.

CASE 15

A 34-year-old lady presented with a swelling in front of the neck for 2 years duration (Fig. 1). There were no symptoms of thyroid dysfunction or compressive symptoms (dysphagia, dyspnea or hoarseness of voice). There was no significant past history or family history.

On examination the swelling moved up with deglutition but not with protrusion of the tongue. The swelling was smooth-surfaced and firm in consistency. It was not fixed to the surrounding structures. There were no other clinical findings.

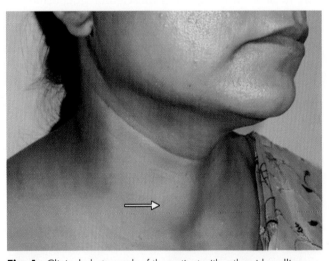

Fig. 1: Clinical photograph of the patient with a thyroid swelling.

An ultrasonography of the thyroid swelling was done (Figs. 2A and B) and the thyroid function tests were normal.

WHAT IS THE PROBABLE DIAGNOSIS?

Ultrasound showed a well defined, solid, isoechoic nodule with positive halo sign (thin hypoechoic rim around the lesion) in the right lobe of thyroid. These are features of probably benign thyroid nodule. There were other small colloid nodules in both lobes. A radionuclide scan was done and revealed a cold nodule in the right lobe (Fig. 3). Thus, dominant nodule in a multinodular goitre is the most likely diagnosis.

DISCUSSION

Nodularity of thyroid tissue is extremely common. In a large population study (Framingham, MA), as an example, clinically apparent thyroid nodules were present in 6.4 percent of women and 1.5 percent of men.

The prevalence of cancer is higher in several groups:

- Children
- Adults less than 30 years or over 60 years old
- Patients with a history of head and neck irradiation
- Patients with a family history of thyroid cancer.

The National Cancer Institute Thyroid Fine Needle Aspiration State of the Science Conference ("Bethesda Conference") suggests the following classification scheme:

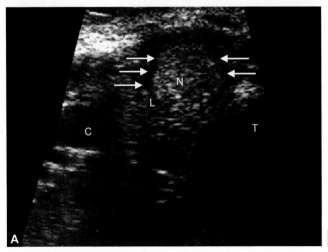

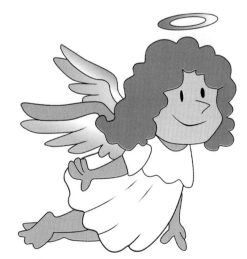

Figs. 2A and B: Halo sign (shown with arrow) on ultrasonography of the thyroid swelling.

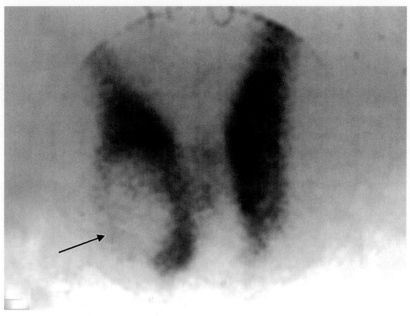

Fig. 3: Cold nodule on thyroid uptake study (shown with arrow).

- Benign—This includes macrofollicular or adenomatoid/hyperplastic nodules, colloid adenomas, nodular goiter, and Hashimoto's thyroiditis
- Follicular lesion or atypia of undetermined significance (FLUS or AUS)—This includes lesions with atypical cells, or mixed macro- and micro-follicular nodules
- Follicular neoplasm—This includes microfollicular nodules, including Hürthle cell lesions
- Suspicious for malignancy
- Malignant
- Nondiagnostic

Preliminary studies suggest the potential use of an imaging staging system similar to that used for breast imaging. The Thyroid Imaging Reporting and Data System (TIRADS) system rates ultrasound findings on a score of 1–6 based upon ultrasonographic characteristics.[1]

Similar to The Breast Imaging-Reporting and Data System (BI-RADS) category, sonographic TIRADS classification is as follows:

- TIRADS 1—normal thyroid gland
- TIRADS 2—benign lesions
- TIRADS 3—probably benign lesions
- TIRADS 4—suspicious lesions (sub classified as 4a, 4b, and later 4c with increasing risk of malignancy)
- TIRADS 5—probably malignant lesions (more than 80% risk of malignancy)
- TIRADS 6—biopsy proven malignancy

For benign nodules, surgery is indicated if any of the following are present:[2]

- Reaccumulation in the cystic nodule despite 3–4 repeated FNACs
- Size more than 4 cm in some cases
- Compressive symptoms (dyspnea, dysphagia)
- Signs of malignancy (vocal cord dysfunction, lymphadenopathy.

REFERENCES

1. Russ G, Bigorgne C, Royer B, et al. Bienvenu-Perrard M. [The Thyroid Imaging Reporting and Data System (TIRADS) for ultrasound of the thyroid]. J Radiol. 2011;92(7-8):701-13.
2. Ko SY, Lee HS, Kim E-K, et al. Application of the Thyroid Imaging Reporting and Data System in thyroid ultrasonography interpretation by less experienced physicians. Ultrasonography. 2014;33(1):49-57.

CASE 16

A 72-year-old, Mrs. E from Meghalaya was seen in the endocrinology OPD with a history of swelling in front of the neck for 50 years. She had been operated in 1972, with a probable subtotal thyroidectomy, for the swelling. Ten years after the surgery, she noticed a similar neck swelling, which had gradually progressed to the present size (Figs. 1A and B). She had symptoms of dyspnea and hoarseness of voice. She also complained of dysphagia. There were no other symptoms suggestive of hyperthyroidism or hypothyroidism.

On examination, a large thyroid gland was palpable which had an irregular surface. It was firm in consistency and had a size of 16 × 15 cm. The lower border was not palpable. Pemberton's sign was positive (Fig. 1B). Upper and mid cervical palpable lymph nodes were also palpable.

Plain radiograph a lateral view of the neck was done to assess the degree of tracheal compression (Fig. 2).

An ultrasound of the neck swelling showed multiple solid, isoechoic nodules with a positive halo sign, coarse calcifications and peripheral vascularity in both lobes of the thyroid gland (TIRADS 3) (Figs. 3 to 5).

WHAT IS THE DIAGNOSIS?

Fine needle aspiration (FNA) smears from the right thyroid nodule were suggestive of benign follicular nodule. In view of the large thyroid mass and compressive symptoms, she underwent total thyroidectomy. The surgical specimen on examination showed features of nodular hyperplasia. So the diagnosis of recurrent symptomatic benign nodular hyperplasia of thyroid was made. She was advised total thyroidectomy inview of the size and compressive symptoms.

DISCUSSION

Nodularity of thyroid tissue is extremely common. In a large population study (Framingham, MA), as an example, clinically apparent thyroid nodules were present in 6.4 percent of women and 1.5 percent of men.

The prevalence of cancer is higher in several groups:

- Children
- Adults less than 30 years or over 60 years old
- Patients with a history of head and neck irradiation
- Patients with a family history of thyroid cancer.

The National Cancer Institute Thyroid Fine Needle Aspiration State of the Science Conference ("Bethesda Conference") suggests the following classification scheme:

- Benign—This includes macrofollicular or adenomatoid/hyperplastic nodules, colloid adenomas, nodular goiter, and Hashimoto's thyroiditis
- Follicular lesion or atypia of undetermined significance (FLUS or AUS)—This includes lesions with atypical cells, or mixed macro- and micro-follicular nodules
- Follicular neoplasm—This includes microfollicular nodules, including Hürthle cell lesions

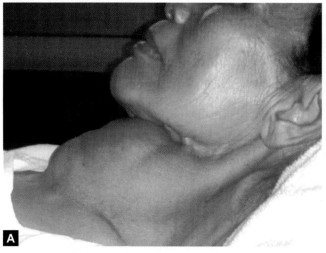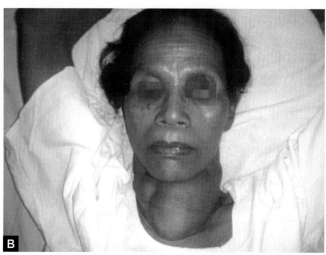

Figs. 1A and B: Massive thyroid swelling with a positive Pemberton's sign.

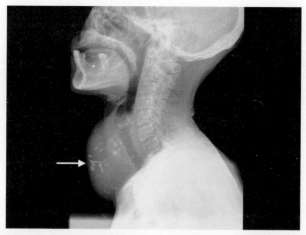

Fig. 2: Lateral radiograph of the neck showing a large goitre with macrocalcifications (shown with arrow). There was no significant tracheal compression.

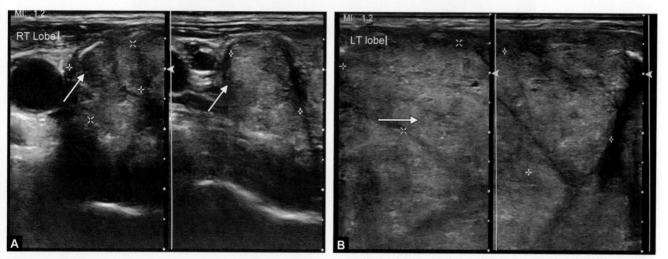

Figs. 3A and B: USG thyroid showing multiple well defined, solid, isoechoic nodules in both lobes of the thyroid (shown with arrow).

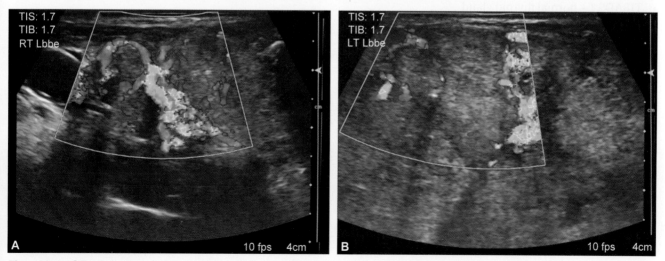

Figs. 4A and B: Color Doppler examination revealing peripheral vascularity in the thyroid nodules.

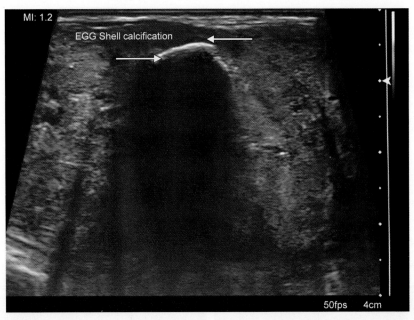

Fig. 5: Egg shell calcification.

- Suspicious for malignancy
- Malignant
- Nondiagnostic

Preliminary studies suggest the potential use of an imaging staging system similar to that used for breast imaging. The Thyroid Imaging Reporting and Data System (TIRADS) system rates ultrasound findings on a score of 1–6 based upon ultrasonographic characteristics.[1]

Similar to The Breast Imaging-Reporting and Data System (BI-RADS) category, sonographic TIRADS classification is as follows:

- TIRADS 1—normal thyroid gland
- TIRADS 2—benign lesions
- TIRADS 3—probably benign lesions
- TIRADS 4—suspicious lesions (sub classified as 4a, 4b, and later 4c with increasing risk of malignancy)
- TIRADS 5—probably malignant lesions (more than 80% risk of malignancy)
- TIRADS 6—biopsy proven malignancy

For benign nodules, surgery is indicated if any of the following are present:[2]

- Reaccumulation in cystic the nodule despite 3–4 repeated FNACs
- Size more than 4 cm in some cases
- Compressive symptoms (dyspnea, dysphagia)
- Signs of malignancy (vocal cord dysfunction, lymphadenopathy.

REFERENCES

1. Russ G, Bigorgne C, Royer B, et al. Bienvenu-Perrard M. [The Thyroid Imaging Reporting and Data System (TIRADS) for ultrasound of the thyroid]. J Radiol. 2011;92(7-8): 701–13.
2. Ko SY, Lee HS, Kim E-K, et al. Application of the Thyroid Imaging Reporting and Data System in thyroid ultrasonography interpretation by less experienced physicians. Ultrasonography. 2014;33(1):49–57.

CASE 17

A 72-year-old lady, presented with the history of low back-ache which had worsened over the past ten days and a progressively increasing neck swelling for the past 2 years. Previously, she had undergone a right hemi-thyroidectomy in 1990 for a solitary thyroid nodule.

On examination, the left lobe of thyroid was just palpable. The trachea was central and both carotids were normal. There was no enlargement of the cervical lymph nodes. There was a palpable sacral mass that was firm and nontender.

An ultrasound of the neck was done and showed a hypoechoic thyroid mass with calcifications and an absent peripheral halo (Figs.1A and B).

Figure 1B shows color Doppler with an increased vascularity.

WHAT IS THE PROBABLE DIAGNOSIS?

Magnetic resonance imaging (MRI) of the spine (Figs. 2A to C) was done and it showed a sacral mass which was suggestive of metastasis. A whole body iodine uptake scan was done and showed similar evidence of sacral metastasis.

A bone scan was done and it showed an increased uptake in the sacral region suggestive of metastasis (Figs. 3A and B).

Her bone scan and whole body uptake scan showed an increased tracer uptake in the sacral region (Figs. 3 and 4). However, there were no uptake in the thyroid bed area. She underwent partial excision of the sacral mass in 2012 and the biopsy report at that time revealed metastatic papillary thyroid carcinoma (Figs. 5A and B). She was given I[131]

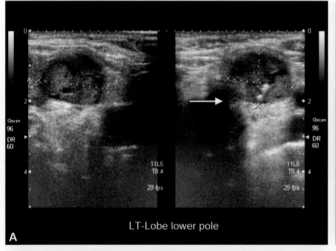

LT-Lobe lower pole

A

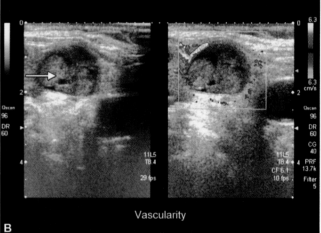

Vascularity

B

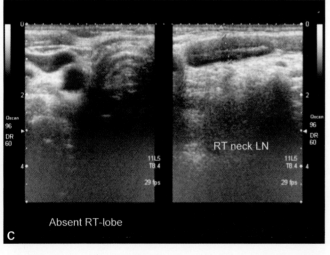

RT neck LN

Absent RT-lobe

C

Figs. 1A to C Ultrasound of the neck showing an absent right lobe (postoperative status), a solid, round, hypoechoic, heterogeneous nodule with vascularity in the lower pole of left lobe of thyroid. There were few benign right sided neck nodes.

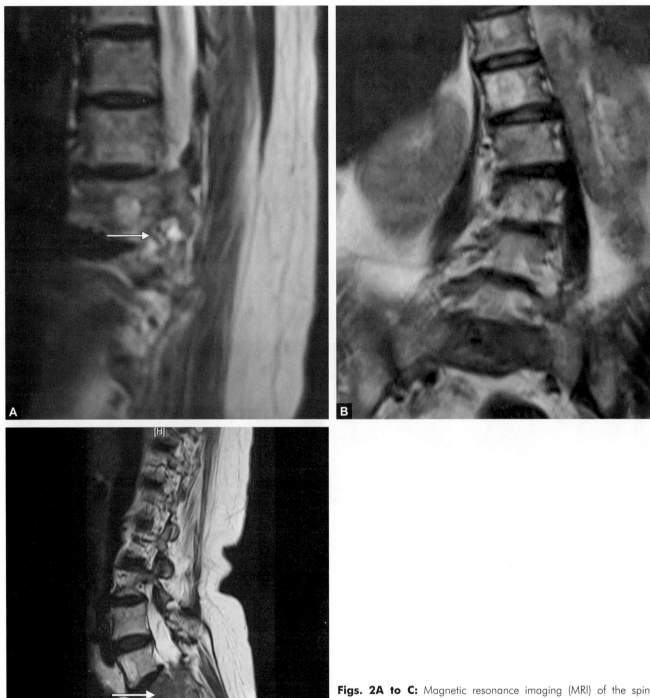

Figs. 2A to C: Magnetic resonance imaging (MRI) of the spine showing a hypointense ill-defined mass (shown with arrow) replacing marrow and destroying sacral bone suggestive of metastasis.

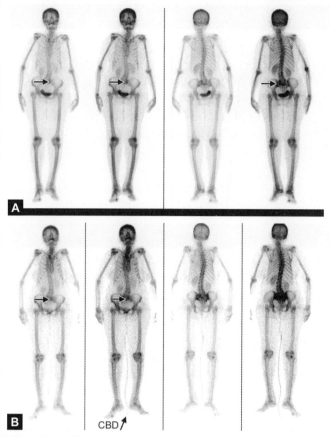

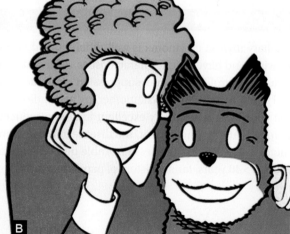

Fig. 4: I^131 whole body scintigraphy post-ablation scan showing metastasis in the region of lumbar spine (shown with arrow). (SSN: Supra Sternal Notch).

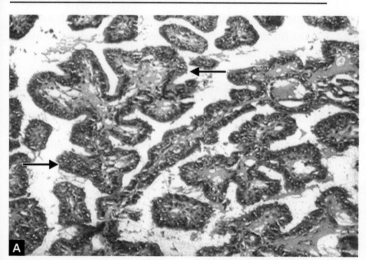

Figs. 3A and B: Bone scan showing an increased uptake in the sacral region suggestive of sacral metastasis (shown with arrow). (CBD: Continuous Bladder Drainage).

Figs. 5A and B: Orphan Annie eye nuclei (shown with arrow) in papillary carcinoma of thyroid, the nuclei looked similar to the eyes of all the characters of the American comic strip, Little Orphan Annie.

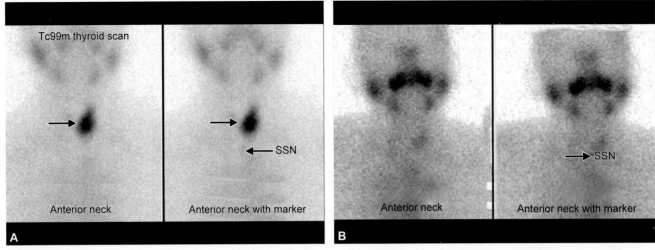

Figs. 6A and B: (A) Thyroid uptake study done before completion thyroidectomy showing an increased uptake in the left side of the thyroid region (shown with arrow), (B) Thyroid uptake study done after completion thyroidectomy showing no uptake in the thyroid bed. (SSN: Supra Sternal Notch).

100 mCi ablation and advised to come for follow-up after 6 months.

The follow-up whole body uptake scan after one year revealed an increased uptake in the thyroid region (Fig. 6A). The subsequent ultrasound thyroid confirmed 2 cm size recurrence of the thyroid tumor. She underwent a completion thyroidectomy. The surgical specimen showed multifocal papillary microcarcinoma (follicular variant). She also was given I^{131} 100 mCi ablation following surgery (Fig. 6B).

DISCUSSION

Papillary thyroid carcinoma is well-differentiated and slow growing, and have unique characteristics. Adjuvant therapy includes thyroid hormone suppression and radioiodine (^{131}I) therapy rather than chemotherapy and radiotherapy. The prognosis is generally excellent and is influenced by factors related to the patient, the disease and the therapy. Factors associated with a less favorable outcome are male sex, age >40 years, family history of papillary cancer, tumor diameter >4 cm, lymph node or distant metastases and invasive nature or poorly differentiated tumor. After total thyroidectomy and ^{131}I ablation, the follow-up includes a diagnostic radioiodine scan and serum thyroglobulin estimation (after thyroxine withdrawal) at six months. Further long term follow-up includes clinical examination, TSH monitoring to ensure adequate suppression and serum thyroglobulin measurement.[1] If thyroglobulin becomes detectable in a patient taking thyroxine then thyroxine is withdrawn, a diagnostic whole body scan is performed and the thyroglobulin measurement is repeated. Recombinant human TSH administration can be used to avoid the need for thyroxine withdrawal.[2]

REFERENCES

1. Jones MK. Management of papillary and follicular thyroid cancer. J R Soc Med. 2002;95(7):325–6.
2. Unnikrishnan AG, Kalra S, Baruah M, et al. Endocrine Society of India management guidelines for patients with thyroid nodules: A position statement. Indian J Endocrinol Metab. 2011;15(1):2–8.

CASE 18

A 54-year-old Mr. G was seen in the Endocrinology OPD with history of progressive swelling in neck for 5 years, associated with history of pain in neck. He was clinically and biochemically euthyroid. He had no other compressive symptoms. On examination, there was a 6 × 5 cm firm to hard swelling more on the left than the right side, which moved up with deglutition. The trachea was deviated to the right. Computed tomography (CT) scan of the neck is shown in Figures 1 and 2. He underwent a total thyroidectomy and the specimen were sent for histopathological examination (Figs. 3 and 4).

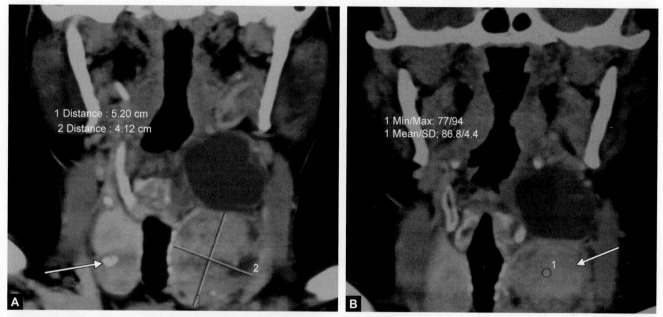

Figs. 1A and B: CT scan (coronal view) showing a heterogeneously enhancing large left thyroid nodule (arrow in 1B) with tracheal deviation to the right and a smaller nodule in the right lobe of thyroid with calcification (arrow in 1A).

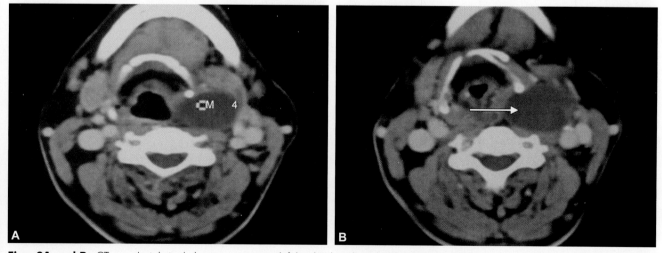

Figs. 2A and B: CT scan (axial view) showing a necrotic left level III lymph node (shown with arrow).

WHAT IS THE PROBABLE DIAGNOSIS?

The surgical specimen was evaluated and was found to have multifocal classical papillary thyroid carcinoma.

The follow-up Iodine[131] whole body survey revealed a residual thyroid and lymph nodal metastases (Fig. 5). He underwent Iodine[131] ablation a few months later. He was started on suppressive doses of Thyroxine and was followed up on a regular basis.

A few months later, he presented with progressive weakness of both lower limbs for ten days. He also had decreased sensation in both the lower limbs, more on the right than the left. There was no history of urinary or faecal incontinence. Shown below is the MRI of the spine (Fig. 6). His chest X-ray shown heterogeneous infiltrates with CT thorax also confirming the same (Figs. 7 and 8).

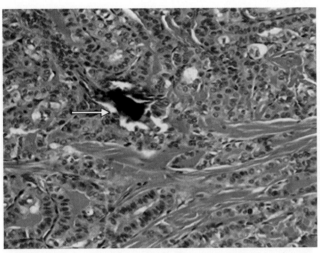

Fig. 3: Psammoma body in Papillary carcinoma of thyroid (shown with arrow).

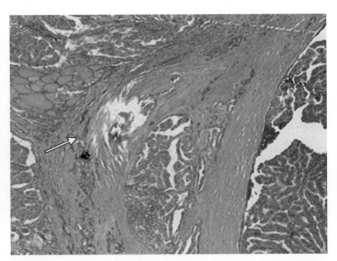

Fig. 4: Capsular invasion and extracapsular disease, a classical feature of Papillary carcinoma of thyroid (shown with arrow).

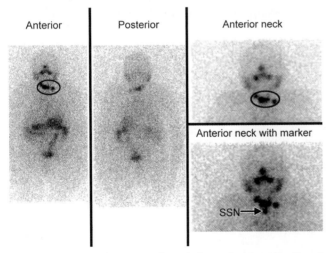

Fig. 5: Thyroid scintigraphy revealing a bulky residual thyroid and lymph node metastasis (shown with circle). (SSN: Supra Sternal Notch).

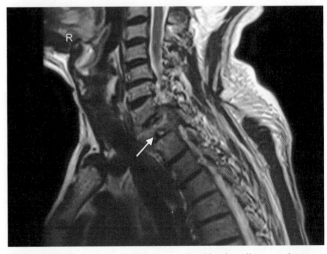

Fig. 6: MRI of spine revealing T1 vertebral body collapse with posterior bulge and cord compression (shown with arrow).

WHAT DO YOU THINK HAPPENED?

Mr G was evaluated for rapidly progressing paraparesis. A MRI spine showed features of skeletal metastases in multiple vertebrae. First thoracic vertebra showed collapse and epidural component causing cord compression (Fig. 6). A CT scan of the thorax also revealed multiple nodules in both the lungs (Fig. 8). He was planned for palliative radiotherapy to the spine. He was also referred to the spine surgery department for urgent decompressive surgery.

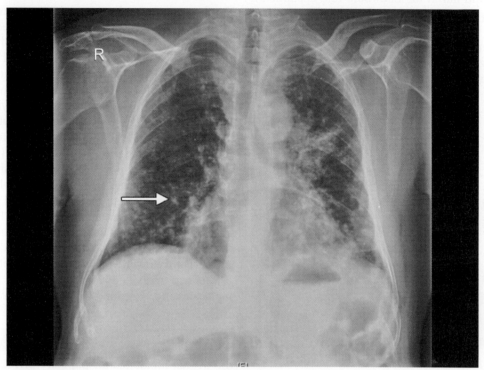

Fig. 7: Chest radiograph showing numerous basal predominant bilateral lung nodules of varying sizes (metastases, shown with arrow).

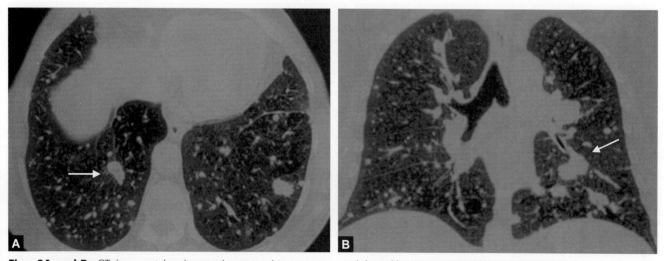

Figs. 8A and B: CT thorax axial and coronal sections showing numerous bilateral lung metastases (shown with arrow).

CASE 19

A 61-year-old, Mrs S presented to the casualty with history of slip and fall in the bathroom and sustained a closed injury to her left thigh. She had undergone a total thyroidectomy and Sistrunk's operation few months earlier. On examination she had swelling and tenderness over the left thigh with an abnormal mobility and crepitus. The X-ray of the left femur is shown below.

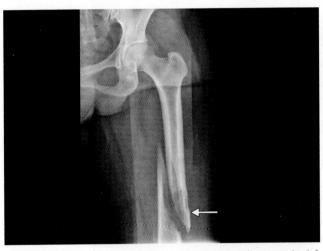

Fig. 1: Radiograph of the left femur showing a lytic lesion in the left mid shaft of femur with pathological fracture (shown with arrow).

WHAT IS THE DIAGNOSIS?

Mrs S was diagnosed to have papillary carcinoma thyroid who underwent a total thyroidectomy elsewhere came to our centre for further management. She developed a pathological fracture of the left femur and she underwent intramedullary nailing and fixation for the same (Fig. 1). The histopathology from the left femur was reported as metastatic adenocarcinoma and the thyroid pathology slides reviewed was reported as classical papillary carcinoma thyroid. Chest X-ray and Computed tomography (CT) thorax revealed features of metastasis (Figs. 2A and B). Computed tomography (CT) abdomen showed a metastasis in the vertebrae (Fig. 3). The I_{131} whole body scan showed an increased uptake in the thyroid residue (Fig. 4).

She was further evaluated with a PET CT for the disease status and was found to have disseminated metastatic disease (Figs. 5A to D). She was planned for diagnostic iodine scan followed by a therapeutic radioiodine ablation.

She was managed conservatively in the ward with analgesics and symptomatic, palliative care.

DISCUSSION

The overall incidence for papillary thyroid cancer (PTC) is 16.3/100,000 for women and 5.6/100,000 for men.

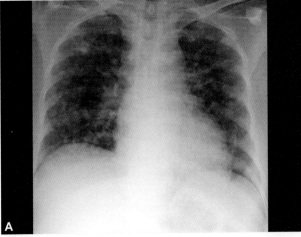

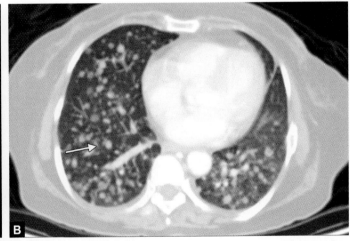

Figs. 2A and B: Chest radiograph and CT of thorax showing multiple lung metastasis (canon ball appearance, shown with arrow).

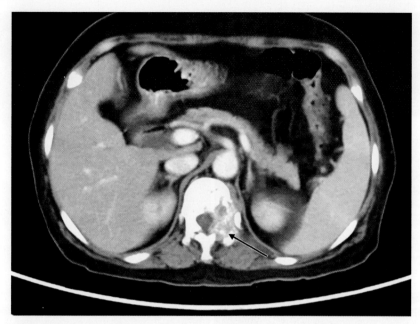

Fig. 3: Computed tomography of the abdomen showing a vertebral metastasis (shown with arrow).

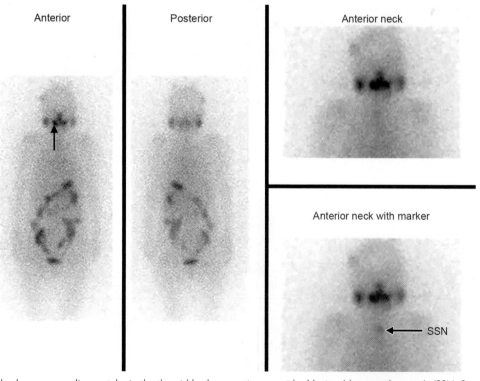

Fig. 4: I^{131} Whole body scan revealing uptake in the thyroid bed suggesting a residual lesion (shown with arrow). (SSN: Supra Sternal Notch).

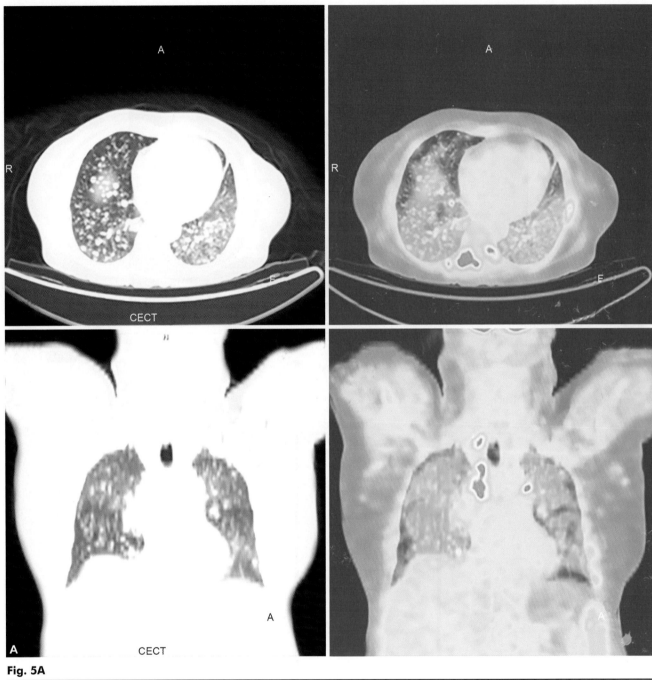

Fig. 5A

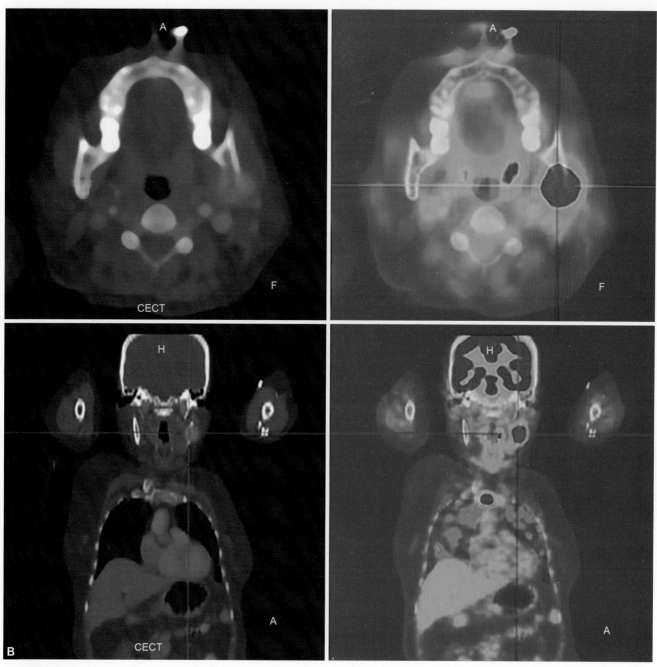

Fig. 5B

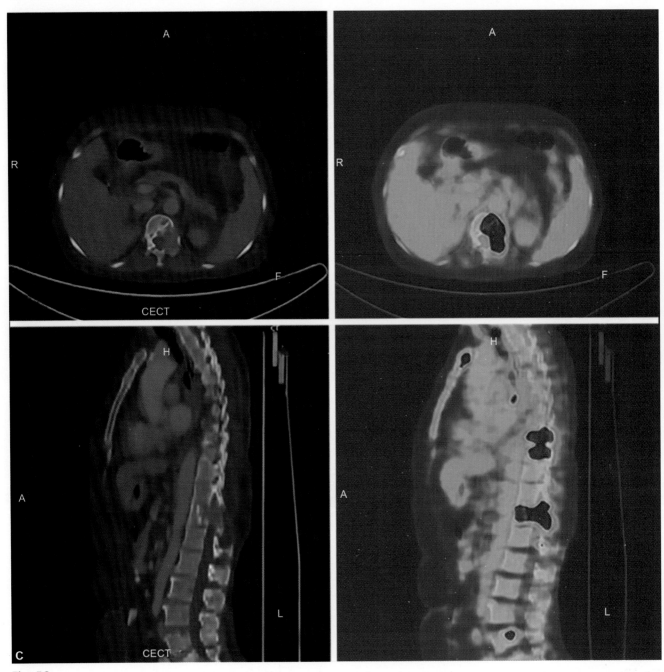

Fig. 5C

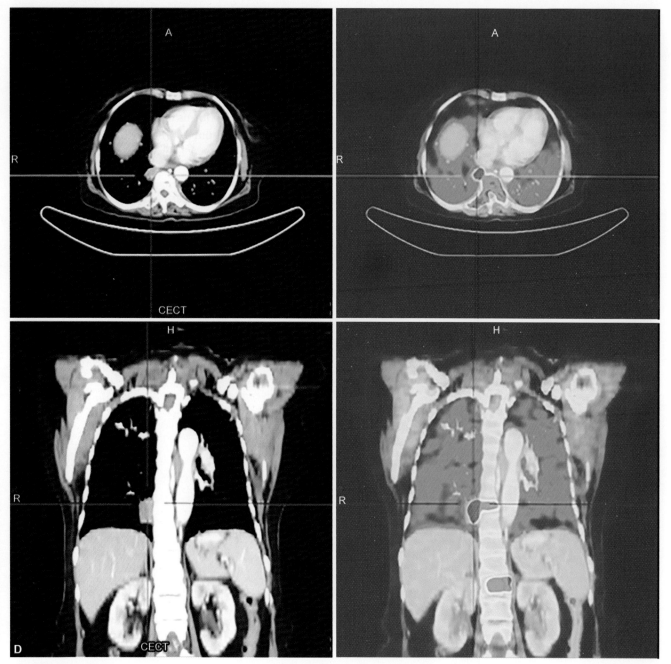

Figs. 5A to D: PET CT showing various areas of metastases including metastatic neck and mediastinal nodes, bone and lung metastases (areas in red indicate areas of increased FDG-uptake).

A history of rapid growth, a thyroid nodule or fixation of the nodule to surrounding tissues, and compressive symptoms like new onset hoarseness or vocal cord paralysis, dysphagia or dyspnea or the presence of ipsilateral cervical lymphadenopathy should raise the suspicion that a nodule may be malignant. Risk factors for PTC include a history of radiation exposure during childhood, a history of thyroid cancer in a first-degree relative, or a family history of a thyroid cancer.[1]

Mutations in the genes encoding for the proteins in the mitogen-activated protein kinase (MAPK) pathway are critical to the development and progression of differentiated thyroid cancer. Mutations in RET/PTC, neurotropic tyrosine kinase receptor type 1 (NTRK1), Ras, or BRAF occur in as many as 70 percent of well differentiated thyroid cancers.

Papillary cancers are typically unencapsulated and may be partially cystic. Microscopically, most are characterized by the presence of papillae consisting of one or two layers of tumor cells surrounding a well-defined fibro-vascular core; follicles and colloid are typically absent. Orphan Annie eye nuclear inclusions (nuclei with uniform staining, which appear empty) and psammoma bodies seen on light microscopy are characteristic for PTC. The former is useful in identifying the follicular variant of papillary thyroid carcinomas. The morphologic diagnosis is based upon an aggregate of typical cytologic features which itself is a pathognomonic feature of PTC. The nuclei are large, oval, and appear crowded and overlapping on microscopic sections. They may contain hypodense powdery chromatin, cytoplasmic pseudo inclusions due to a redundant nuclear membrane, or nuclear grooves. Lymphatic spread is more common than haematogenous spread. The so-called lateral aberrant thyroid is actually a lymph node metastasis from papillary thyroid carcinoma.

Most patients with papillary cancer do not succumb to disease itself. Variant forms of papillary cancer include the follicular variant (about 10%) and the tall-cell variant (a more aggressive tumor, 1%).[2]

REFERENCES

1. DM, TMK, Khan DM, Raman R T. Follicular variant of papillary thyroid carcinoma: cytological indicators of diagnostic value. J Clin Diagn Res. 2014;8(3):46-8.
2. Schneider AB, Sarne DH. Long-term risks for thyroid cancer and other neoplasms after exposure to radiation. Nat Clin Pract Endocrinol Metab 2005;1:82.

CASE **20**

A 75-year-old lady, presented with a progressive swelling in front of the neck for 30 years. There was no history of hyperthyroidism or hypothyroidism. There were no pressure symptoms like dysphagia or hoarseness of voice. She complained of a choking feeling for the past 2 years, when she lies flat. Her husband and three of her children were taking medicines for hypothyroidism. On examination, she had a 10 × 8 cm size, firm swelling in front of the neck which was more on the right side, which moved up with deglutition. There was no retrosternal extension but the trachea was deviated to left side.

WHAT IS THE PRELIMINARY DIAGNOSIS? WHAT ARE THE DIFFERENTIAL DIAGNOSES?

The diagnosis was that of a dominant nodule in a multinodular goitre. The patient underwent a total thyroidectomy and the surgical specimen was diagnosed to be a follicular variant of papillary carcinoma involving left lobe. Hurthle cell nodules were also evident in the left lobe. Post surgery she was put on suppressive doses of thyroxine.

The following year an ultrasound neck was done which showed enlarged lymph nodes (Fig. 1). she underwent Iodine[131] whole body scan which revealed a residual thyroid (Fig. 2). She was then admitted for Iodine[131] ablation.

After 6 months she was found to have elevated serum thyroglobulin and a repeat I[131] whole body scan there was an increased tracer activity in the left thyroid region and T6 thoracic vertebrae which is highly suggestive of skeletal metastases (Fig. 3).

This patient was given 100 mci of I[131] and then kept on suppressive dose of thyroxine, with regular follow-up.

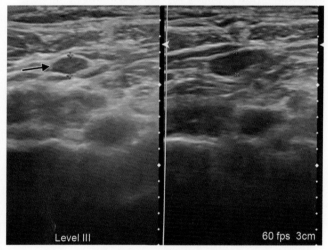

Fig. 1: Postoperative ultrasonography (USG) of the neck showing level 3 cervical lymph nodes (shown with arrow).

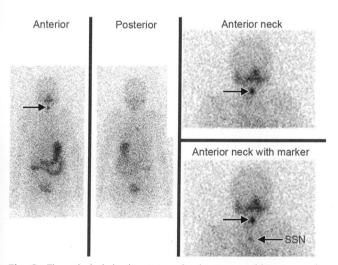

Fig. 2: Thyroid whole body scintigraphy showing a mild tracer uptake in the thyroid bed suggestive of mild residual thyroid (shown with arrow). (SSN: Supra Sternal Notch).

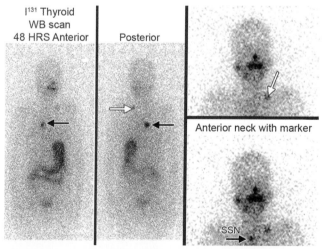

Fig. 3: Thyroid whole body scintigraphy done 6 months later, showing tracer accumulation in the left side of the neck and in the region of the T6 vertebra, suggestive of functioning metastases to the left supraclavicular lymph node (shown with white arrow) and the T6 vertebra (shown with black arrow).

DISCUSSION

The overall incidence for papillary thyroid cancer (PTC) is 16.3/100,000 for women and 5.6/100,000 for men. A history of rapid growth, a thyroid nodule or fixation of the nodule to surrounding tissues, and compressive symptoms like new onset hoarseness or vocal cord paralysis, dysphagia or dyspnea or the presence of ipsilateral cervical lymphadenopathy should raise the suspicion that a nodule may be malignant. Risk factors for PTC include a history of radiation exposure during childhood, a history of thyroid cancer in a first-degree relative, or a family history of a thyroid cancer.[1]

Mutations in the genes encoding for the proteins in the mitogen-activated protein kinase (MAPK) pathway are critical to the development and progression of differentiated thyroid cancer. Mutations in RET/PTC, neurotropic tyrosine kinase receptor type 1 (NTRK1), Ras, or (proto oncogene BRAF or V-RAF murine sarcoma viral oncogene hemoglobin) occur in as many as 70 percent of well differentiated thyroid cancers.

Papillary cancers are typically unencapsulated and may be partially cystic. Microscopically, most are characterized by the presence of papillae consisting of one or two layers of tumor cells surrounding a well-defined fibro-vascular core; follicles and colloid are typically absent. Orphan Annie eye nuclear inclusions (nuclei with uniform staining, which appear empty) and psammoma bodies seen on light microscopy are characteristic for PTC. The former is useful in identifying the follicular variant of papillary thyroid carcinomas. The morphologic diagnosis is based upon an aggregate of typical cytologic features which by itself is a pathognomonic feature of PTC. The nuclei are large, oval, and appear crowded and overlapping on microscopic sections. They may contain hypodense powdery chromatin, cytoplasmic pseudo inclusions due to a redundant nuclear membrane, or nuclear grooves. Lymphatic spread is more common than haematogenous spread. The so-called lateral aberrant thyroid is actually a lymph node metastasis from papillary thyroid carcinoma.

Most patients with papillary cancer do not succumb to disease itself. Variant forms of papillary cancer include the follicular variant (about 10%) and the tall-cell variant (a more aggressive tumor, 1%).[2]

REFERENCES

1. DM, TMK, Khan DM, Raman R T. Follicular variant of papillary thyroid carcinoma: cytological indicators of diagnostic value. J Clin Diagn Res. 2014;8(3):46-8.
2. Schneider AB, Sarne DH. Long-term risks for thyroid cancer and other neoplasms after exposure to radiation. Nat Clin Pract Endocrinol Metab. 2005;1:82.

CASE 21

A 60-year-old lady presented with swellings on head for the past 2 years and in front of her neck for the past 6 years. (Fig. 1)

WHAT IS YOUR PRELIMINARY DIAGNOSIS?

On further history she had symptoms of hypothyroidism (lethargy, tiredness) and complained of pain in the swelling of the head. She also complained of lower back ache.

On examination, the neck swelling moved up with deglutition and was bilateral and diffusely enlarged, the surface of which was irregular. She also had multiple enlarged cervical lymph nodes.

On investigations, the Chest X-ray showed multiple well defined infiltrates bilaterally (Fig. 2). Whole body uptake scan showed increased uptake in both the lungs (Fig. 3). The clinical picture was highly suggestive of a thyroid primary malignancy with distant metastases. A fine needle aspiration (FNA) biopsy revealed epithelial cells arranged in a pattern of microfollicles, scant or absent colloid, and few macrophages and defined the lesion of follicular lesion of undetermined significance.

With the clinical picture and investigations she was diagnosed with follicular thyroid carcinoma with distant metastasis.

DISCUSSION

Follicular thyroid cancer is the second most common type of thyroid cancer after papillary thyroid cancer.[1] Follicular thyroid cancer typically spreads via hematogeneous dissemination. Common sites of distant metastases are bone (with lytic lesions) and lung and, less commonly, the brain, liver, bladder, and skin. Unlike papillary thyroid cancer, FNA biopsy cannot diagnose or distinguish between the follicular adenomas and cancers. Microscopically, the diagnosis of follicular cancer requires distinguishing

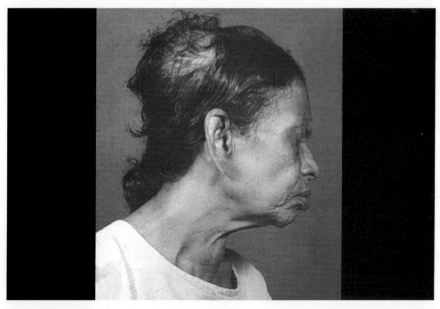

Fig. 1: Clinical picture of the patient with skull and neck swellings.

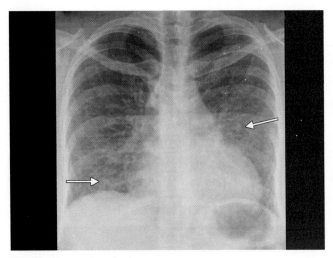

Fig. 2: Metastasis to the lungs.

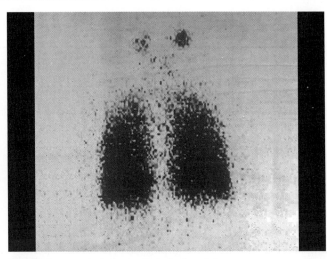

Fig. 3: Lung metastasis on whole body uptake scan.

adenoma from cancer, through identification of tumor extension through the tumor capsule and/or vascular invasion, given the fact that follicular cancer commonly occurs in older patients and is more often associated with an aggressive clinical course and distant metastases. It has higher mortality than papillary thyroid cancer.[2]

REFERENCES

1. D'Avanzo A, Treseler P, Ituarte PHG, et al. Follicular thyroid carcinoma: histology and prognosis. Cancer. 2004; 15;100(6):1123–9.
2. Machens A, Holzhausen H-J, Dralle H. The prognostic value of primary tumor size in papillary and follicular thyroid carcinoma. Cancer. 2005;1;103(11):2269–73.

CASE 22

A 48-year-old lady presented to our clinic with a history of progressive, painless swelling in front of the neck over the past 25 years. However, more recently, she had developed dyspnea on exertion with hoarseness of her voice. She was not a hypertensive and did not have any associated skin lesions.

On examination she was found to have thyroid swelling of 10 × 7 cm which was of variegated consistency. She had stridor on palpation of the gland (Fig. 1A). Pemberton's sign was positive (Fig. 1B). There were no other clinical features.

An ultrasound of the neck revealed bilateral thyroid masses with heterogeneous echotexture, central pattern of vascularity, macro and micro calcifications. Chest X-ray showed deviated trachea with probable compression or infiltration of the trachea (Fig. 2). Fine needle aspiration cytology (FNAC) of the thyroid showed amyloid deposits in the background of colloid and the cells were positive for calcitonin (Figs. 3 and 4).

Computed tomography (CT) scan neck showed a thyroid mass with infiltration of the trachea (Fig. 5).

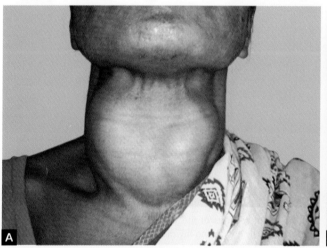 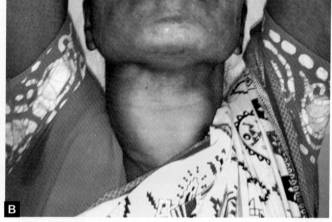

Figs. 1A and B: (A) Thyroid swelling, (B) Pemberton's sign.

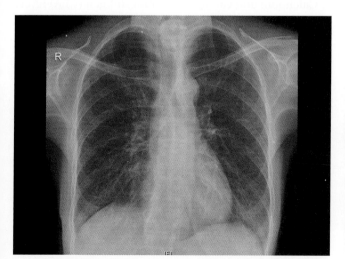 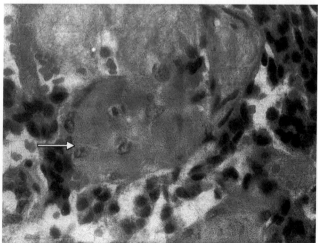

Fig. 2: Chest X-ray showing deviation of the trachea to the right side.

Fig. 3: Amyloid deposits in the background of colloid.

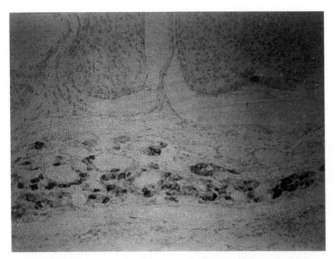

Fig. 4: Well demarcated collections of calcitonin staining cells.

WHAT IS THE DIAGNOSIS?

Based on the clinical, pathological and radiological findings she was diagnosed with medullary thyroid carcinoma with tracheal invasion.

Subsequently, she underwent total thyroidectomy with central compartment dissection and resection and anastamosis of the tracheal infiltration segment.

DISCUSSION

Medullary thyroid carcinoma (MTC) is an uncommon neuroendocrine malignancy that accounts for 5% of all the thyroid cancers.[1] Medullary thyroid carcinoma (MTC) presents in sporadic and familial forms (multiple endocrine neoplasia (MEN) 2A, MEN 2B, or familial MTC syndromes). The familial forms are secondary to germline mutations in the REarranged during Transfection (RET) proto-oncogene. Early diagnosis and treatment is most important. Genetic testing has made possible, the early detection in asymptomatic carriers and high-risk patients, with early or prophylactic surgery being curative in many. All carriers of an RET mutation should be evaluated and treated surgically for MTC. The primary treatment in all patients diagnosed with MTC is total thyroidectomy with central lymph node dissection.[2]

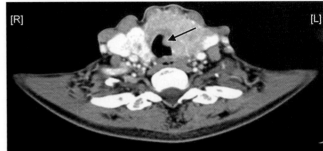

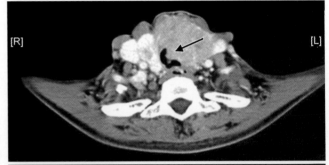

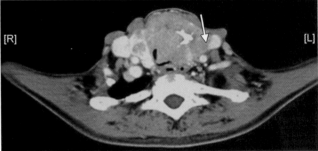

Fig. 5: Serial sections of the CT scan of the neck showing a large heterogeneously enhancing thyroid mass infiltrating the trachea (black arrow) and left internal jugular vein (white arrow).

Calcitonin and carcinoembryonic antigen (CEA) levels can be used as prognostic factors and as tumor markers. If elevated, further investigation, including use of imaging modalities, may be necessary for evaluation of metastatic disease.

REFERENCES

1. Finny P, Jacob JJ, Thomas N, et al. Medullary thyroid carcinoma: a 20-year experience from a centre in South India. ANZ J Surg. 2007;77(3):130-4.
2. Griebeler ML, Gharib H, Thompson GB. Medullary thyroid carcinoma. Endocr Pract. 2013;19(4):703-11.

CASE 23

A 34-year-old lady presented with an insidious onset and slowly progressive neck swelling for over 12 years. She did not have features suggestive of either hypothyroidism or hyperthyroidism. There was no previous history of pressure symptoms.

On physical examination there was a 3 cm × 4 cm submental swelling which moved on deglutition and protrusion of the tongue (Figs. 1A and B). The swelling was variegated in consistency with cystic and few firm areas. She did not have any lymph nodal enlargement.

Her thyroid function tests were normal. Ultrasound of the neck showed a complex cystic lesion with an irregular papillary solid component with microcalcifications in the midline of the neck at the level of hyoid bone. The normal thyroid gland was separately seen.

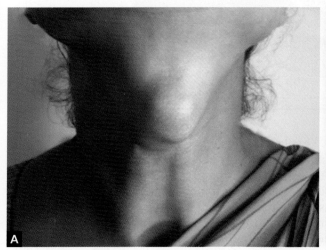
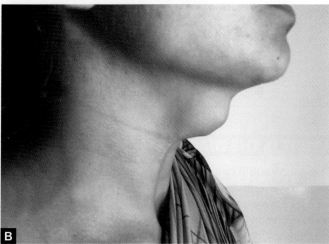

Figs. 1A and B: Submental neck swelling.

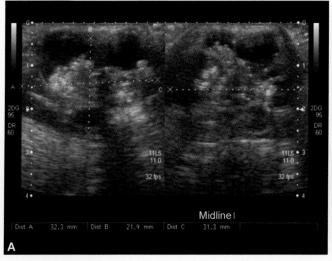
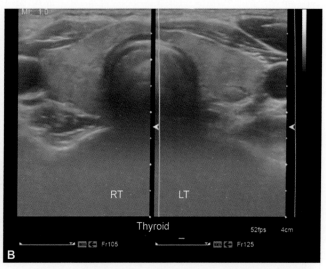

Figs. 2A and B: Ultrasound of the neck (A) Midline subhyoid complex cystic lesion with irregular solid component and microcalcification, (B) Normal thyroid gland.

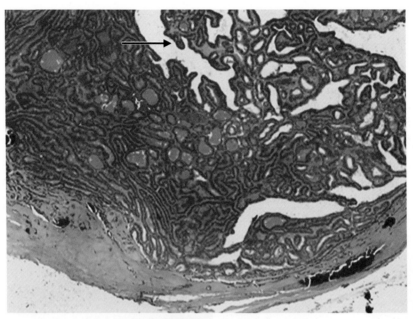

Fig. 3: Papillae (finger like projections) suggestive of Papillary carcinoma of thyroid.

WHAT IS THE DIAGNOSIS?

Figures 2A and B could represent malignancy in a thyroglossal cyst. Subsequently, she underwent FNA cytology which showed clusters of colloid and psammoma bodies with occasional follicular cells suggestive of Papillary carcinoma thyroid in a thyroglossal cyst (Fig. 3).

She underwent a Sistrunk operation with total thyroidectomy for the swelling and was put on replacement doses of thyroxine.

DISCUSSION

The thyroglossal duct cyst (TGDC) is the most common anomaly associated with thyroid development. The thyroid gland descends from the foramen caecum to a point below the thyroid cartilage and leaves an epithelial tract known as the thyroglossal tract. The tract disappears during the 5th to the 10th gestational week. Incomplete atrophy of the tract forms the basis of origin of the cyst.[1]

Malignancy within a thyroglossal duct cyst is rare and occurs in only about 1.5% of cases, and diagnosis is usually made postoperatively as clinically it may be difficult to distinguish from benign neoplasms. Features that should arouse suspicion of malignancy include large or increasing size, hardness, fixity, irregular shape and previous exposure to ionizing radiation. There is no role for routine FNAC of a thyroglossal duct cyst in the absence of suspicious features.[2]

REFERENCES

1. Aculate NR, Jones HB, Bansal A, et al. Papillary carcinoma within a thyroglossal duct cyst: significance of a central solid component on ultrasound imaging. Br J Oral Maxillofac Surg. 2014;52(3):277-8. doi:10.1016/j.bjoms.2013.10.003. Epub 2013 Nov 5. PubMed PMID: 24210780.
2. Senthilkumar R, Neville JF, Aravind R. Malignant thyroglossal duct cyst with synchronous occult thyroid gland papillary carcinoma. Indian J Endocrinol Metab. 2013;17 (5):936-8. doi: 10.4103/2230-8210.117229.

CASE 24

A 56-year-old non-smoking farmer presented to our Thyroid clinic with the rapid progression of the thyroid swelling over the past 20 days with simultaneous hoarseness of voice during the same period. He had a thyroid swelling for the past 20 years whose size was static in nature (Fig. 1).

Clinical examination showed a massive deviation of the trachea to the left side with a predominant right lobe thyroid enlargement. Chest X-ray image is shown in Figure 2.

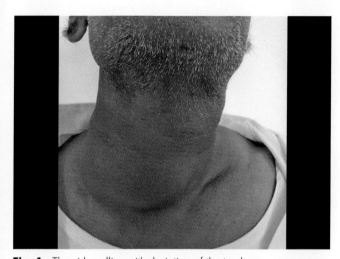

Fig. 1: Thyroid swelling with deviation of the trachea.

WHAT COULD BE THE PROBABLE CLINICAL DIAGNOSIS?

This gentleman had probable anaplastic carcinoma clinically in view of the rapid progression of the symptoms. The hoarseness of voice could be well due to the external laryngeal nerve involvement. The Chest X-ray showed a massive deviation of trachea to the left side.

The computed tomography (CT) scan neck and thorax showed a large heterogeneously enhancing mass with chunky calcifications in the right lobe of thyroid measuring 5.9 × 8 × 12 cm (Fig. 3).

The patient underwent a trucut biopsy of the right lobe of thyroid which was also suggestive of a possible anaplastic carcinoma of the thyroid and the patient was advised external beam radiotherapy.

DISCUSSION

Anaplastic thyroid cancers are undifferentiated tumors of the thyroid follicular epithelium. In marked contrast to the differentiated thyroid cancers, anaplastic cancers are extremely aggressive, with a disease-specific mortality approaching 95 percent. The few exceptions are patients whose tumors are small and who are treated very aggressively. Approximately 20 percent of patients have a history

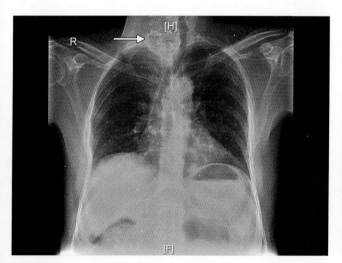

Fig. 2: Chest radiograph showing a large soft tissue density mass in the right side of the neck causing compression and deviation of the trachea to the left side.

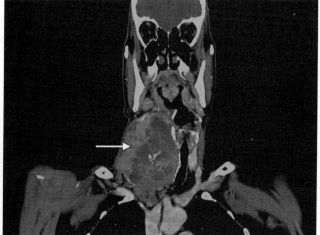

Fig. 3: Computed tomography (CT) showing a large right thyroid mass (shown with arrow) with areas of necrosis and calcifications.

of differentiated thyroid cancer and 20–30 percent have a coexisting differentiated cancer. The primary symptom of anaplastic cancer is a rapidly enlarging neck mass, occurring in about 85 percent of patients.[1]

The diagnosis of anaplastic cancer is usually established by cytologic examination of cells which show spindle cells, pleomorphic giant cells, and/or squamoid. Many anaplastic thyroid cancers have a mixed morphology of two or all three patterns.

For patients with a small intrathyroidal anaplastic cancer associated with a differentiated thyroid cancer, we suggest total thyroidectomy. Total thyroidectomy will facilitate subsequent treatment of the differentiated thyroid cancer. However, for the rare patients with intrathyroidal anaplastic thyroid cancer, without a co-existent well differentiated thyroid cancer component, thyroid lobectomy with wide margins of adjacent soft tissue by the side of the tumor is an appropriately aggressive alternative surgical approach.[2]

REFERENCES

1. Neff RL, Farrar WB, Kloos RT, et al. Anaplastic thyroid cancer. Endocrinol Metab Clin North Am. 2008;37:525.
2. Smallridge RC, Copland JA. Anaplastic thyroid carcinoma: pathogenesis and emerging therapies. Clin Oncol (R Coll Radiol). 2010;22:486.

CASE 25

A 46-year-old lady presented to us with complaints of multiple swellings in front of the neck for a period of 4 years. There were no specific symptoms of thyroid disturbances but she complained of difficulty in swallowing. There were complaints of change in voice.

On examination, she was found to have enlargement of lymph nodes in many levels of the neck including a thyroid swelling (Fig. 1).

An ultrasound of the neck was done and it revealed multiple lymph node swellings with loss of fatty hilum (Fig. 2).

WHAT IS THE DIAGNOSIS?

This patient most likely had a malignant thyroid swelling with nodular metastasis. A fine needle aspiration cytology (FNAC) should be done to confirm the diagnosis.

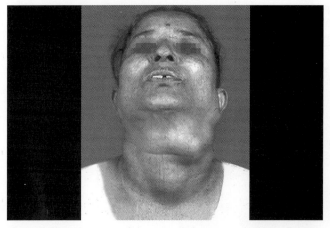

Fig. 1: Clinical picture of the patient showing multiple swellings in front of the neck.

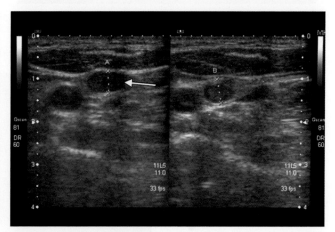

Fig. 2: Lymph node showing loss of fatty hilum suggestive of malignant nature (shown with arrow).

CLINICAL IMAGES OF THYROID SWELLINGS (FIGS. 3 TO 8)

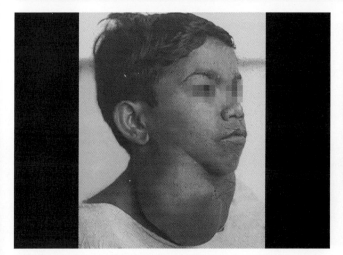

Fig. 3: An 8-year-old boy present with a massive thyroid swelling which was most probably due to lack of Iodine in diet. Goitres are endemic in certain areas of India. Differentials like lympho-proliferative disorders, must be considered for massive neck swellings like this.

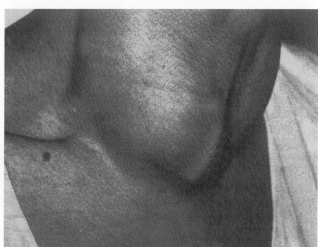

Fig. 4: Unilateral thyroid swelling, most probably a dominant nodule of a multinodular goiter. The left lobe is just visible.

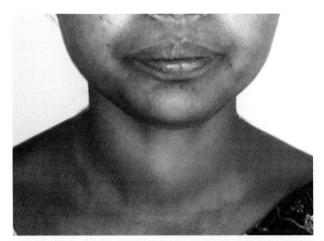

Fig. 5: A 23-year-old lady presented with symptoms suggestive of hypothyroidism, on examination a diffuse thyroid swelling was palpable. She most probably had Hashimoto's thyroiditis clinically.

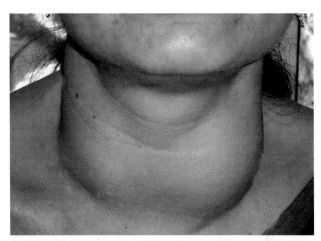

Fig. 6: A 37-year-old lady presented with a bilateral thyroid swelling. She had no symptoms suggestive of thyroid illness. FNAC of the swelling revealed it to be a benign swelling.

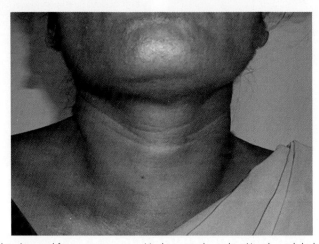

Fig. 7: Diffuse thyroid swelling with biochemical features suggesting Hashimotos thyroiditis (Antithyroglobulin and Anti Thyroid Peroxidase > 400).

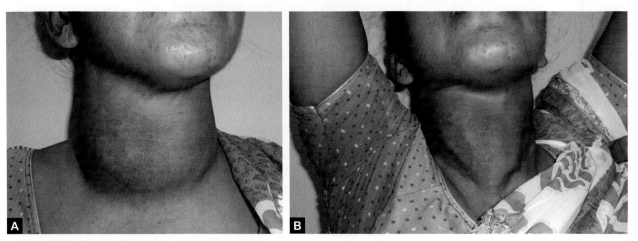

Figs. 8A and B: Positive Pemberton's sign: Dilated veins on the anterior surface of the neck on raising the hands. This lady presented with a massive neck swelling that was extending retrosternally that pressed upon the superior vena cava on raising the hands, thereby causing dilatation of the veins in the upper part of the body.

ULTRASONOGRAPHY OF THYROID (FIGS. 9 TO 19)

Ultrasound of the thyroid is done with high frequency (7 to 13 MHz) transducers. Ultrasonography is highly operator dependent. It is done for detection of non palpable nodules, characterization of nodule, therapeutic purposes and for monitoring of nodule size. The risk of malignancy with respect to the echogenecity are:

- Hyperechoic lesion—4%;
- Isoechoic lesion—26%;
- Hypoechoic lesion—63%.

Lesions with a complete halo around them are usually benign. (Halo sign was described earlier in the chapter).

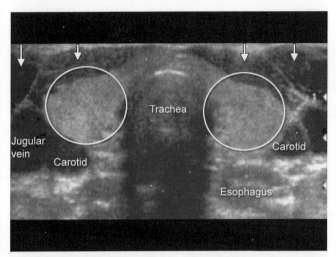

Fig. 9: Ultrasound of the neck showing a normal thyroid.

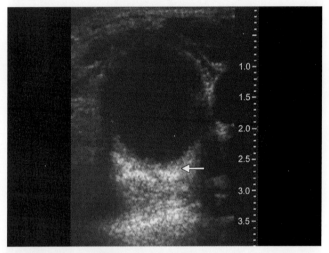

Fig. 10: A cystic nodule in the thyroid.

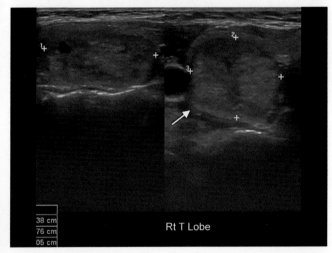

Fig. 11: Ultrasound thyroid showing a well defined iso-echoic nodule with a peripheral halo. This patient presented with a neck swelling on the right side for the past 3 months. She did not have any toxic or hypothyroid symptoms. FNAC revealed a benign pathology.

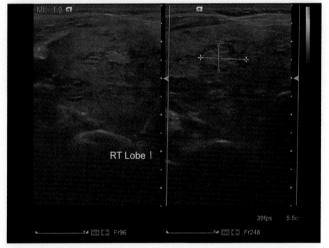

Fig. 12: Well defined isoechoic nodule in the right lobe with honey comb appearance suggestive of a benign (colloid) thyroid nodule.

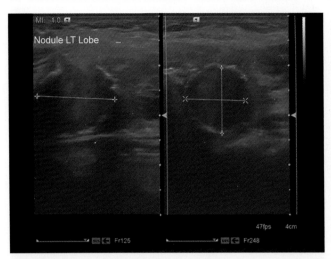

Fig. 13: Ultrasound of thyroid showing a curvilinear peripheral calcification which is a benign finding.

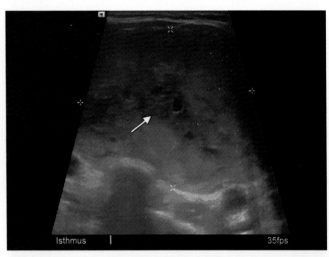

Fig. 14: A large predominantly solid heterogenous nodule with cystic appearance (probably benign).

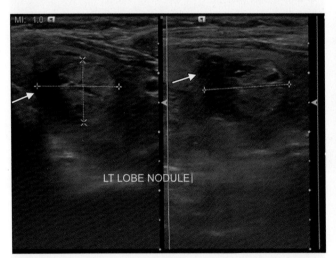

Fig. 15: Ultrasound thyroid showing a heterogeneous isoechoic nodule with eccentric hypoechoic component and an ill-defined lobulated margins, suggestive of malignant potential. This is a 40 year old lady who presented with bilateral neck swelling more prominent on the left side. Clinically, she had a dominant nodule out of a multinodular goitre.

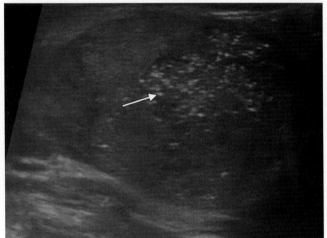

Fig. 16: Thyroid ultrasound showing microcalcification (shown with arrow), a feature of thyroid cancer. This patient, a 55-year-old patient presented with neck swelling, progressively increasing in size, weight loss and loss of appetite. FNAC of the thyroid was suggestive of papillary carcinoma of thyroid.

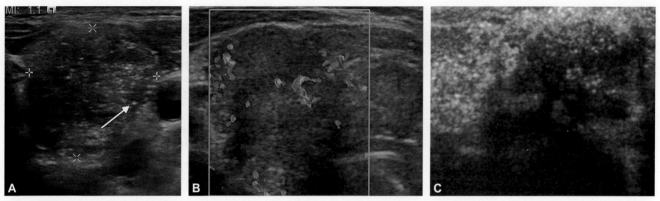

Figs. 17A to C: This patient presented with a thyroid swelling and symptoms suggestive of malignancy. The Ultrasound of the neck showed multiple ill-defined, solid, markedly hypoechoic nodules, taller than wide in shape with microcalcifications and central vascularity. These features are highly suggestive of malignancy.

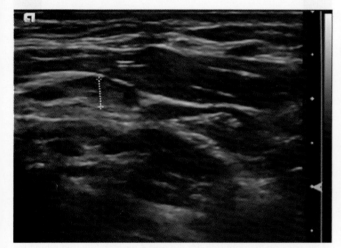

Fig. 18: Normal lymph node with a preserved fatty hilum.

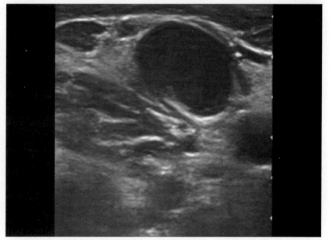

Fig. 19: Malignant node with necrosis and lost fatty hilum. Malignant metastatic lymph nodes from the carcinoma of thyroid gland may also have microcalcifications.

DOPPLER STUDIES OF THYROID (FIG. 20)

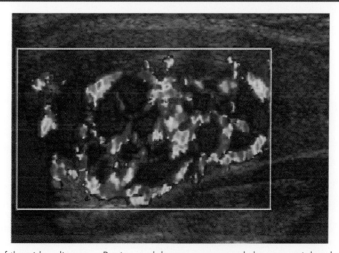

Fig. 20: Central vascularity suggestive of thyroid malignancy. Benign nodules more commonly have a peripheral vascularity.

RADIONUCLIDE SCANNING IMAGES (FIGS. 21 AND 22)

This works on the principle of differential uptake of radio-active isotopes. Risk of malignancy is:

• Cold—16%
• Indeterminate—10%
• Hot—<1%

WHAT DO YOU THINK IS THE DIAGNOSIS OF THE PATIENT?

The patient was diagnosed to have a malignancy in the thyroid swelling. There is an increased risk of malignancy in swellings that are 'cold' on radionuclide scanning.

WHAT IS YOUR DIAGNOSIS?

The patient has a hot nodule (Fig. 22, shown with circle) and the risk of malignancy in such nodules is low ~<1%.

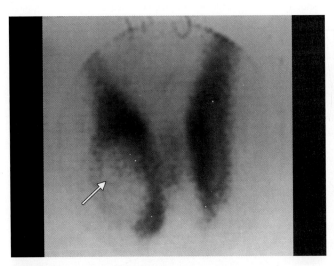

Fig. 21: A 48-year-old gentleman presented with a neck swelling for the past 8 months. He had no symptoms suggestive of hyperthyroidism or hypothyroidism. There was a history of mild change in voice over the past month. The figure above is a radionuclide scan of the patient showing a cold nodule in the right side (shown with arrow).

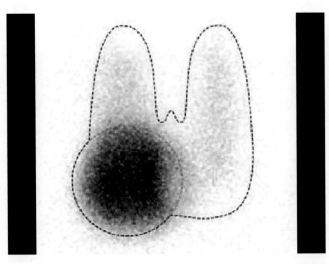

Fig. 22: A 45-year-old lady presented with a nodular swelling in front of the neck on the right side, for the past 4 months. She had symptoms suggestive of hyperthyroidism and a radionuclide scan was done (see figure above).

MULTIPLE CHOICE QUESTIONS

1. A 26-year-old lady presents with recurrent episodes of palpitations over a period of 3 years. Clinical examination reveals a smooth symmetrical goiter, just visible in the anterior part of the neck. Biochemical tests show a total T4 of 19.0 µg/dL (Normal 4.5–11.5 µg/dL) and a TSH of 8.0mIU/mL (Normal 0.5–4.5 mIU/mL). Which of the following is *FALSE:*
   A. It could be a TSH producing tumor
   B. It could be thyroid hormone receptor resistance
   C. The biochemical values could be present in a euthyroid normal pregnancy
   D. A visual field test may be indicated

2. All of the following are associated with normal/raised radioactive iodine uptake activity over the neck with an intact thyroid, *EXCEPT:*
   A. Graves disease
   B. Trophoblastic disease
   C. Thyroid hormone resistance
   D. Excessive metastasis from thyroid cancer

3. All of the following therapies are useful in the management of Thyroid Eye Disease, *EXCEPT:*
   A. Azathioprine
   B. Etanercept
   C. Selenium
   D. Chromium

4. All of the following drugs are associated with thyroiditis, *EXCEPT:*
   A. Amiodarone
   B. Interferon alpha
   C. Interleukin-2
   D. Amitriptyline

5. All of the following mutations are described in follicular carcinoma, *EXCEPT:*
   A. RAS
   B. PAX8
   C. PPAR Gamma
   D. BRAF

6. Hyperthyroidism in children, all of the following statements are true *EXCEPT:*
   A. Sufficient I-131 therapy is advisable for GD management as a single dose to reach a state of hypothyroidism
   B. Pediatric patients with Graves disease who are not in remission following 1–2 years of methimazole therapy should be considered for treatment with RAI therapy/thyroidectomy
   C. I-131 therapy should be completely avoided in children less than 5 years.

D. PTU is associated with a lower number of reported side effects pertaining to hepatotoxicity in children

7. All of the following drugs are associated with thyroiditis, *EXCEPT:*
   A. Amiodarone
   B. Interferon alpha
   C. Interleukin-2
   D. Amitriptyline

8. All of the following can be secreted by Medullary carcinoma thyroid *EXCEPT:*
   A. Carcinoma embryonic antigen
   B. Somatostatin
   C. Cortisol
   D. TRH

9. A 23-year-old lady presented with features suggestive of thyrotoxicosis. Her evaluation for the same with blood investigations and nuclear medicine studies are suggestive of thyrotoxicosis factitia. Which one of the following is not a feature of thyrotoxicosis factitia?
   A. Suppressed—TSH, and elevated T4 and FT4
   B. Elevated thyroglobulin level
   C. Low radioiodine uptake
   D. Absent thyroid auto-antibodies

10. A 25-year-old lady with bipolar disorder has been on lithium therapy since 2 years. She is married for 4 years and has not conceived yet. She has also a recent history of polydipsia, weight loss and palpitation. She was referred by psychiatry department for further evaluation. Which of the following endocrine disorder is not common with long-term lithium therapy?
    A. Hypothyroidism
    B. Thyrotoxicosis
    C. Nephrogenic diabetes insipidus
    D. Hypocalcemia

11. An 18-year-old lady presented with painful thyroid swelling since 2 weeks. On examination she has a grade-2 thyroid swelling with tenderness. Her blood investigation revealed TSH – 0.34 µIU/ml (Normal 0.5–4.5 mIU/mL). T4 of -12.5 µg/dL (Normal 4.5–11.5 µg/dL) and FT4 for 1.8 ng/dL (Normal 0.8–1.8 ng/dL and a high ESR. Radioiodine uptake study showed 10% uptake at 24 hours. She was initially treated with naproxen 1 tab twice daily for 1 week. However, she continued to have pain, so later on she was treated with prednisone. All of the following are the indications of prednisolone (steroid) therapy in thyroid disorders *EXCEPT:*

A. Hashimoto's encephalopathy
B. Thyrotoxicosis storm
C. Myxedema coma
D. Prior to radioiodine therapy in the absence of eye disease

12. All of the following clinical condition are associated with increase in radioiodine uptake in the region of thyroid *EXCEPT*:
A. Graves' disease
B. Metastatic thyroid cancer
C. Choriocarcinoma
D. Struma ovarii

13. A 60-year-old lady, a known patient of Hashimoto's thyroiditis, primary hypothyroidisms presented with rapidly increasing thyroid swelling since 3 months. The thyroid swelling was associated with pressure symptoms and pain. On examination, both lobes of the thyroid were enlarged (right was larger than left). FNAC of the thyroid was suggestive of lymphoma. Which type of lymphoma is more common in the setting of Hashimoto's thyroiditis?
A. Adult T-cell lymphoma
B. Mixed cellularity Hodgkin's lymphoma
C. Hairy cell leukemia
D. MALT lymphoma

14. A 34-year-old lady teacher by profession presented with history of a thyroid swelling since 2 years. On examination, the thyroid swelling appears firm to hard in consistency and there were no palpable lymph nodes. The FNAC of thyroid nodule was suggestive of medullary carcinoma. She had no prior family history of thyroid carcinoma. She is married with 3 children. Her genetic analysis showed mutation at codon 609. Monitoring of kindred with positive for RET mutation include all *EXCEPT*:
A. Annual monitoring of stimulated calcitonin
B. Annual monitoring of urinary metanephrines and normetanephrines
C. 1–2 yearly monitoring of serum calcium and iPTH levels
D. Annual monitoring of prolactin level

15. A 45-year-old gentleman presented with thyroid swelling since 5 years. Patients noticed, that the size of swelling increased 1 and ½ times recently. On examination, there was a large nodule of size >3 cm on the right upper pole of thyroid and clinically there was no significant lymph node enlargement. His ultrasound of the thyroid showed a TIRAD score of 4C. Which of the following is not a feature of this scoring system?
A. Solid component
B. Markedly hyper-echoic nodule
C. Taller than wider shaped nodule
D. Microcalcification

16. All of the following clinical conditions can be associated with an increase in radioiodine uptake *EXCEPT*:

A. Graves' disease
B. Metastatic thyroid cancer
C. Choriocarcinoma
D. Struma ovarii

17. A 34-year-old lady, a known case of Graves' disease diagnosed since 3 years, but on irregular treatment with anti-thyroid drugs. Simultaneously she had developed prominence of her both eye balls which was associated with redness off and on. Since last 1month she noticed rapid deterioration of her vision in her right eye. All of the following are the causes of rapid deterioration of vision in Graves' opthalmopathy *EXCEPT*:
A. Globe sub-luxation
B. Exposure keratitis
C. Central serous retinopathy
D. Optic nerve compression

18. A 23-year-old male was evaluated for his thyroid disorders. His thyroid function revealed TSH - 8μIU/mL, T4 of 15.2 μg/dL (Normal 4.5-11.5 μg/dL) and Ft4 of 3.2 ng/mL (Normal 0.8–1.8 ng/mL). He had no history of prior medication. He was diagnosed with Refetoff syndrome based on clinical features and biochemical evidence. In which clinical condition does thyroid hormone function simulate like a thyroid hormone resistance syndrome?
A. Sick euthyroid syndrome
B. Thyrotoxicosis factitia
C. TSH secreting pituitary tumor
D. Grave's thyrotoxicosis

19. Mark *True/False* for the following statements on management of thyroid nodules during pregnancy:
A. Surgery for suspected PTC detected during pregnancy is best operated around 24 weeks. *True/False*
B. It may be beneficial to use thyroxine in a suppressive dose to maintain TSH between 0.1–1 Miu/L. *True/False*
C. TSH levels if suppressed in first trimester, will require a RAI uptake study after delivery. *True/False*
D. TSH receptor antibody is useful in differentiating Graves' disease Vs thyroiditis. *True/False*

20. Mark *True/False* on the following statements on thyroid nodules:
A. Thyroglobulin is a sensitive and specific test for diagnosis of thyroid carcinoma. *True/False*
B. The risk of malignancy in FNAC cytology reported as suggestive of malignancy could be as high as 96%. *True/False*
C. Ultrasound Guided FNAC is recommended for those nodules that are non-palpable, cystic and anteriorly placed. *True/False*
D. Molecular markers like Galectin-3 can be used to identify high risk patients with indeterminate cytology. *True/False*

CHAPTER 2

Diabolical Diabetes
(Diabetes Mellitus)

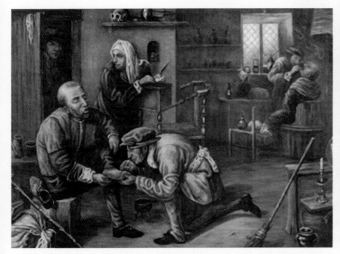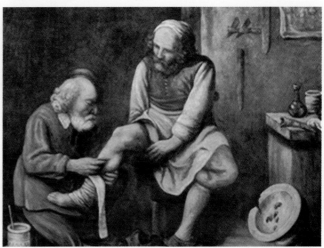

"The Foot is a masterpiece of engineering and a work of art"

—*Leonardo da Vinci*

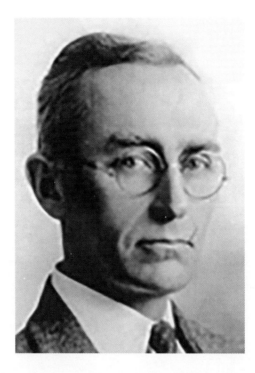

Allen Oldfather Whipple (September 2, 1881—April 6, 1963) was an American surgeon who is known for the pancreatic cancer operation which bears his name (the Whipple procedure) as well as Whipple's triad.

Whipple was born to missionary parents William Levi Whipple and Mary Louise Whipple (née Allen), in Urmia, Persia. He attended Princeton University and received his MD from the Columbia University College of Physicians and Surgeons in 1908, and started practice in the state of New York on February 4, 1910. He was the Professor of Surgery at Columbia University for 20 years where he began his work on the procedure for resection of the pancreas (pancreaticoduodenectomy) in 1935. In 1940, he shortened the procedure into a one-stage process.

He also is known for developing the diagnostic triad for insulinoma, known as Whipple's triad. Whipple became President of the American College of Physicians and Surgeons, later on becoming the trustee of Princeton University and was awarded with Woodrow Wilson Award in 1956.

CASE 1

Ms. A, aged 17 years, presented to the emergency room with complaints of progressive weight loss and fever, with an abscess over her back. She gave history of 8–9 kg of weight loss over the past two months in spite of a good appetite. For the past 7 days, she has been very ill, fatigued and bed ridden with fever and a painful swelling on her mid upper back.

Upon arrival, her vital signs revealed a pulse rate of 126 beats/min and a blood pressure of 80/50 mm Hg. She had a respiratory rate of 27 breaths per min and her oxygen saturation was 89%. She also had a temperature of 39.4°C.

Her investigations revealed a capillary blood glucose of 359 mg/dL. The arterial blood gas analysis showed metabolic acidosis with a pH of 7.0, bicarbonate of 13 mEq/l (18–25 mEq/l), sodium of 129 mEq/l, potassium of 4.0 mEq/l and a creatinine of 1.5 mg/dL.

WHAT IS THE DIAGNOSIS?

Concluding a diagnosis of diabetic ketoacidosis, bolus intravenous fluids were given for rehydration; insulin infusion was started once blood pressure picked up. A repeat blood gas sample revealed normalization of pH and a bicarbonate of 20 mEq/L.

Once stabilized, she was shifted to the ward. In retrospect, she attained menarche at 14 years of age, but has had only one period at onset, and has been amenorrheic since then. She had very sparse axillary hair and her secondary sexual characteristics were underdeveloped (breasts: Tanner stage 2; pubic hair: Tanner stage 2). She had hepatomegaly and was malnourished. Her height was 142 cm (mean parental height – 158 cm), (Fig. 1) and she had an elder sister who was well built and healthy.

WHAT WOULD THE COMPLETE DIAGNOSIS BE NOW?

She had newly detected Type 1 diabetes mellitus (T1DM) with diabetic ketoacidosis; secondary to the abscess on her back; hypothalamic amenorrhea, probable Mauriac Syndrome.

DISCUSSION

Mauriac syndrome occurs in children with poorly controlled T1DM, and is characterized by growth attenuation,

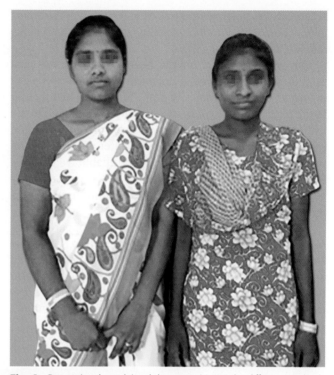

Fig. 1: Patient (on the right) with her sister. Notice the difference in body structure.

delayed puberty and hepatomegaly with abnormal glycogen storage. Some of them may also have Cushingoid features. In recent times, this syndrome is rarely found due to early diagnosis of T1DM and intensive insulin therapy, but it is still occasionally reported. The mechanisms of Mauriac syndrome are not well understood, but may involve hypercortisolemia induced by episodes of hyperglycemia and ketosis. Catch-up growth generally occurs if diabetic control is restored. However, individuals who are quickly restored to acceptable glucose levels may have worsening of retinopathy, and should be monitored closely.[1,2]

REFERENCES

1. Franzese A, Iorio R, Buono P, et. al. Mauriac syndrome still exists. Diabetes Res Clin Pract. 2001;54(3):219-21.
2. Elder CJ, Natarajan A. Mauriac syndrome–a modern reality. J Pediatr Endocrinol Metab. 2010;23(3):311-3.

CASE 2

A 56-year-old, postmenopausal, Mrs. B arrived at the emergency room with complaints of high grade fever with chills and left flank pain for 4 days.

She gave history of having been unwell for the past month when she noticed an increase in frequency of passing urine, during the day and night. She gave a history that in the past, once she voids, ants usually get attracted to the urine. She had also noticed excessive thirst and hunger, in spite of a significant increase in water and diet intake respectively. She had noticed unquantifiable weight loss. She complained of blurring of vision. She also gave a history of having burning micturition once in 3 months with fever for which she was not on any medications.

On examination, she was dehydrated, appeared malnourished and had an altered sensorium (Glasgow Coma Scale-GCS: 11). Her general examination revealed acanthosis nigricans (Fig. 1) and a BMI of 33.4kg/m². Her blood pressure was 107/60 mm Hg and she had tachycardia and was febrile (38.2°C). Physical examination revealed left flank tenderness.

AT THIS STAGE OF EVALUATION, WHAT IS THE WORKING DIAGNOSIS? WHAT INVESTIGATIONS SHOULD BE DONE?

On investigating, her random plasma glucose level was found to be 257 mg/dL. Urine was cloudy and ketones were detected (1+). An ECG was done and showed sinus tachycardia. The chest X-ray was normal.

Her ABG analysis revealed mild metabolic acidosis. Total WBC count was 36,000/mm³. Serum electrolytes were: sodium 146 mEq/l, potassium 4.2 mEq/l, bicarbonate 16 mEq/l, chloride 110 mEq/l. The anion gap was 24.2 (normal: 12–20). Plasma osmolality was 564.1 mosm/kg (normal: 285–295). Her glycated hemoglobin levels were 8.9%.

Kidney function tests revealed a blood urea of 67 mEq/l and a serum creatinine of 1.8 mg/dL.

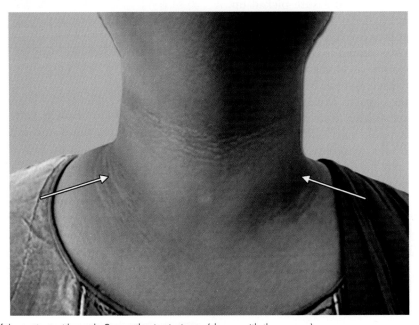

Fig. 1: Clinical picture of the patient with grade 2 acanthosis nigricans (shown with the arrows).

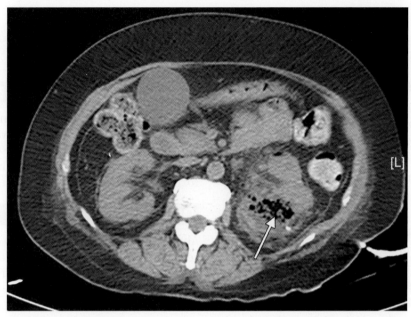

Fig. 2: CT scan of the abdomen showing multiple air pockets (shown with arrow) in the renal pelvis due to necrotising gas-producing bacterial infection.

A CT (computerised tomography) scan of the abdomen was done and revealed an enlarged kidney with multiple air pockets in the renal parenchyma and in the perinephric space. There was perinephric stranding and thickening of the pararenal fascia (Fig. 2).

Her diagnosis was Type 2 Diabetes with insulin resistance, Hyperglycemic hyperosmolar non-ketotic coma (HONK) Hyperosmolar state with dehydration causing hypotension, left sided emphysematous pyelonephritis with renal dysfunction, Postmenopausal state with recurrent urinary tract infections.

She was initiated on intravenous antibiotics, was well hydrated, and was put on anticoagulant therapy (in view of HONK being a pro coagulant state). Her sugar levels were normalized with intravenous infusion of insulin, alongside and have with potassium replacement as required.

As her sensorium improved, she and her family were educated on self management of diabetes, including the use of a mud pot to store insulin (electricity being a luxury she could not afford), she was taught about food care as well. She was also advised estradiol vaginal cream to decrease the incidence of further episodes of urinary tract infections.

DISCUSSION

Emphysematous urinary tract infections (UTIs) are infections of the lower or upper urinary tract associated with gas formation. They may manifest as cystitis, pyelitis, or pyelonephritis. Diabetes mellitus is a major risk factor for these infections and is also associated with an increased risk of asymptomatic bacteriuria and certain symptomatic UTIs such as cystitis, renal and perinephric abscess, and Candida infections.

Emphysematous pyelonephritis is a gas-producing, necrotizing infection involving the renal parenchyma and, in some cases, perirenal tissue. Emphysematous pyelitis (i.e., gas in the renal pelvis) or cystitis can occur with or without associated emphysematous pyelonephritis. These infections are usually due to Escherichia coli or Klebsiella pneumonia. Candida is a rare cause.[1,2]

REFERENCES

1. Ronald A, Ludwig E. Urinary tract infections in adults with diabetes. Int J Antimicrob Agents. 2001;17:287.
2. Geerlings SE, Stolk RP, Camps MJ, et al. Risk factors for symptomatic urinary tract infection in women with diabetes. Diabetes Care. 2000;23:1737.

CASE 3

Mrs. R, a 36-year-old lady, who was detected to have diabetes (T2DM) 2 years ago, presented to the endocrinology clinic with complaints of weight gain, constipation and cold intolerance. Over the past 3 months she noticed hypopigmented patches over her fingers and face (Fig. 1). She was on maximum doses of 3 oral glucose-lowering agents (metformin, glimepiride and voglibose).

She was found to have persistently elevated HbA1c levels of 11.4%. She was further evaluated and was found to have hypothyroidism with a TSH of 42.3 µIU/mL, total thyroxine levels of 4 µg/dL and free thyroxine levels of 0.34 µg/dL. She was also found to be positive for glutamic decarboxylase (GAD) anitbody positive. Her serum 8 AM cortisol and vitamin B12 levels were found to be normal.

WHAT IS THE DIAGNOSIS?

A diagnosis of Latent Onset Autoimmune diabetes in the Adult (LADA) was made, and she was initiated on insulin for glycemic control, and the dose of oral agents was reduced. She was also advised to be started on levothyroxine and regular follow up with her physician.

DISCUSSION

About 1–7% of all diabetic patients have vitiligo as opposed to 0.2–1% of the general population. The mechanism behind the association has not been elucidated, although some have suggested polyglandular autoimmune syndrome (PAS), a rare immune endocrinopathy characterized by the coexistence of at least two endocrine gland insufficiencies that are based on autoimmune mechanisms.[1,2]

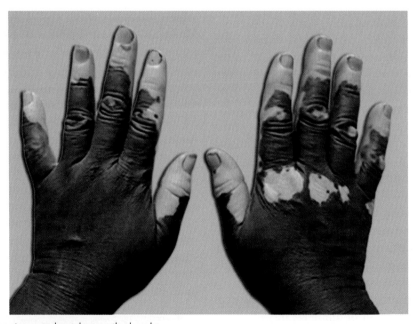

Fig. 1: Acral vitiligo: hypopigmented patches on the hands.

REFERENCES

1. Forschner T, Buchholtz S, Stockfleth E. Current state of vitiligo therapy-evidence-based analysis of the literature. J Dtsch Dermatol Ges. 2007;5:467-75.

2. Kahaly GJ. Polyglandular autoimmune syndromes. Eur J Endocrinol July 1, 2009;161:11-20

CASE 4

At the age of 15 years, Mr. P was detected to have diabetes mellitus. Upon onset of his symptoms he had weight loss and increased frequency of micturition. His plasma glucose at the time of initial presentation was 490 mg/dL. There was no evidence of ketosis in the past. Since childhood he recalls having recurrent left subcostal pain, requiring admissions and intravenous pain killer therapy. He also gave history of associated bulky oily stools, especially following spicy, oily meals and he learned to avoid the same.

Currently aged 32 years, he presented to the Diabetes Out Patient Department (OPD) with complaints of poor glycemic control with pre mixed insulin and failure to gain weight and was looking into prospects of marriage and worried about his sexual function. Upon probing, he also had complaints of muscular pains, and mild difficulty in climbing upstairs – he required minimal support to do so.

His BMI was 17.1 kg/m². He did not have any signs of insulin resistance. Fundus examination did not show any evidence of diabetic retinopathy. He did not have evidence of other complications of diabetes either. He had mild lower limb proximal myopathy, with no other significant signs on neurological examination. There were no Bitot's spots.

WHAT IS THE DIAGNOSIS?

Considering his history, Fibrocalculous pancreatic diabetes (FCPD) was suspected, and was confirmed upon abdominal imaging.

Imaging was done and the plain X-ray of the abdomen revealed calcification on either side of D11-L1 vertebrae (Fig. 1). A Computerized tomography of abdomen showed multiple ductal as well as parenchymal calcification (Figs. 2A and B, shown with arrow).

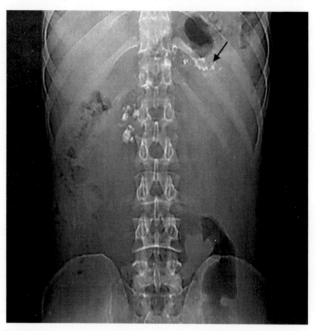

Fig. 1: X-ray of the abdomen revealing pancreatic calculi (shown with arrow).

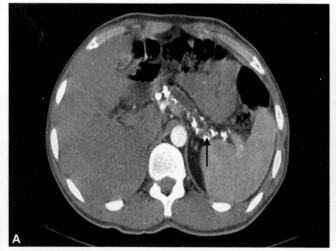

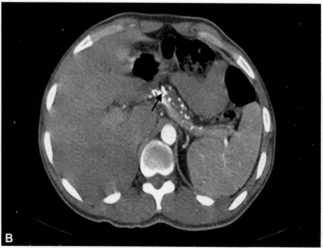

Figs. 2A and B: CT scan of the abdomen.

The patient was also confirmed to have steatorrhea with a 72 hour stool fat of 25 g (normal <18 g). The diagnosis of Fibrocalculous pancreatic disease (FCPD) was confirmed.

The patient was managed with basal bolus insulin regimen for glycemic control and pancreatic enzyme supplementation. He was given intramuscular vitamin D injection.

DISCUSSION

In approximately 1–5% of diabetic patient, the diabetes may be secondary to other disorders. In this group, the most common are the disorders of the pancreas. Various disorders such as pancreatic infections, inflammation, neoplasms, cystic fibrosis and hemochromatosis can present with diabetes. However chronic pancreatitis is the most common pancreatic disorder associated with diabetes; with world wide prevalence of alcoholism a leading cause for pancreatitis. However, in Indian sub-continent, the etiology includes "tropical chronic pancreatitis" and the diabetes mellitus associated with the condition has been termed "fibrocalcific pancreatic diabetes" (FCPD).[1,2]

REFERENCES

1. Dasgupta R, Naik D, Thomas N. Emerging concepts in the pathogenesis of diabetes in fibrocalculous pancreatic diabetes. J Diabetes. 2015;23.
2. Behera KK, Joseph M, Shetty SK, et al. Resting energy expenditure in subjects with fibro-calculous pancreatic diabetes. J Diabetes. 2014;6(2):158-63.

CASE 5

A 32-year-old lady presented with a history of diabetes mellitus which was diagnosed during her second pregnancy. She gave a history of episodic upper abdominal pain associated with vomiting and loose stools during her childhood. She required oral glucose-lowering medications initially but was later started on insulin therapy. An X-ray and a CT scan of the abdomen were done.

WHAT IS THE DIAGNOSIS?

The X-ray of the abdomen demonstrated calcification along the main pancreatic duct and CT scan of the abdomen showed calcification in the pancreatic duct (Figs. 1 and 2). This is consistent with fibrocalcific pancreatic disease (FCPD). The cause for the diabetes in this patient is due to damage to both the exocrine and endocrine parts of the pancreas.

DISCUSSION

FCPD is a unique form of juvenile onset, non-alcoholic, chronic pancreatitis peculiar to the tropical countries. It represents about 1% of all diabetics and 4% of young diabetes with age of onset below 30 years. It has a marked male preponderance. Most patients require Insulin for glycemic control. The classic radiological finding is the presence of pancreatic calculi on a plain X-ray of the abdomen, mostly situated to the right of first or second lumbar vertebrae. CT and MRCP can be used to confirm the diagnosis. The calculi tend to be rounded and intraductal in location. Ultrasonography can be normal, but is a useful initial tool especially in those who present with advanced disease. There are generally ketosis resistant and most have both exocrine and endocrine insufficiency.[1,2]

REFERENCES

1. Mohan V, Nagalotimath SJ, Yajnik CS, et al. Fibrocalculous pancreatic diabetes. Diabetes Metab Rev. 1998;14(2):153-70.
2. Rajesh G, Nair AS, Narayanan VA, et al. Tropical pancreatitis and fibrocalculous pancreatic diabetes–two sides of the same coin? Trop Gastroenterol. 2008;29(3):175-6.

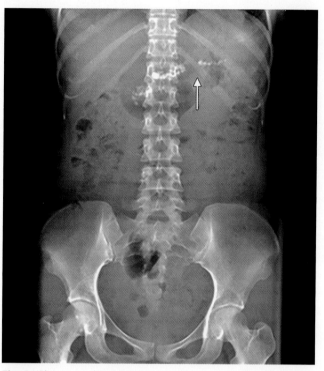

Fig. 1: Plain X-ray of the abdomen showing minute calcific areas (shown with arrow).

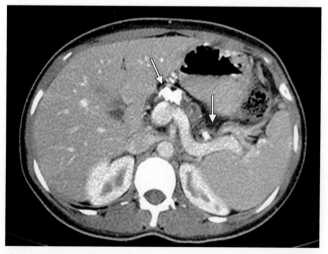

Fig. 2: CT Scan of the abdomen showing calcific areas in the pancreatic duct (shown with the arrows).

CASE 6

GENETICS AND DIABETES

A 23-year-old gentleman, a known patient with diabetes, had presented with uncontrolled sugars. He had osmotic symptoms with excessive thirst, increased urinary frequency and weight loss at the age of 21 years. At that time he had no ketosis. Now, on oral medications, his HbA1c was 8.3%. His grandfather, father, and 4 out of father's 7 siblings had diabetes with two of them having been diagnosed before 35 years of age (*see* Fig. 1). All were managed with oral medications, sulphonylureas. His BMI was 23 kg/m^2 and on physical examination, he had no acanthosis nigricans. Systemic examination was normal. On evaluation post-meal C-peptide was 3.54 ng/mL (>0.6 ng/mL). GAD antibody and Islet Cell antibody (IA2) were negative.

WHAT IS THE LIKELY DIAGNOSIS? WHAT TYPE OF DIABETES DOES THIS PATIENT HAVE?

An autosomal dominant pattern of inheritance of diabetes was noticed and he was screened for *MODY* gene defects using next generation sequencing techniques. His genetic analysis revealed a mutation in the *HNF4α* gene. He has Maturity Onset of Diabetes in Young (MODY1). Shown below are data acquired from the gene sequencer.

MODY is characterized by an autosomal dominant inheritance of diabetes and onset of diabetes usually age less than 25 years, though some have onset at 30–45 years of age. It accounts for 2–5% of all diabetes. It has overlapping clinical features with type 1 or type 2 diabetes, though some have specific phenotypes. Most are misdiagnosed as type 1 or type 2 diabetes.

MODY 1 accounts for 5–10% of the 13 currently described forms of MODY. It is caused by a mutation in the HNF4α (hepatocyte nuclear factor) gene located on chromosome 20q13 (Figs. 2 and 3). HNFα gene plays a role in the early development of the pancreas, liver, and intestines and specifically influences expression of the principal glucose transporter (GLUT 2) in the pancreas. Patients with MODY1 mutation respond very well to sulphonylureas and rarely require insulin until late stages.

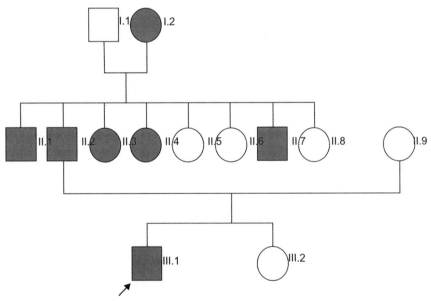

Fig. 1: Pedigree chart of the patient showing 3 generations of diabetes.

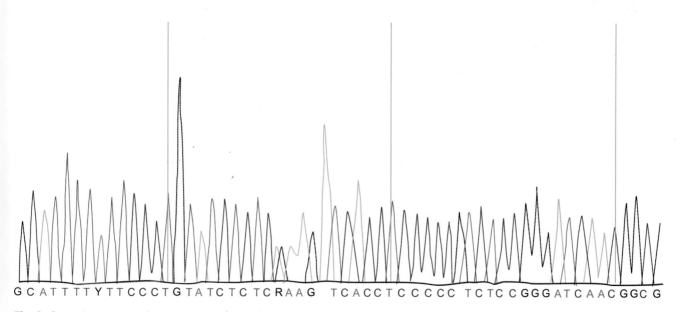

Fig. 2: Second generation genetic analysis by Ion Torrent Next Generation Sequencer.
(PGM: Personal genome machine).
a: IVS4-nt20 C to T, b: IVS4-nt4 G to A, c: Exon 5(V199L)

G C A T T T T Y T T C C C T G T A T C T C T C R A A G   T C A C C T C C C C C T C T C C G G G A T C A A C G G C G

Fig. 3: Sanger's sequencing chromatogram confirming the above defect.

CASE 7

An 8-year-old girl, a newly diagnosed to have diabetes mellitus, was brought to clinic on regular follow up with a strong family history of diabetes. Many members in her family were diagnosed to have diabetes at very young ages. All of her father's siblings have diabetes. On investigating, her fasting plasma glucose level was 135 mg/dL. Antibodies to GAD and IA2 were <5. Shown below in the Pedigree Chart (Fig. 1).

WHAT IS YOUR IMPRESSION? WHAT WOULD YOU LOOK FOR IN THIS PATIENT?

An autosomal dominant pattern of inheritance of diabetes was noticed and she was screened for *MODY* gene defects using next generation sequencing techniques. Shown below are the gene mapping data and the chromatogram.

After next generation sequencing she was found to have a glucokinase (GCK) mutation (Figs. 2 and 3).

MODY2 mutations are seen in 30–70% of the cases. Such patients usually present with a strong family history and have a persistent fasting hyperglycemia. These patients do not require oral antidiabetic agents (OADs) and do well with diet modification and exercise. But some of them need insulin during pregnancy for good glycemic control.

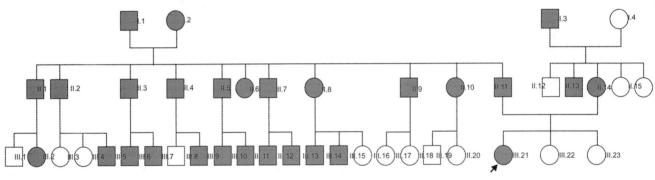

Fig. 1: Pedigree chart of the patient.

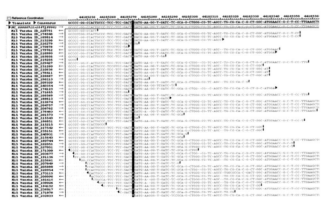

Fig. 2: Gene sequencing data mutation in exon 10.

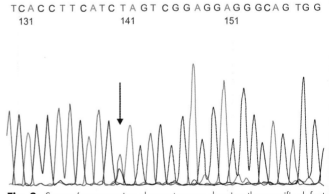

TCACCTTCATCTAGTCGGAGGAGGGCAGTGG
131   141   151

Fig. 3: Sanger's sequencing chromatogram showing the specific defect (shown with arrow).

CASE 8

A 28-year-old male presented to the out patient department (OPD) with osmotic symptoms (thirst, dry mouth, weakness). He was known to have diabetes mellitus for the past 2 years. He had 2 episodes of diabetic ketoacidosis in the past. He was on self adjusting doses of insulin and home based glucose monitoring with regular hospital follow up visits. On further evaluation, his random plasma glucose levels were 265 mg/dL. The glycated hemoglobin of this patient was 8.5%. He had a significant family history of diabetes in his family, more on the patient's maternal side. Shown below in the pedigree chart (Fig. 1).

WHAT WOULD YOU SUSPECT IN THIS PATIENT?

From the pedigree chart (Fig. 1) we can see that the patient had a significant family history of diabetes. MODY (Maturity Onset of Diabetes in Young) was suspected and he was counselled to undergo screening of the various gene defects.

Next generation sequencing was done and was found to have a mutation in the *PDX1* gene (e.g.: PDX1 c.302C>T. p.P101L). *PDX 1* gene (Insulin promoter factor, IPF 1 homeobox gene) is found on chromosome 13 and its mutation is seen in *MODY4.*

In MODY4, homozygous mutations of the *PDX1* gene cause pancreatic agenesis, which is extremely rare, while heterozygous mutations cause IDDM (insulin dependent diabetes mellitus. Patients with either variant of the disease may require lifelong insulin therapy.

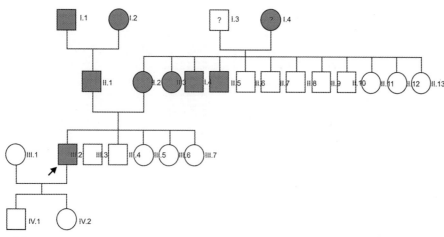

Fig. 1: Pedigree chart of the patient.

CASE 9

A 30-year-old lady was referred to the endocrinology out patient department from her antenatal clinic with a history of first trimester abortion and previous gestational diabetes mellitus at the age of 25. On further history, she has a sister who also had gestational diabetes mellitus and relatives on her father's side with diabetes type 2 (Fig. 1). She was on oral glucose-lowering agents (Metformin and Glibenclamide) but her glucose levels weren't under control with that medication.

On evaluation she was found to have an HbA1c of 7.6%. An ultrasound of the abdomen was done and showed a renal cyst of her right kidney. With the given clinical picture and a strong family history of diabetes, Maturity Onset Disease of the Young (MODY) was suspected and she was evaluated for the same. Shown below in the pedigree chart and the gene sequencing data (Figs. 2 and 3).

On next generation gene sequencing, she was found to have HNF1β mutation (in this case: HNF1β L92F).

WHAT IS THE DIAGNOSIS?

The HNF1β mutation is typical of MODY 5 (Maturity Onset of Diabetes in Young).

She was started on insulin and her glycemic control improved.

MODY 5 is found to be associated with pancreatic hypoplasia/atrophy and severe forms of renal disease like genito-urinary anomalies and renal cysts. MODY 5 is one of the less common forms of MODY and is seen in 5% to 10% of the cases. These patients may require lifelong insulin therapy for good glycemic control.

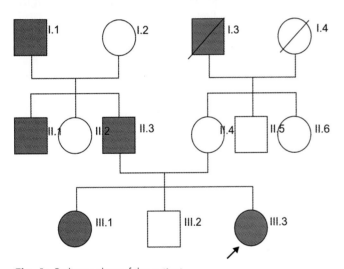

Fig. 1: Pedigree chart of the patient.

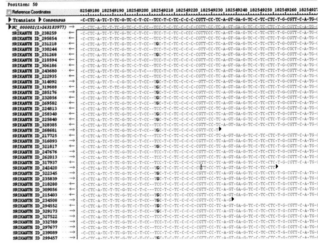

Fig. 2: Gene sequencing data.

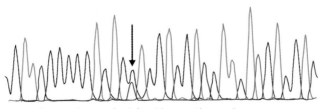

GGAACGGGGGAGAGCAGGAGGACGAAGATGAGGAC

221   232   243   254

Fig. 3: Sanger's sequencing chromatogram showing the specific defect (shown with arrow).

CASE 10

A 30-year-old man, a known patient with diabetes mellitus for the past 3 months was evaluated for MODY (Maturity Onset of Diabetes in Young) by next generation gene sequencing due to a significant history of diabetes in the family for three generations. One of his siblings had an early onset of the disease (Fig. 1). Glycated hemoglobin levels were 8.4%. Shown below in the pedigree chart and the gene sequencing data.

His test results showed a mutation in the gene for the transcription factor referred to as neurogenic differentiation 1 (NEURO D1), specifically E59Q, a novel variant (Figs. 2 and 3).

WHAT IS THE DIAGNOSIS?

The NEURO D1 mutation is seen in MODY6. They usually do not present with diabetic complications.

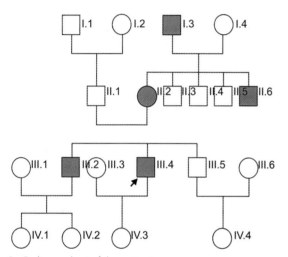

Fig. 1: Pedigree chart of the patient.

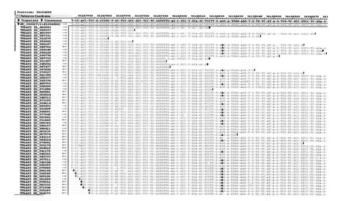

Fig. 2: Gene sequencing data.

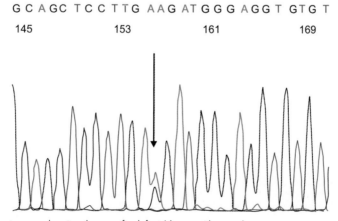

Fig. 3: Sanger's sequencing chromatogram showing the specific defect (shown with arrow).

CASE 11

A 35-year-old lady, a known patient with diabetes on oral glucose lowering agents for the past 5 years was evaluated for MODY (Maturity Onset of Diabetes in Young), as most of the relatives on her father's side had diabetes (Fig. 1). She had a HbA1c of 7.1%. She had no diabetic complications.

On next generation gene sequencing she was found to have a heterozygous mutation in the *KLF11* (Kruppel like factor) gene on chromosome 2p25. In this patient specifically, KLF11 c.49A > G p.I17V was present.

WHERE IS KLF MUTATION SEEN?

This mutation is typical of *MODY 7*.

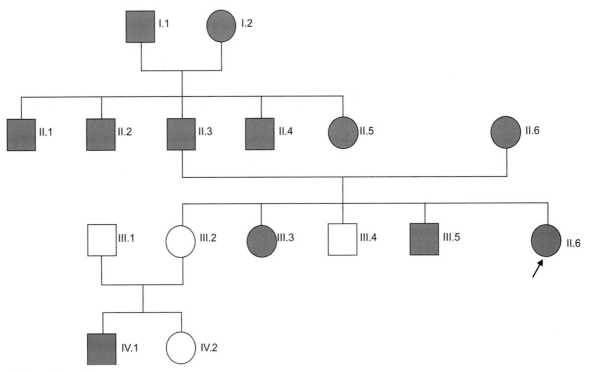

Fig. 1: Pedigree chart of the patient.

CASE 12

A 32-year-old lady, a known patient with diabetes for 3 years, was evaluated for MODY (Maturity Onset of Diabetes in Young) as she had multiple siblings with diabetes at a young age (Fig. 1). Her HbA1c was 8.0%. An Ultrasound of the abdomen showed a hypoplastic pancreas.

On gene sequencing, she was found to have a heterozygous mutation in the CEL gene on chromosome 9q34, specifically, CEL c.248T>C p.F83S. This gene encodes for Bile salt dependent lipase.

CEL GENE MUTATIONS ARE SEEN IN WHAT TYPE OF MODY?

MODY 8 also called diabetes-pancreatic exocrine dysfunction syndrome is a very rare condition and only a few cases have been reported. It is associated with exocrine pancreatic dysfunction.

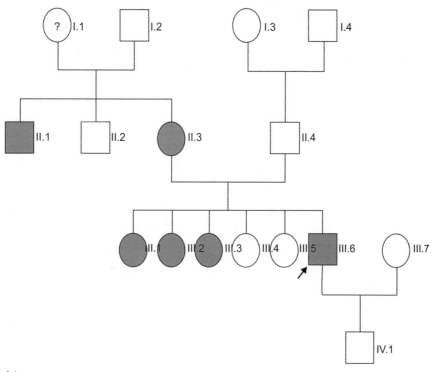

Fig. 1: Pedigree chart of the patient.

CASE 13

A 17-year-old gentleman who is a known patient with diabetes for the past 3 years, presented with severe osmotic symptoms but no ketosis. He is currently on premixed insulin. His family members too had diabetes upto 3 generations (Fig. 1). His HbA1c was 9.5%. He had no diabetic complications.

On evaluation he was found to have a heterozygous mutation in the *PAX4* gene on chromosome 7q32, specifically PAX4 c.92G>T p.Arg31Leu. This is seen in MODY9.

MODY9 is also a rare condition.

DISCUSSION

Maturity Onset Diabetes of the Young (MODY) is a monogenic disorder with an autosomal dominant inheritance pattern, characterized by β-Cell dysfunction. An overlap of clinical features with the more common polygenic diabetes makes differentiation of MODY a diagnostic challenge. MODY is classically characterized by:

a. Diabetes mellitus with an age of onset less than 25 years
b. Three generation family history with sibling involvement
c. Patients generally being non-insulin requiring[1,2]

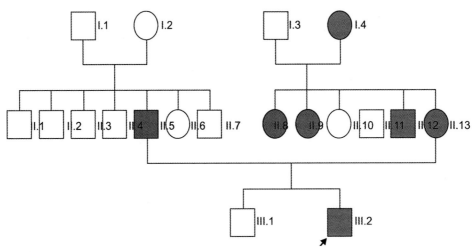

Fig. 1: Pedigree chart of the patient.

MODY	Defect	Associated features	Treatment
MODY1	HNF 4α	Macrosomia common	OADs → Insulin
MODY2	Glucokinase	Persistent fasting hyperglycemia (100–144 mg/dL)	Diet modification and insulin during pregnancy
MODY3	HNF 1α	Progressive hyperglycemia with age Low renal threshold Sensitive to sulfonylureas	OADs
MODY4	*PDX1* homeobox gene on chromosome 13 (IPF1)	Homozygous mutations cause pancreatic agenesis Heterozygous mutations cause diabetes	OADs → Insulin
MODY5	HNF 1β	Pancreatic hypoplasia Genitourinary anomalies Renal cysts	OADs → Insulin
MODY6	Neuro D1	Obesity Found to be common in Indian population	

Contd...

Contd...

MODY	Defect	Associated features	Treatment
MODY7	Kruppel-like factor 11 (KLF11)		
MODY8	Bile salt dependant lipase	Bile salt dependent lipase (CEL) has been associated with a form of diabetes. It is associated with exocrine pancreatic dysfunction.	
MODY9	PAX4		
MODY10	Insulin gene (*INS*) chromosome 11p15.5.	Neonatal diabetes	
MODY11	Mutated B-lymphocyte tyrosine kinase (*BLK* gene)		
MODY12	ABCC8	Hyperinsulinemic hypoglycemia of infancy followed by diabetes in adults Neonatal diabetes	
MODY13	KCNJ11	Permanent neonatal diabetes	

REFERENCES

1. Chapla A, Mahesh DM, Varghese D, et al. Next Generation Sequencing Coupled with a Novel Multiplex PCR Protocol for Comprehensive Genetic Screening of Maturity Onset Diabetes of the Young in India; (Poster 2526T). Accepted at the 63nd Annual Meeting of The American Society of Human Genetics, October 22-24, 2013 in Boston.

2. Chapla A, Mruthyunjaya MD, Asha HS, et al. Maturity onset diabetes of the young in India. A distinctive mutation pattern identified through targeted next-Generation Sequencing. Clin Endocrinol. (OXF). 2015;82(4): 533-42.

CASE 14

Ms. K, a 22-year-old lady was detected to have diabetes mellitus and hypertriglyceridemia at the age of 15 years. She presented to the Out Patient Department (OPD) with poor glycemic control in spite of requiring 31 IU/kg of body weight of insulin. She has been on premixed insulin since the onset of the disease but was recently shifted on to a basal bolus regimen. There was no history of diabetic ketoacidosis. There was a significant history of diabetes on her maternal side and the affected individuals had similar fat distribution.

These were the similarities found between the patient and her mother (Figs. 1 to 3):

- Diabetes detected before 30 years of age.
- Glycemic control required insulin therapy from the time of diagnosis
- No history of Diabetic ketoacidosis
- Hypertriglyceridemia
- Cushingoid facies
- Acanthosis nigricans
- Phlebomegaly—prominent veins on the limbs, more so in upper limbs
- Prominence of calf muscles and deltoid muscles
- Hypertrophic Valvular fat
- Hepatomegaly

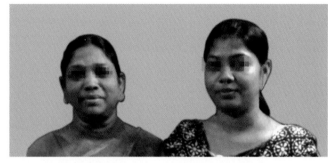

Fig. 1: The patient on the right, with her mother. Notice pattern of fat distribution on the faces.

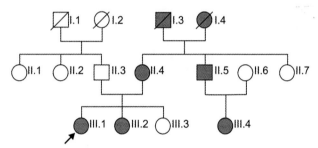

Fig. 2: Pedigree chart of the affected daughter.

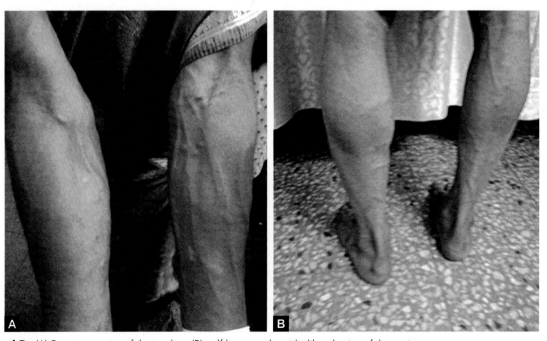

Figs. 3A and B: (A) Prominent veins of the mother; (B) calf hypertrophy with dilated veins of the patient.

Table 1: Investigations of the mother and daughter

Parameters	Mother	Daughter
C-peptide (ng/mL)		
Fasting	3.2	1.43
2h Post-meal	3.6	3.67
Fasting insulin (μIU/mL)	52.5	6.99
HOMA-IR	23.33	3.11
Triglycerides (mg/dL)	118 (on treatment)	1070

(HOMA-IR: Homeostatic model assessment of insulin resistance).

Table 2: Limbs and trunk had very less fat with increased fat in the head

Region	Fat (gm)	% Fat
Lt Arm	249.6	13.7
Rt Arm	295	15
Trunk	3361.2	14.2
Lt Leg	837.7	12.0
Rt Leg	1053	14.3
Head	833	20.3
Total	**6629.5**	**89.5**

Dual energy X-ray absorptiometry in the patient and her mother showed an increased fat in the head and truncal region with decreased limb fat confirming the fat redistribution (Fig. 5).

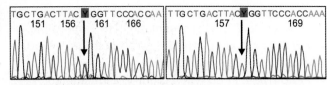

Fig. 4: Sanger's sequencing chromatogram.

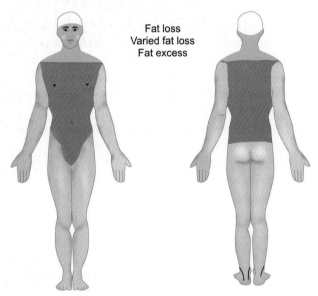

Fat loss
Varied fat loss
Fat excess

Fig. 5: Fat distribution in FPLD2.

WHAT IS THE DIAGNOSIS?

The presentation of this patient fits into a probable diagnosis of familial partial lipodystrophy (FPLD). Next gene sequencing (*NGS*) was done to confirm the same. On NGS, she was found to have a mutation in the LMNA gene (Chr 1q21.1), a gene which encodes nuclear lamins A and C, nuclear envelope proteins that organize nuclear architecture through structural attachments that vary during the cell cycle and cell differentiation. She was found to be heterozygous for a reported c.1444C > T missense mutation (substitution of the Arginine at residue 482 by a Tryptophan). This identified mutation was confirmed by Sanger sequencing (Fig. 4).

This mutation is seen in familial partial lipodystrophy (FPLD) type 2, also called Dunnigan's syndrome. FPLD2 is associated with fat loss from the extremities, abdomen, and thorax, and excess subcutaneous fat in the chin and supraclavicular area. The locus for the autosomal dominant form is located on chromosome 1q21-22.

There patients have normal adipose tissue in childhood, but lose subcutaneous adipose tissue from the extremities later, usually with the onset of puberty. The syndrome is associated with increased muscularity, not merely the appearance of increased muscularity that occurs with loss of subcutaneous fat, which makes it relatively easier to recognize in women. The distribution of fat is characteristic (as shown in the picture).

DISCUSSION

FPLD syndromes are rare syndromes that are characterized by regional fat loss and are associated with a simultaneous hypertrophy of adipose tissue in nonatrophic areas, that occurs during childhood, puberty, or young adulthood. They are associated with metabolic complications, and in some cases, cardiomyopathy, conduction disturbances, and congestive heart failure.

- *FPLD type 1*: FPLD type 1 (Kobberling's syndrome). There is significant fat loss from the extremities. The genetic defect is unknown
- *FPLD type 2*: FPLD type 2 (Dunnigan's syndrome) is associated with fat loss from the extremities, abdomen,

and thorax, and adipose hypertrophy in the head and neck region. *LMNA* gene mutations are responsible.

- *FPLD type 3*: FPLD type 3 is associated with heterozygous *PPAR-G* gene mutations.
- *FPLD type 4*: FPLD type 4 is due to a mutation of *AKT2* (protein kinase B).
- *FPLD type 5*: Familial lipodystrophy due to *PLIN1* mutation.

Congenital generalized lipodystrophy (CGL) is inherited as an autosomal recessive trait, with frequent parental consanguinity. A few molecularly distinct forms of CGL have been defined, with the mutations of AGPAT2 and BSCL2 being responsible for 95 percent of reported cases of CGL (Figs. 6 and 7).

Clinical features of patients with lipodystrophic disorders include

- Lipodystrophy
- Acanthosis nigricans (associated with severe hyperinsulinemia)
- Muscle hypertrophy, prominent veins
- Hepatomegaly
  - Fatty liver
  - Cirrhosis
- Hypertrichosis, hirsutism (occasionally)

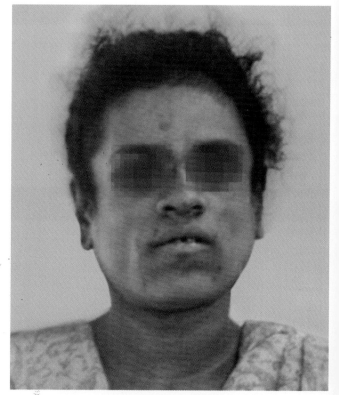

Fig. 6: A patient with congenital generalized lipodystrophy.

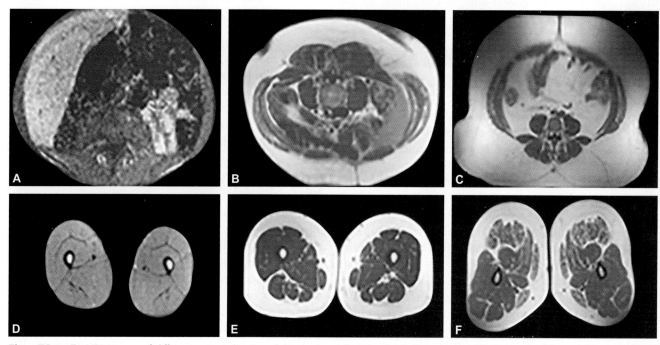

Figs. 7A to F: MRI images of different patient showing abdominal and limb fat distribution: (A and D): Generalized lipoatrophy (associated with severe insulin resistance), (B and E): Normal fat distribution (normal insulin sensitivity) and (C and F): Generalized obesity (associated with severe insulin resistance).

- Cardiomegaly due to hypertrophic cardiomyopathy (occasionally)
- Mental retardation (occasionally)
- Metabolic abnormalities[1,2]
  - Hyperglycemia, without ketosis
  - Insulin resistance
  - Hypertriglyceridemia
  - Increased basal metabolic rate

REFERENCES

1. Garg A. Clinical review: Lipodystrophies: genetic and acquired body fat disorders. J Clin Endocrinol Metab 2011; 96:3313.
2. Asha HS, Chapla A, Shetty S, et al. Next-Generation Sequencing-Based Genetic Testing For Familial Partial Lipodystrophy. AACE clinical case reports: Winter 2015, Vol. no., 1, pp:828-31.

CASE **15**

A 25-year-old woman was known to have diabetes for 6 years, well controlled on sulphonylurea therapy with an HbA1c of 6.5%. She presented with complaints of sticky stools, muscle aches, weakness in the lower limbs and weight loss of 5 kg over one year. She also had a history of intermittent abdominal pain for 5 years.

On examination, her BMI was 17.5 kg/m² with normal blood pressure. There was diffuse darkening of skin with no clinical features of insulin resistance. She appeared "lipoatrophic". Systemic examination revealed no anomalies. She had fat malabsorption with a 72 hour stool fat of 41 g (normal < 18 g) while her hemogram, liver and renal function tests were normal. Ultrasonography of the abdomen was reported to be normal. Her Magnetic resonance imaging (MRI) of abdomen is shown in Figures 1A and B.

Hemochromatosis, adrenal insufficiency and also vitamin B_{12} deficiency, were ruled out after biochemical investigations. The serum ferritin was 41.2 ng/mL (normal: 10 to 290 ng/mL), the vitamin B_{12} level was 731 pg/mL (normal: 200 to 950 pg/mL) and the 8 am serum cortisol was 11.79 mcg/dL (normal mL: 5–23 mcg/dL).

WHAT IS THE DIAGNOSIS?

MR images of the pancreas demonstrated an atrophic pancreas with total fat replacement. There was no dilatation of intrahepatic biliary radicals or common bile duct. This patient was diagnosed to have Lipomatous pseudohypertrophy of the pancreas or total pancreatic lipomatosis.

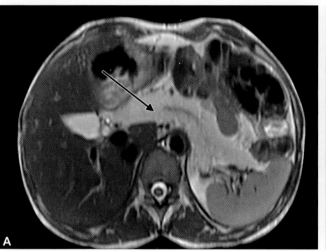 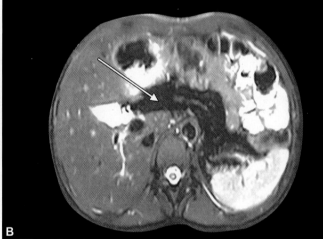

Figs. 1A and B: MRI of the abdomen showing a fat replaced pancreas in (A) T1W and (B) fat suppression (shown with arrow).

CASE 16

A 35-year-old lady, who is a known patient with diabetes mellitus on insulin, presented with complaints of darkening of skin, weight loss, pain in the lower limbs and fatigue since 1 year. She also had history of intermittent abdominal pain and steatorrhea. She had an elevated stool fat and urine xylose levels. Her CT abdomen images are displayed in Figures 1A and B.

WHAT IS THE DIAGNOSIS?

CT abdomen showed a completely fat replaced pancreatic parenchyma with non dilated main pancreatic duct. The features are suggestive of pancreatic lipomatosis (Figs. 1A and B, shown with arrow).

DISCUSSION

Lipomatous pseudohypertrophy of the pancreas or total pancreatic lipomatosis is a rare disorder characterized by the disappearance of pancreatic exocrine tissue due to adipose tissue replacement, although the pancreatic duct and islets remain intact. Though initially described by Hantelmann as early as 1903, the specific etiology remains unknown. Several predisposing factors have been suggested; mainly obesity, diabetes and age-related pancreatic fat infiltration. However, the imaging characteristics of these patients revealed a remnant pancreatic parenchyma with uneven fat infiltration, different from the uniform fatty replacement in the present case. On the basis of the findings demonstrated in the images above, the diagnosis of diffuse pancreatic lipomatosis leading to fat malabsorption was made. The role of sonology in the diagnosis is limited. Chemical shift MRI has an advantage over the CT in confirming the presence of focal fatty replacement of the pancreas. It is a benign disorder, but considerable pancreatic exocrine dysfunction is occasionally present.

Pancreatic enzyme supplementation in combination with dietary counselling is the mainstay of therapy. Clinicians should keep total pancreatic lipomatosis as a possible differential diagnosis in a patient with malabsorption. CT/MRI abdomen can reliably confirm the disease.[1,2]

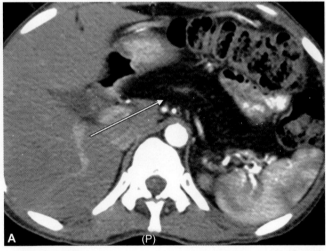 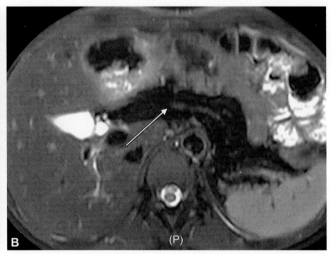

Figs. 1A and B: CT and MRI of the abdomen.

REFERENCES

1. Yasuda M, Niina Y, Uchida M, et al. A case of lipomatous pseudohypertrophy of the pancreas diagnosed by typical imaging. J Pancreas. 2010;11:385-8.

2. Olsen TS. Lipomatosis of the pancreas in autopsy material and its relation to age and overweight. Acta Pathol Microbiol Scand A. 1978;86:367-73.

CASE 17

Mrs. S, a 28-year-old known patient with diabetes since her 16 years of age, presented to the OPD with complaints of swelling of the body for the past 1 year. She also complained of occasional paresthesias on the feet. A further history revealed that she also had hearing loss for the past 3 years with multiple episodes of discharge from the ear. She had bilateral ptosis since birth. She had no documented evidence of ketosis in the past. Despite being on increasing doses of insulin she had poor glycemic control. She had a strong family history with her grandmother, mother and her brothers and sisters being diagnosed with diabetes. Shown below is the pedigree chart (Fig. 1).

On examination, she had epicanthic folds with up-slanting eyes, a broad nose and a high arched palate (Fig. 2). Her BMI was 28.2 kg/m². She had signs of diabetic dermopathy. She had bilateral neuropathy with symptomatic painful paraesthesias.

On further evaluation, she had microvascular complications like bilateral proliferative retinopathy. She underwent an audiometry which showed bilateral mixed hearing loss.

WHAT IS THE DIAGNOSIS?

With the history of young onset diabetes, hearing loss and significant maternal pattern of inheritance, she was suspected to have Mitochondrial diabetes with bilateral mixed hearing loss and with bilateral proliferative diabetic retinopathy.

Buccal swab was tested to detect mutations in the mitochondrial DNA by real time PCR. The reports showed an m.3243A > G mutation of the mitochondrial DNA. This is characteristic of maternally inherited diabetes and deafness (MIDD) syndrome.

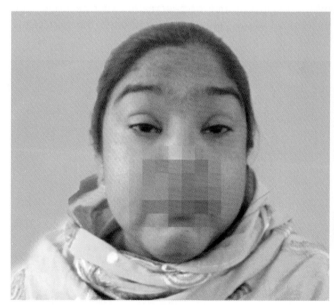

Fig. 2: Clinical picture of the patient.

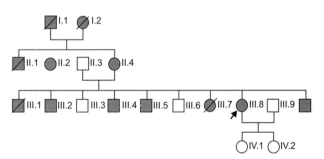

Fig. 1: Pedigree analysis chart showing significant maternal family members been affected.

CASE 18

A 23-year-old Mr S, born of a non-consanguineous marriage, presented to the outpatient clinic with uncontrolled plasma glucose levels. There was no evidence of ketosis. He was treated for bilateral childhood cataract for which he was operated within 2 years of age. (Figs. 1A and B). He was on self-adjusting doses of insulin. He also had a strong history of diabetes in his family especially on the maternal side of the family. General and systemic examination was grossly normal.

WHAT IS YOUR DIAGNOSIS?

This patient was tested for mitochondrial DNA mutations and was found to be positive for it. He was then diagnosed to have mitochondrial diabetes.

DISCUSSION

About 1% of all cases of diabetes are due to mutations in the mitochondrial DNA (mtDNA). The commonest mutation is the m.3243A>G, associated with the maternally inherited diabetes and deafness (MIDD) syndrome or commonly mitochondrial diabetes when classical deafness is absent.

Mitochondrial diabetes was first described in 1992 by van den Ouweland et al. in a Dutch family and by Reardon et al. in a UK family. This syndrome results from an A to G substitution at the conserved position 3243 (m.3243A>G) of the mitochondrial DNA.

Patients with MIDD are often misclassified as type 2 or type 1 diabetes by physicians unaware of the syndrome. Typically these patients present with diabetes, deafness and a family history in maternal relatives, although other features (psychiatric disorders, eye, muscular and cardiac involvement) may coexist. The classical symptoms should raise suspicion of MIDD and genetic testing should be done in view of the implications for personalized management and genetic counselling for patients and relatives. Diabetes in these patients is typically early in onset. Diabetes is treated initially with oral hypoglycemic agents, but an early use of insulin is commonly required due to the presence of insulin deficiency.[1,2]

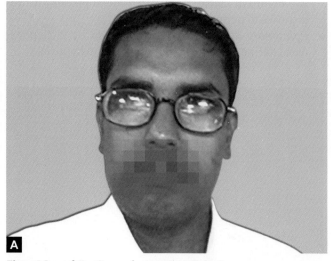 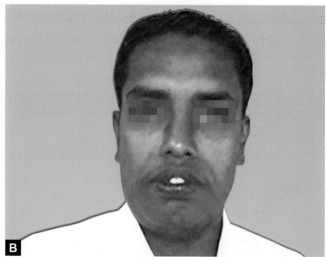

Figs. 1A and B: Coarse facies with aphakic lenses.

REFERENCES

1. Murphy R, et al., Clinical features, diagnosis and management of maternally inherited diabetes and deafness (MIDD) associated with the 3243A>G mitochondrial point mutation. Diabet Med. 2008. 25(4): pp. 383-99.

2. van den Ouweland, JM, et al., Mutation in mitochondrial tRNA(Leu)(UUR) gene in a large pedigree with maternally transmitted type II diabetes mellitus and deafness. Nat Genet, 1992. 1(5): pp. 368-71.

CASE 19

Mrs. J, a 25-year-old lady, married for 3 years, presented with infertility due to polycystic ovarian disease. Her BMI was 29.4 kg/m². She subsequently conceived after 6 months, but within 14 weeks of gestation, had a miscarriage. An year after the miscarriage she conceived again and came for her first antenatal check up during 16 weeks of gestation. She was asked to undergo a 75 g oral glucose tolerance test (OGTT). The results were 157 mg/dL, 240 mg/dL and 218 mg/dL at 0, 1 and 2 hour respectively.

WHAT IS THE DIAGNOSIS?

She was diagnosed to have overt diabetes mellitus and was advised insulin therapy and 5 mg of folic acid daily.

On consequent visits, a further detailed history revealed that her plasma glucose values were 112 mg/dL (fasting) and 138 mg/dL (post-prandial) during an antenatal visit for the previous pregnancy, 2 years ago. However, she had not received any treatment or advice for her impaired fasting glucose state at that time.

WHAT IS THE DIAGNOSIS NOW?

So, her diagnosis was $G_2 A_1$ with pregestational diabetes mellitus and was at high risk for fetal anomalies.

A ultrasonography at 18 weeks gestation revealed findings of caudal regression (Figs. 1 and 2). Mrs. J was counselled accordingly and she elected for termination of pregnancy.

She was later advised on the need for strict glycemic control and folate on a daily basis as she was planning for pregnancy. She was continued on insulin and was advised contraception till her HbA1c levels were less than 6.5%.

DISCUSSION

Infants of mothers with diabetes have experienced, nearly, a 30-fold decrease in morbidity and mortality rates since the development of specialized maternal, fetal, and neonatal care. Before that, fetal and neonatal mortality rates were as high as 65%.

The complications that are seen in infants of mothers with diabetes are many and may include:

- *Fetal macrosomia (> 3.45 kgs)*: This occurs in 15–45% of pregnancies, a consequence of maternal hyperglycemia.
- *Impaired fetal growth*: Maternal renovascular disease is a common cause of impaired foetal growth. It predisposes to perinatal asphyxia.
- *Pulmonary disease*: It is accompanied by tachypnea, nasal flaring, intercostal retractions, and hypoxia.

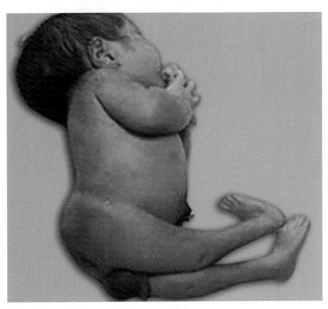

Fig. 1: Clinical image showing caudal regression.
(*Courtesy*: Dr Niranjan Thomas, Professor, Department of Neonatology, CMC, Vellore, Tamil Nadu, India).

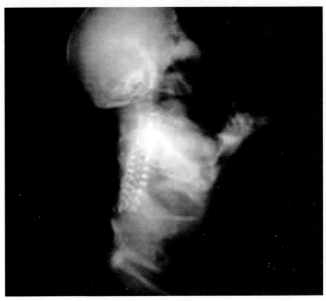

Fig. 2: X-ray spine showing caudal regression.

- *Metabolic and electrolyte abnormalities*: Hypoglycemia, hypocalcemia or hypomagnesemia may present within the first few hours of life
- *Hematologic problems*: Polycythemia predisposes the infant to persistent pulmonary hypertension of the newborn.
- *Cardiovascular anomalies*: Cardiomyopathy with ventricular hypertrophy and outflow tract obstruction are also seen. These infants are also at an increased risk of developing congenital heart defects, including:
  - Ventricular septal defects
  - Transposition of the great arteries
  - Atrial septal defects
  - Coarctation of the aorta.
- *Central nervous system (CNS)* malformations are 16 times more likely to occur. In particular, the risk of anencephaly is 13 times higher, whereas the risk of spina bifida is 20 times higher. The risk of caudal dysplasia is up to 600 times higher in these infants.
- *Renal complications*: Hydronephrosis, renal agenesis and ureteral duplication have also been observed.
- *Gastrointestinal complications*: Duodenal or anorectal atresia, small left colon syndrome

- *Others*: Thrombocytopenia, hyperbilirubinemia

Caudal regression syndrome and caudal dysgenesis syndrome are broad terms that refer to a heterogenous constellation of congenital caudal anomalies affecting the caudal spine and spinal cord, the hindgut, the urogenital system, and the lower limbs. About 15–25% of mothers of children with caudal regression syndrome have insulin-dependent diabetes mellitus. It is associated with complete absence of the sacrum and lower vertebrae with multiple congenital anomalies, agenesis of the distal sacral or coccygeal segments, hemisacral dysgenesis with presacral teratoma, and hemisacral dysgenesis with anterior meningocele. A detailed examination of fetal anatomy revealed a sudden termination of spine at lumbar level in this case and fixed lower extremities with club feet.

REFERENCES

1. Nold JL, Georgieff MK. Infants of diabetic mothers. Pediatr Clin North Am. 2004;51(3):619-37, viii. Review.
2. Mills JL. Malformations in infants of diabetic mothers. Teratology. 1982;25(3):385-94.

THE FOOT IN DIABETES

Our feet carry us throughout our life without problems. Upon the onset of diabetes; they are at a higher risk of developing complications apart from the other more commonly looked into difficulties they face. Foot ulceration affects about 25% of patients with diabetes during their lifetime. Over 85% of lower limb amputations are preceded by foot ulcers and diabetes remains the most common cause of non-traumatic amputation in western countries (Figs. 1 to 3).

Fortunately, most of these complications can be prevented with careful foot care and appropriate footwear. If complications do occur, daily attention will ensure that they are detected before they become more serious. It may take time and effort to build good foot care habits, but self-care is essential.

But, unfortunately, several studies have found that primary care physicians infrequently perform foot examinations in diabetic patients during routine visits to the hospital.

When a patient with diabetes is being evaluated, one must pay importance to the foot during clinical examination. On inspection, one must look for swelling, erythema, joint deformities, abnormal pressure-bearing areas, callosities, fissures and ulcers (Figs. 1 to 4). On palpation of the feet, look for warmth, check for peripheral pulses and adjacent lymphadenopathy. After general examination of the feet, we must test for various objective aspects.

Pathobiology of Foot Ulcers

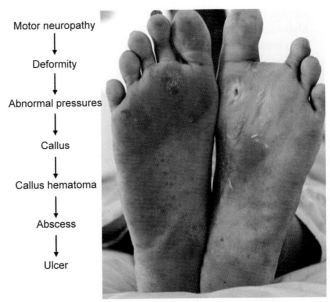

Fig. 1: Progression/Pathophysiology of an ulcer: the "callous story".

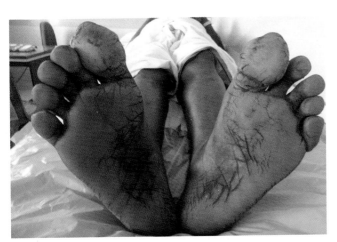

Fig. 2: Progression/Pathophysiology of an ulcer: the "fissure story".

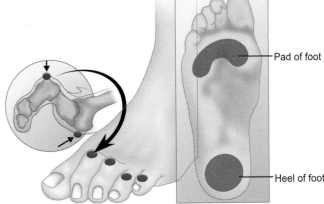

Fig 3: Usual locations of ulcers in the diabetic foot: dorsal portion of the toes, the plantar aspect of the metatarsal heads and the heel.

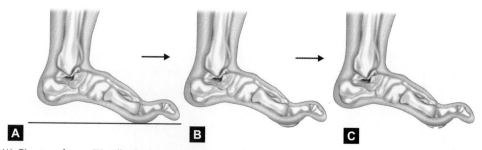

Figs. 4A to C: (A) Clawing of toes, (B) callus built up due to increased pressure, which results in subcutaneous hemorrhage, (C) skin breakdown.

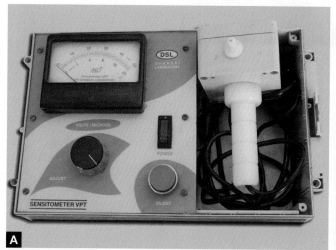
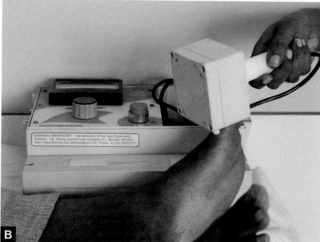

Figs. 5A and B: (A) Biothesiometer. (B) Biothesiometer while examining.

Evaluation of the Foot in Diabetes

A thorough evaluation of any ulcer is critical to plan management. An adequate description of ulcer characteristics is important for mapping the progress during treatment.

A. Quantitative Sensory Testing

Although a tuning fork of 128 Hz is handy, quantitative evaluation of vibration sense as part of neuropathy work up is indispensible. Vibration threshold measurements are typically done using a *biothesiometer* (Figs. 5A and B). Vibration is assessed in a graded manner using the dial up to a maximum of 50 mV. The grading is as follows:

- *Vibration felt less than 15V*: Normal
- *Vibration felt between 15 and 25V*: Mild neuropathy
- *Vibration felt between 25–40V*: moderate neuropathy
- *Vibration felt beyond 40V*: Severe neuropathy

The Semmes-Weinstein (SW) Monofilament Test (Figs. 6A to C)

Gently apply the nylon monofilament over 9 points on the plantar aspect of the foot and one point over dorsum of the foot, avoiding areas of thickened skin. The filament should be used perpendicular to the skin, and pressure to allow the filament to just about buckle is adequate for one second. Recognition of one or more of 3 applications is considered acceptable. The existence of more than four insensitive sites out of 10 (excluding heel) is considered as loss of protective sensation.

The nylon monofilaments are color coded:

- *Purple*: 2 grams
- *Red*: 4 grams
- *Orange*: 10 grams

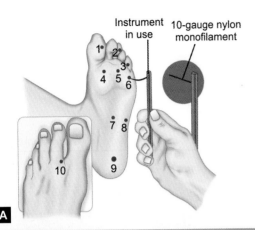

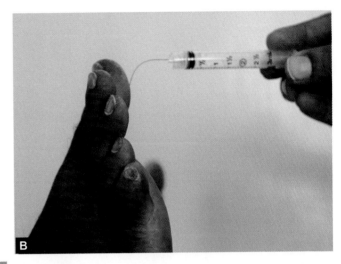

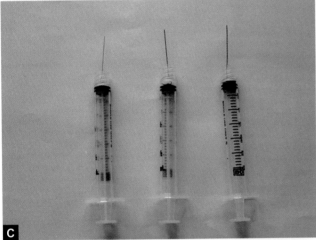

Figs. 6A to C: (A) The SW monofilament test for protective sensation. (B and C) The SW monofilament test.

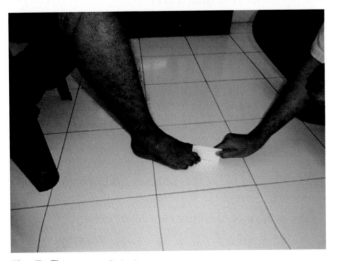

Fig. 7: The paper grip test.

B. Plantar Pressure Assessment

This assessment helps to detect areas of abnormal and high pressures in the foot. This helps determine areas at risk for ulceration (Fig. 7).

Harris Mat Assessment

The Harris mat is a rubber mat, which has ridges of graduated heights, forming squares of varying size. The rubber mat is evenly inked over with printer's ink on a rubber roller to spread the ink uniformly. The inked mat is then laid carefully face up on a white sheet of paper. Ask the patient to walk over the mat to leave an impression of his foot on the paper (Figs. 8 A to D). Figure 8B depicts the quantification of plantar pressure using this mat. This is a semi-quantitative and fairly reliable, inexpensive.

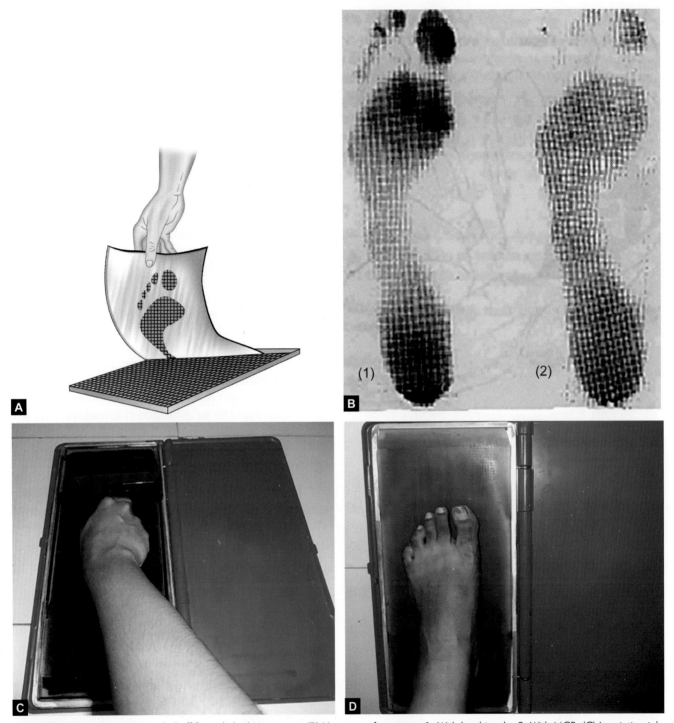

Figs. 8A to D: (A) A paper peeled off from, linked Harris mat. (B) Harris mat foot prints. 1: With hard insole. 2: With MCR. (C) Imprinting ink on the Harris mat (D) Patient steps over the Harris mat with ink beneath the mat for the foot imprints.

Computer Assessments

Plantar pressure assessment is now possible with at least six well-known computer software programs and pressure appreciating sensors that are commercially available. This is a quantitative assessment. In our experience, it is of more use in research than in day-to-day clinical practice. There are two types of sensors; one in which the sensor is placed inside the footwear and another where the subject is asked to walk barefoot on a mat containing sensors. The results are presented as a two-dimensional figure in different colors, corresponding to the different levels of pressure. Three-dimensional figures can also be obtained with colors and "peaks" as shown in Figures 9A and B.

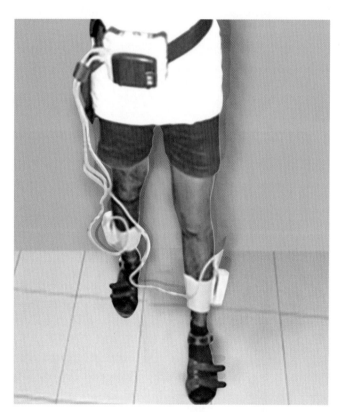

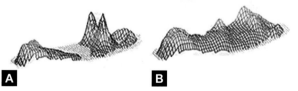

Figs. 9A and B: Three-dimensional view of the foot pressure distribution. (A) foot pressure distribution with a hard flat insole. (B) moulded hard insole.

C. Vascular Assessment

A small hand-held Doppler can be used to quantify the vascular status. Used in conjunction with a sphygmomanometer, the brachial systolic pressure and ankle systolic pressure can be measured, and the pressure index (ABPI), which is the ratio of ankle systolic pressure to brachial systolic pressure, can be calculated. In normal subjects, the pressure index is 1.

Thus, absent pulses and an ABPI less than 1 usually confirms ischemia. Conversely, the presence of pulses and an ABPI more than 1 rules out ischemia; it may suggest, that macrovascular disease is not an important factor and further vascular investigations are not required. Many diabetic patients have intima medial arterial calcification, giving an artificially elevated systolic pressure, even in the presence of ischaemia. The other explanation why pulses are absent in spite of an ABPI more 1 is missed pulses, particularly in an oedematous foot. In such cases one should palpate the foot after the arteries have been located by Doppler ultrasound.

It is then necessary to use other methods to assess flow in the arteries of the foot, such as examining the pattern of the Doppler arterial waveform or measuring trans-cutaneous oxygen tension or toe systolic pressures. Absence of foot pulses would be an indication to investigate popliteal and femoral arteries (Fig. 10).

D. Skin Temperature

It is helpful to follow-up the clinical assessment of skin temperature with the use of a digital skin thermometer. An infrared thermometer is ideal and skin temperatures

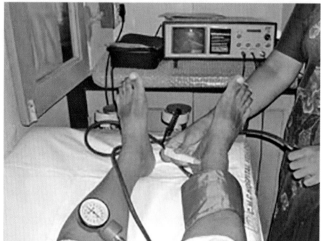

Fig. 10: ABPI measurement.

are compared between similar areas on each foot. This is particularly helpful in the management of the Charcot foot when the affected foot is 2–6°C higher than the contra-lateral foot.

E. Laboratory Investigations

Laboratory investigations are determined by clinical findings, but the following investigations are useful as a baseline in most patients:

- Full blood count (to detect anemia or polycythaemia), and white blood cell count (to reflect the presence of infection)
- Serum electrolytes, urea and creatinine (to assess baseline renal function)
- Serum bilirubin, alkaline phosphatase, gamma-glutamyl transferase, aspartate transaminase (to assess baseline liver function)
- Plasma glucose and HbA1c (to assess glycemic control)
- Serum cholesterol and triglycerides (to assess arterial disease risk factors)
- C-reactive protein (as an acute inflammatory marker).

F. Radiological Assessment

The need for radiological investigation will be determined by the clinical presentation, and may not always be necessary. However, in most cases, an X-ray of the foot will be required to detect:

- Osteomyelitis
- Fracture/dislocation
- Grading of Charcot's foot

- Gas in soft tissues
- Foreign body.

Podiatrists

Podiatrists, man the clinic's emergency service throughout the week, and undertake specialist wound care of ulcers, including debridement, and plaster casting for indolent ulcers and Charcot's osteoarthropathy. The podiatrists play a part in diagnosing problems, involving other members of the team, as appropriate, and also educate the patients, their families and friends and other healthcare professionals. They also provide routine preventive foot care.

G. Foot Care and Foot Wear in Diabetes (Figs. 11A and B)

In a patient with diabetes, the foot must be examined thoroughly. But examination of the footwear is equally important.

a. Examination of patient's footwear includes the following:
   1. Is the size of the shoe right?
   2. Is the toe box broad and deep enough?
   3. Are the heels low (below 5 cm)?
   4. Does the shoe fasten tight enough? with a lace or strap? Slip-ons are unsuitable for everyday wear—they cause friction
   5. Is the sole thick enough to prevent Injury from the unders surface of the shoe?
   6. The shoe lining is intact and is smooth enough? Does it require replacement?

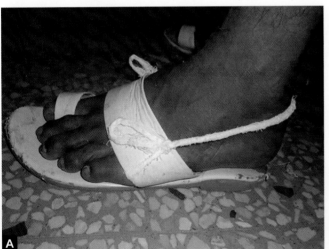
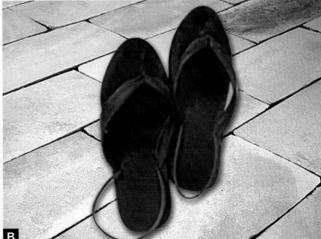

Figs. 11A and B: What is wrong with this footwear? This patient with diabetic neuropathy ingeniously tied a cord for a strap to prevent his footwear from slipping off.

7. Are there foreign bodies within the shoes?
8. Does the shoe avoid pressure points over the toes or margins of the feet?
9. Does the heel cup fit snugly round the heel?
10. What other types of shoes does the patient wear and when? Patients should be advised to wear MCR footwear even inside the house.

b. Examination of patient's socks includes the following:

1. Are the socks large enough?
2. Are the seams too prominent?
3. Is there a tight band at the top?
4. Are the socks in good repair no holes or lumpy darns?
5. Are the socks made of absorbent material?
6. Are the socks very thick, taking up too much space in the shoe?

While it is known that appropriate footwear is a key method in the treatment and prevention of development of a foot ulcer, self management and self foot care is equally important. Here are some key points:

- Taking care of skin by keeping it clean and dry
- Inspection of feet on a daily basis and more importantly inspecting footwear for foreign bodies
- Nail care
- Regular/continuous use of the appropriate footwear
- Regular evaluation of neuropathy and arterial perfusion
- Knowing the red flags for cellulitis and gangrene
- Having a "treatment seeking" behavior.

MICROCELLULAR RUBBER (MCR)

More than 40 years of experience have shown that a shore value between 10-15 (MCR) gives satisfactory results in both preventing ulcers and ulcer recurrence in majority of patients with anesthetic feet. MCR is a specially processed rubber material with 15 chemicals, where pockets of air are introduced into the rubber, creating millions of "micro cells" containing air. These micro-sized closed cells resemble fat filled cells under the sole of the foot.

MCR is a self-moulding material, which increases the area of contact and distributes weight evenly as illustrated in Figure 1. It is also an excellent replacement for fat pad loss and small muscle atrophy in the sole, which results in thinning of plantar padding due to nerve damage (Figs. 1 and 2).

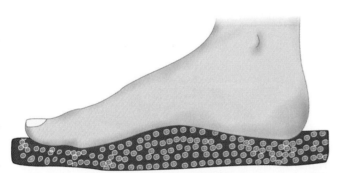

Fig. 1: The individually enclosed airspaces in the micro-porous compound of MCR gives it the elasticity and "springiness" which allows the foot to "float" on it.

Generally a pair of good MCR sandals will last for 8-12 months. It has the following qualities if maintained adequately :

1. MCR withstands friction while walking and still maintains its thickness
2. Its property of elastic recoiling moulds the foot instantly to its shape; thus the area of the foot weight bearing is increased. (Compression of the rubber indicates that the air spaces in the MCR are weak and it is not able to recoil)
3. Good quality microcellular rubber will not tear if it is hand stitched or cut to insert straps.

It is important to check the above three qualities of MCR and there are two ways to do it. One is a simple manual pinch test by pinching a piece of rubber between the finger and thumb. A firm pinch of average strength should be able to squeeze the rubber to half its resting thickness as shown in Figure 3. Flattening more than this indicates that the MCR is too soft; less than this, it is too firm.

Another method is by using an instrument called Durometer which measures the degree of hardness of MCR in shores. Good footwear requires a shore value of 10–15° (Figs. 4A and B). MCR is manufactured in two thicknesses—10 mm thickness used in manufacturing open sandals, and 3 mm used inside closed shoes.

1. Patients with Forefoot Ulcers/Deformities

The forefoot may present with a wide range of deformities and ulcers, as the pressures over the metatarsal heads and the big toe are highest during the toe-off of the gait cycle.

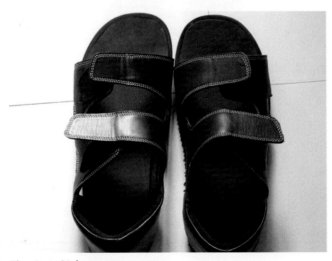

Fig. 2: MCR footwear.

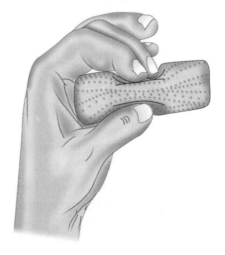

Fig. 3: The pinch test.

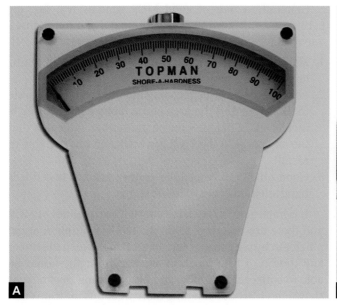

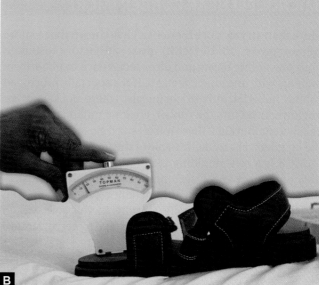

Figs. 4A and B: Durometer being used to test the shore value of the sole of the footwear.

Hammer Toe, Mallet Toe and Claw Toe

These deformities result from intrinsic muscle weakness, subsequent muscle imbalance and improper footwear.

a. *Hammer toe (Fig. 5)*: Associated with hyperextension of the metatarsophalangeal (MTP) joint with flexion at the proximal interphalangeal (PIP) joint. This deformity predisposes to injury over the dorsum of the PIP joint as well as the MTP joint.

b. *Mallet toe (Fig. 6)*: Associated with flexion deformity of the distal interphalangeal joint.

c. *Claw toe (Fig. 7)*: Associated with flexion deformities of the PIP and the DIP joints.

The add-ons that may be given for the above are:

- Silicone toe caps or toe sleeve for protection of the PIP joint (Figs. 8 and 9).
- *Silicone toe prop or elevator* reduces contact of the pulp of the toes with the footwear.
- *A metata*rsal pad (Fig. 10) can be given to take pressure off the metatarsal heads.

Alternatively a metatarsal bar in the footwear, placed just proximal to the metatarsal head reduces the forefoot pressure by decreasing the time taken in toe-off during the gait cycle (Figs. 11A to C).

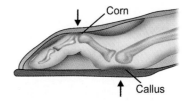

Fig. 5: Hammer toe.

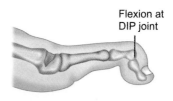

Fig. 6: Mallet toe.

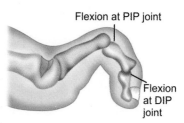

Fig. 7: Claw toe.

Rocker-bottom Sole (Fig. 12)

This is an add-on, given for long standing forefoot problems like superficial ulcers, and callosities after above mentioned measures have failed.

Hallux Valgus (Figs. 13A to C)

In this deformity, there is medial migration of the first metatarsal along with rotation and lateral deviation of the hallux. Eventually, enlargement of the bursa occurs leading to bunion formation which often ulcerates due to increase in pressure.

Bunion caps or shields are used to protect ulceration of the area. To prevent worsening of the valgus deformity, toe separators (Figs. 14A and B) are used in the first web space to maintain the anatomy of the big toe.

Inter Digital Web Space Infection (Figs. 15A and B)

Keeping interdigital web spaces dry, is of utmost importance, lest a fungal infection as shown in Figure 15A sets in. This may lead to secondary bacterial infection which may eventually cause wet gangrene and thereby an amputation. Topical miconazole cream or clotrimazole dusting powder, followed by counselling to prevent further recurrence is necessary.

In the case of overcrowding of toes, a silicon toe seperator may reduce the risk of developing interdigital web space infection.

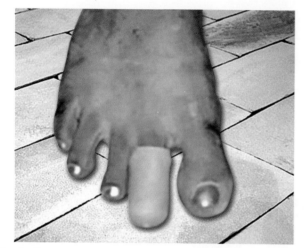

Fig. 8: Toe cap.

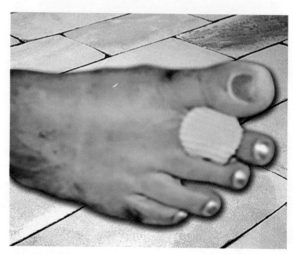

Fig. 9: Toe sleeve.

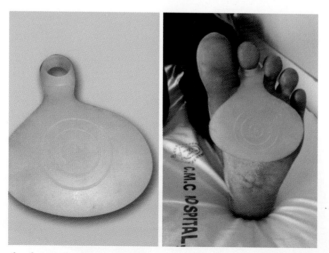

Fig. 10: Metatarsal pad for relieving forefoot pressure.

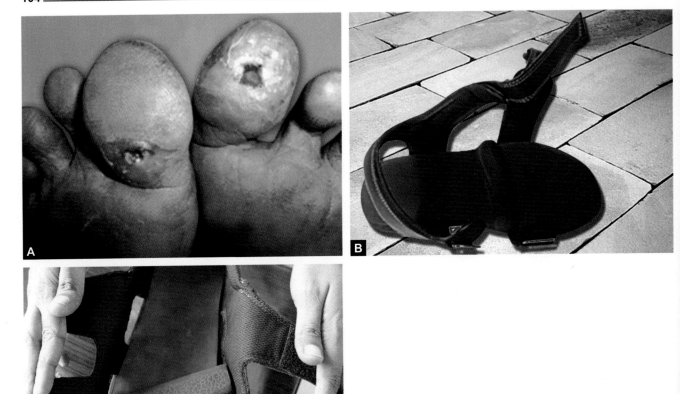

Figs. 11A to C: Forefoot ulcers can heal with complete off-loading the affected areas using a metatarsal bar. The MCR bar is placed just proximal to the metatarsal heads.

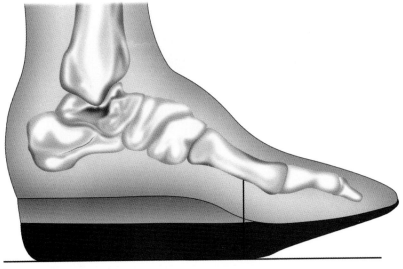

Fig. 12: Rocker-bottom sole.

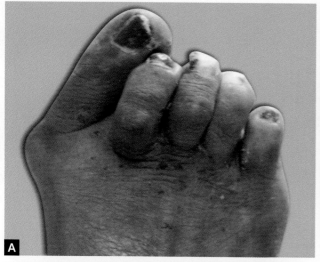

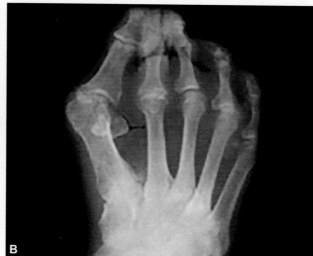

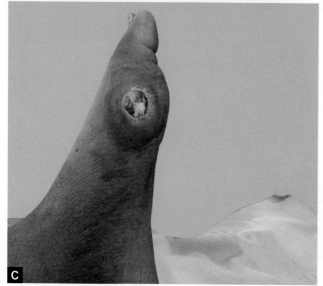

Figs. 13A to C: (A and B) Hallux valgus with radiographical evidence. (C) Ulcerated Bunion

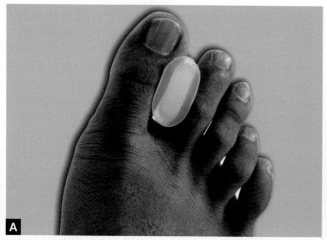

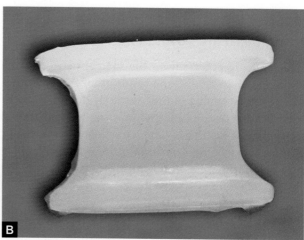

Figs. 14A and B: Toe separator.

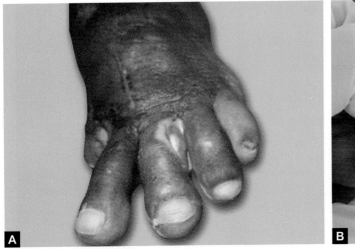
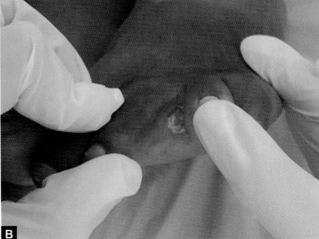

Figs. 15A and B: Inter-digital web space infection.

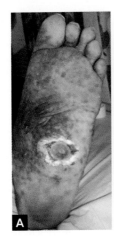
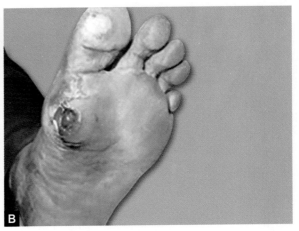

Figs. 16A and B: Mid-foot ulcers.

2. Patients with Mid-Foot Ulcers/Deformities (Figs. 16 and 17)

Mid-foot ulcers especially in the medial aspect of the foot are generally due to the result of an injury from a sharp object. Scooping out the insole is done in case of a superficial ulcer or callosity. In case of deep ulcers, management is preferable with a total contact casting or with the use of a Böhler-iron orthosis. Alternatively, a clog can be given with relief in the outsole for the area of the ulcer (Fig. 17).

Pes Cavus (Fig. 18)

Normally the dorsum of the foot is domed due to the medial longitudinal arch, which extends between the first metatarsal head and the calcaneus. When it is abnormally high, the deformity is called pes cavus and leads to reduction of the area of the foot in contact with the ground during walking. Resulting abnormal distribution of pressure leads to excessive callus formation under the metatarsal heads. This deformity is a sign of a motor neuropathy but may be idiopathic. It is often associated with clawing of lesser toes or a trigger first toe.

A *filler pad* made of MCR is fixed on a similar rubber insole of the patient's footwear. Such footwear should have a back-strap so that the foot does not move away from the pad. This pad fills the empty space between the high arch area and the insole of the footwear, thereby enlarging the weight bearing area of the foot and reducing the pressure on metatarsal heads and heel (Fig. 19).

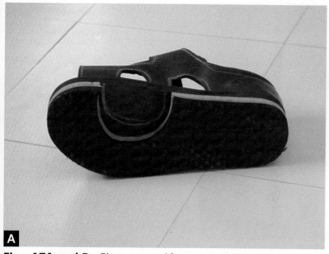

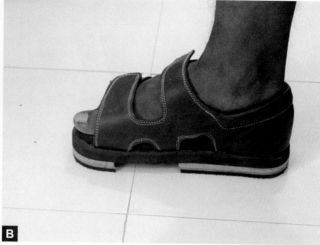

Figs. 17A and B: Clogs are modifications in the outsole given for ulcers in the forefoot, midfoot.

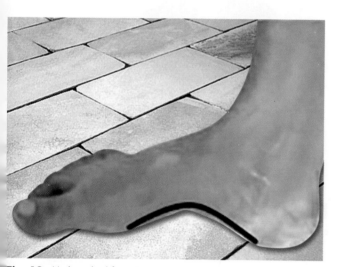

Fig. 18: High arched foot: Pes cavus.

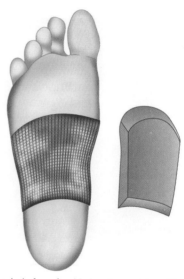

Fig. 19: A tarsal platform fixed below the metatarsal heads and above the heel.

Pes Planus (Fig. 20)

For people with flat feet, a MCR with medical arch support can be given. This helps in supporting and protecting the soft tissue in the medial aspect of the foot and also helps in prevention of plantar fasciitis and metatarsalgia by redistribution of weight.

3. Patients With Hind-Foot Ulcers/Deformities (Figs. 21 and 22)

These ulcers are generally a result of pressure in the heel due to the biomechanical abnormalities. When protective footwear is not used, injury due to sharp objects can also lead to these injuries. One of the more frequent causes of hind-foot ulcers is poor care of the heels. Poor hygiene and contamination can lead to local infection, abscess formation and subsequent ulceration. Other than footwear modification in the form of a clog, Böhler-iron orthosis are the options to off-load the limb of all pressures.

Heel Wedges (Figs. 23A and B)

This could be given for both the supinated and pronated foot. A heel wedge reduces the stress at the subtalar a joint and improves stability by resisting abnormal foot function.

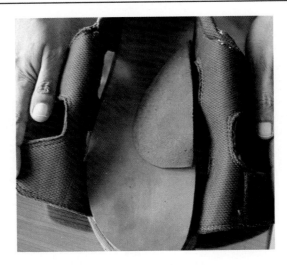

Fig. 20: Medial arch support.

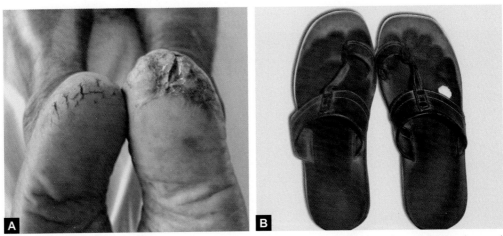

Figs. 21A and B: Hind-foot ulcer due to inappropriate footwear (absence of back straps, insole deformed due to abnormal pressures).

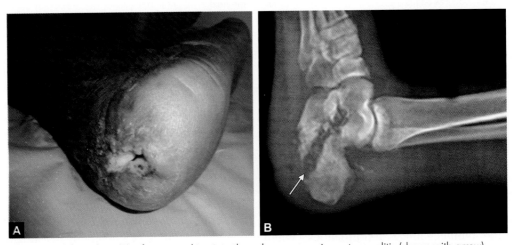

Figs. 22A and B: (A) Hind-foot ulcer, (B) infection tracking into the calcaneus causing osteomyelitis (shown with arrow).

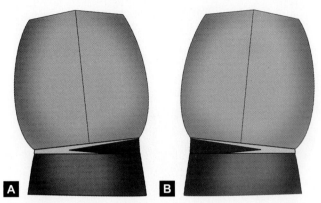

Figs. 23A and B: Both the above illustrations are right sided shoes. (A) the lateral heel wedge in the shoe corrects the excessive supination (B) Medial heel wedge correct the excessive pronation.

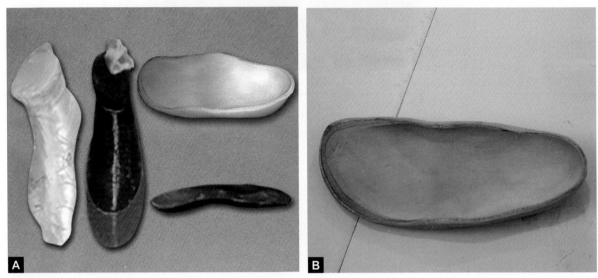

Figs. 24A and B: The three steps involved in the manufacturing moulded insole. The first procedure is making a negative cast (extreme left). This is done by applying Plaster of Paris (PoP) bandage to the patient's foot in a semi-weight bearing position with knee and ankle at 90° angles. Next step is producing a positive cast (middle) by filling the negative cast with PoP paste. This cast is used as a base to make a moulded insole either with leather and cork (right top and Figure B) or ethylene vinyl acetate (right bottom)

4. Patients with "High-Risk" Feet

Moulded Shoes (Figs. 24A and B)

This is prescribed for those who have stable foot and ankle but have extensive scarring in the sole of the foot. Such affected plantar skin is generally incapable of withstanding even the stresses of normal walking and an ulcer may quickly form.

The deciding factor for the use of a moulded shoe is if the patient has less than 50 percent a of normal weight bearing surface.

Moulded shoes consist of two parts: A moulded insole and rigid rocker outer sole (Fig. 25). The function of the moulded insole is to conform to the shape of the foot, enabling the entire plantar surface of the foot to participate in the weight bearing process. This wider distribution of weight bearing reduces the risk of high pressure lesions at vulnerable sites. The rocker sole provides a smooth rocking motion from heel to toe, without requiring either the footwear or the foot itself to bend. This results in very little movement at the metatarsophalangeal joints and subsequently reduces motion at the ankle, subtalar, talonavicular, calcaneocuboid and tarso-metatarsal joints. Studies have shown that the rigid rocker sole can reduce 30 percent of forefoot pressure during the push-off phase of gait by preventing toe hyperextension.

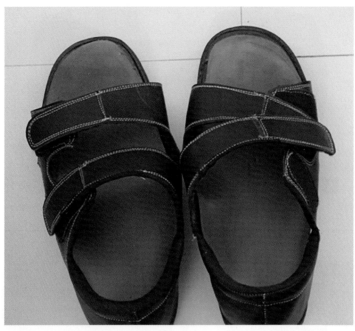

Fig. 25: MCR footwear with moulded insole.

CASE 20

Mr MK was managing his diabetes well for the past 12 years, but gradually noticed decreased sensation in his feet over the past 1 year. Although he was persistently advised against barefoot walking by his doctor, he did not heed.

He was brought to the emergency room with complaints of fever with chills, pain, swelling of the right lower limb up to mid calf and a foul smelling wound over the plantar surface of his foot (Fig. 1). The ulcer was debrided, and he was treated with intravenous antibiotics.

As his wound was not healing, 3 weeks later he presented to the Integrated Diabetes Foot Clinic. On examination, he was found to have an elevated medial longitudinal arch—which was likely the reason that the ulcer was not healing.

WHAT WOULD BE THE ADVICE YOU WOULD GIVE HIM? WHAT FOOTWEAR MODIFICATION WOULD HELP MR. MK?

His foot wear was modified so that the ulcer was offloaded. A clog with a cut out in the outer sole underneath the ulcer was done (Fig. 2).

After 3 months of wearing this footwear, both indoors and outdoors and ulcer care in the form of normal saline dressings done daily, his ulcer gradually healed (Fig. 3). His foot wear was once again re-modified in that the clog was excluded and regular MCR foot wear with back straps was given.

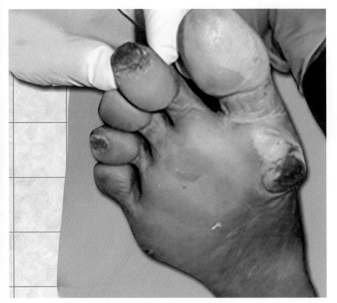

Fig. 1: Non-healing ulcer at the anterior edge of the medial longitudinal arch.

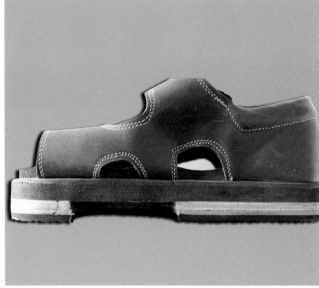

Fig. 2: Clog cut out in the outer sole of his MCR footwear.

To offload the abnormal pressure point due to the elevated medial longitudinal arch, he was given a medial wedge orthoses (Fig. 4). If the medial arch is not greatly elevated, ulcer recurrence in the same region can be prevented by the use of a silicon metatarsal pad (as shown in the previous chapter).

LEARNING POINTS

- Barefoot walking is unadvisable.
- For an ulcer in the plantar aspect of the fore foot, a clog may be provided to offload pressure upon the ulcer, so that healing can occur at a faster rate.
- Even after an ulcer has healed, measures to prevent recurrence of the same should be taken.

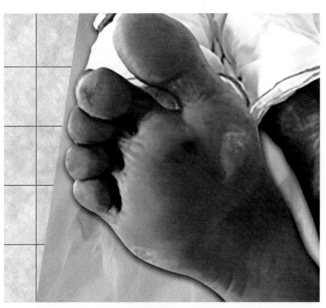

Fig. 3: Healed ulcer as compared to Figure 1.

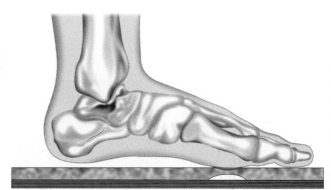

Fig. 4: Diagram showing a partially scooped insole.

CASE 21

Mrs SR with long-standing diabetes (over 10 years) presented to the foot clinic with complaints of a progressive ulcer over the plantar aspect of the foot for the past 1 year (Fig. 1). There was no foul smelling discharge or tenderness. She did not have any constitutional symptoms.

Upon radiological evaluation she had a Types 3 and 4 Charcot foot. She was advised to offload the ulcer by using a Total Contact Cast (TCC) with a window for dressing. But due to the cost and the need for recurrent review for the TCC she refused the same. The next best option of was a Patellar Tendon Bohler-iron brace (PTB), which

she refused as well. Her last option was offloading with crutches (Fig. 2), which she promised to be compliant with.

After 4 months of using the crutches, her ulcer healed (Fig. 3). She was then advised a moulded insole to ensure the abnormal pressure point does not ulcerate further.

LEARNING OBJECTIVES

• This patient has long-standing diabetes with an abnormal pressure point, which gradually ulcerated.

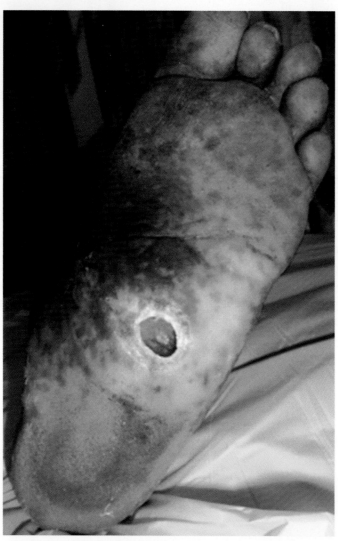

Fig. 1: Non-healing ulcer on the plantar aspect of the left foot.

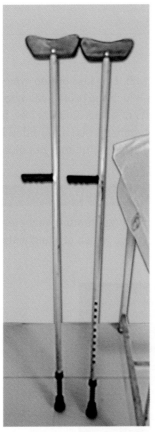

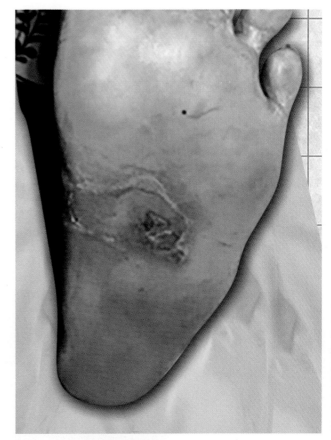

Fig. 2: Crutches given to the patient for complete offloading.

Fig. 3: Ulcer healed with complete offloading, compared to Figure 1.

- For a Charcot foot with an ulcer, a TCC is ideal, but comes with challenges e.g. cost, need for a change every week, window in the cast for dressing an ulcer, inability to use in an acute Charcot's foot. A Patellar tendon Bohler iron is the next best option as it keeps the foot suspended, transmitting the pressure predominantly to the knee, but again mobilization is difficult with the same and also difficult in patients with knee joint osteoarthritis.

- Crutches are best used in an individual with adequate upper body strength to completely or at least partially offload an ulcer in the mid or hind foot. If the ulcer is large,then wheel chair also may be advised for offloading

CASE 22

Mrs K, a 42-year-old lady, known to have diabetes for the past 6 years, recently noticed dryness of the skin and worsening of fissures over the heel of her feet. She was never accustomed to daily foot care and walked bare footed predominantly (Figs. 1 and 2).

HOW DO WE MANAGE MRS. K?

Mrs K underwent fissure debridement in the same outpatient visit and was prescribed 6% salicylic acid for topical application and a petroleum based jelly.

She was also advised daily foot care (self-examination of the feet using a mirror, soaking feet in lukewarm saline water, smoothening out of fissures using a pumice stone). Inter-digital web spaces were to be kept dry.

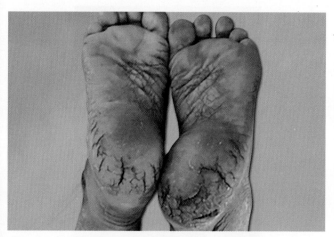

Fig. 1: Fissures in the both feet.

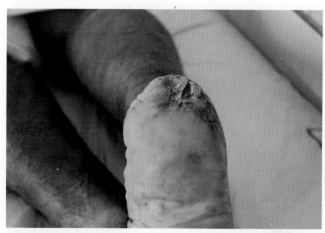

Fig. 2: Fissures leading on to an ulcer in the hind foot.

CASE 23

Mr R is a 42-year-old gentleman—a vegetable vendor by occupation, was diagnosed to have diabetes 6 years ago. He presented to the foot clinic, with complaints of pain in the right foot and a progressive swelling, with discharge from the lateral aspect of his right ankle (Figs. 1 and 2). He sits cross-legged on the floor while at work. He had no constitutional symptoms, e.g. fever, erythema.

He was diagnosed to have infected lateral malleolus bursitis, a commonly occurring affliction in any individual with diabetes who sits cross legged on the floor. The constant pressure over the lateral malleolus leads to callus formation, abscess and eventually ulcerates discharging pus.

He was specifically advised to stop sitting cross legged. Considering his occupation, he was asked to use a small foot stool to sit upon at his work place, so his malleoli are relieved from pressure. He was also given a course of oral antibiotics. It was ensured that he wears MCR footwear with a back strap that is not in contact in contact with the ulcer.

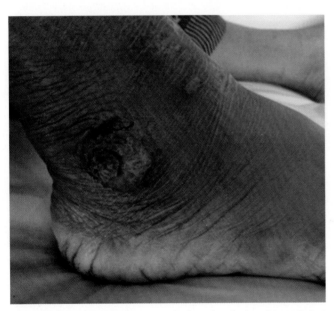

Fig. 1: Swelling and ulceration over the lateral malleolus of the right foot and also fissures in the hind foot.

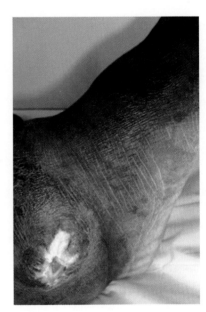

Fig. 2: Healing ulcer and decreased swelling.

CASE 24

Mr. N, a 53-year-old gentleman with history of type 2 diabetes and hypertension for the past 4 years, presented with complaints of swelling of the left foot for the past 5 months. His complaints included decreased sensation of his feet which was progressive for the past 1 year, with difficulty in retaining his footwear. On examination, the left leg was swollen, pigmented and had bounding pulses (Fig. 1). Here is the X-ray of the left foot of the patient (Figs. 2 and 3).

WHAT IS THE DIAGNOSIS?

X-rays showed classical changes suggestive of a Charcot's foot. They included flattening of the foot which include the measurement of two angles: Meary's angle and Calcaneal pitch. This patient was taught off loading and was given orthotic appliances for the same, until the ulcer healed and was later given a suitable footwear.

DISCUSSION

Diabetic neuroarthropathy can be classified according to Sanders and Mrdjenovich (Fig. 3).

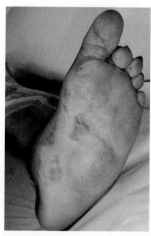

Fig. 1: Deformity of the left foot.

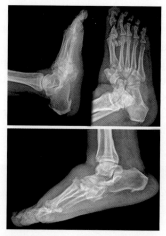

Fig. 2: X-rays of the left foot.

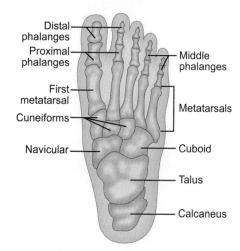

- Pattern 1-Forefoot
- Pattern 2-Lisfranc's joint
- Pattern 3-Lesser tarsus
- Pattern 4-Ankle
- Pattern 5-Calcaneus or posterior pillar

Fig. 3: Sander and Mrdjenovich classification of Charcot's arthropathy.

INVESTIGATIONS FOR CHARCOT'S ARTHROPATHY

I. *Plain radiography*

Plain radiographs are useful to
- Stage the disease
- Determine if active disease is present, or if the joint is stable (Monitor serial radiographs)
- Identify osteopenia, periarticular fragmentation of bone, subluxations, dislocations, fractures, and generalized destruction

Here are some radiological examples of the various types of Charcot's arthropathy. Quite naturally, mixed forms may occur in the same patient.

Pattern 2 neuroarthropathy is the commonest form (Fig. 1). The ideal X-ray that should be taken are an antero-oblique-lateral and standing lateral view. The standard AP view may lead to overlap of the heads of the metatarsals which could obscure dislocations and fractures.

Pattern 4 involves the classical neuroarthropathy with descent of the talonavicular joint (Fig. 2).

Loss of joint position and joint position sensation leads to friction between bones and joints. This leads to atrophy or sclerosis of bones.

The Figure 3 show pattern 1 neuroarthropathy with atrophy of the distal bones of the feet.

The X-rays in Figures 4A and B show pattern 3 and 4 disease with sclerosis (Predominantly hypertrophic).

To diagnose early pattern 4 and 5 disease, a standing lateral X-ray may be taken to identify early collapse of the arches of the foot.

The following two angles may be measured to identify the early arch of foot collapse.

a. In the X-ray (Fig. 5), Meary's angle is measured. If greater than 90°, it is pathological.
b. In the X-ray (Fig. 6), the calcaneal pitch is measured, if it is less than 17°, it is pathological. The X-ray (Figs. 4 and 6) shows clear evidence of a collapse of the longitudinal arch.

The X-ray shows advanced disease with a "rocker-bottom" foot deformity (Fig. 7). There is collapse of the arch and gross descent of the talus. There is also significant pattern 2 and 3 disease.

II. *Bone scan (Figs. 8 and 9)*
- To differentiate between Charcot joint and osteomyelitis. But the results are frequently ambiguous.
- Indium-111 WBC scan is used because it is more specific than the technetium-99 for detecting osteomyelitis. The technetium-99 scan can show positivity even in the presence of Charcot's arthropathy.
- Does not differentiate septic inflammation.

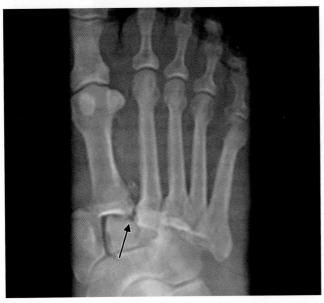

Fig. 1: Neuroarthropathy pattern 2, Lisfranc's dislocation (shown with arrow).

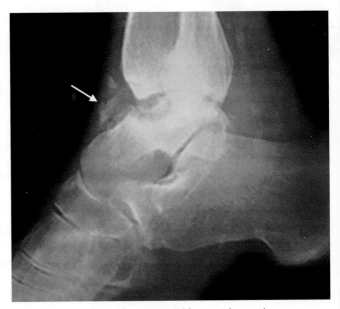

Fig. 2: Neuroarthropathy pattern 4 (shown with arrow).

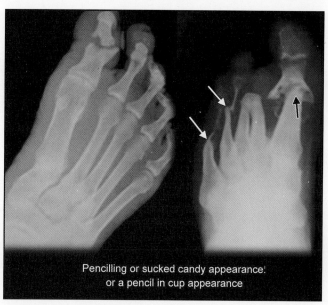

Pencilling or sucked candy appearance:
or a pencil in cup appearance

Fig. 3: Neuroarthropathy 1: Predominantly atrophic (shown with the arrows).

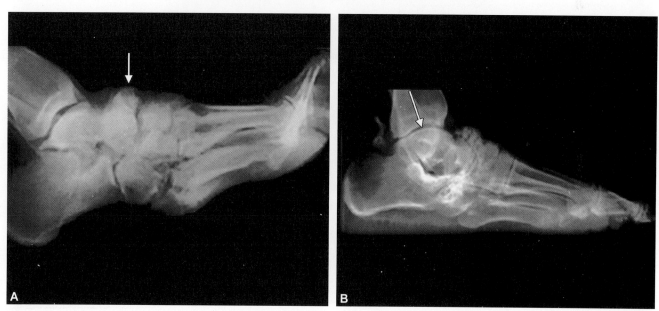

Figs. 4A and B: (A) Neuropathy 3: Predominantly hypertrophic (shown with arrow). (B) Neuropathy 4: Predominantly hypertrophic (shown with arrow).

- Bilateral involvement favors neuropathic disease
- The WBC scan is a triple-phase bone scan often used to help confirm the diagnosis of osteomyelitis (positive in all phases).

III. MRI (Figs. 10 to 12)
- Allows for anatomical imaging of the area
- Has good sensitivity and specificity
- May help distinguish between osteomyelitis and Charcot's joint

IV. Portable infrared dermal thermometry
- Used for skin temperature assessment
- Can be used to monitor active inflammation
- A 2-6 degree difference is generally seen in the acute stage charcots foot

V. Joint aspiration is used to help rule out a septic joint.

VI. Synovial biopsy
- Small fragments of bone and cartilage debris are embedded in the synovium due to joint destruction.

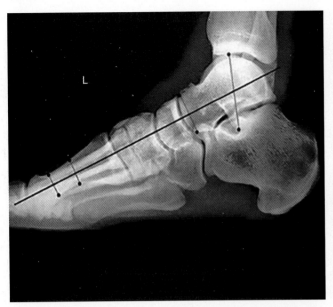

Fig. 5: Measurement of Meary's angle.

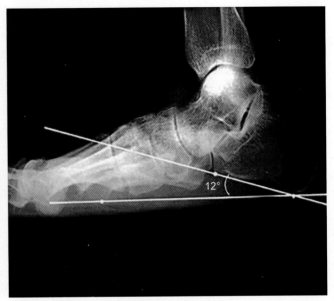

Fig. 6: Measurement of calcaneal pitch.

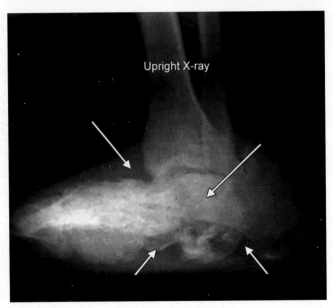

Fig. 7: "Rocker-bottom" foot deformity.

Treatment

Non-Surgical Therapy

Treatment of Charcot arthropathy is primarily non-operative and consists of 2 phases: an acute phase and a post acute phase.

1. Acute Phase

Management of the acute phase includes:

- Immobilization usually is accomplished by casting. Total contact casts have been shown to allow patients to ambulate while preventing the progression of deformity (Fig. 13). Casts must be checked weekly to evaluate for proper fit, and they should be replaced every 1–2 weeks.
- Reduction of stress is accomplished by decreasing the amount of weight bearing on the affected extremity, either by total non-weight bearing (NWB) or partial

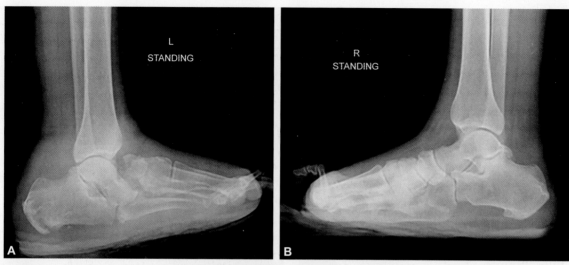

Figs. 8A and B: X-ray images of a patient with bilateral Charcot's foot.

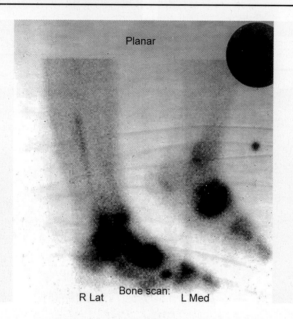

Fig. 9: Technetium 99m Bone scan.

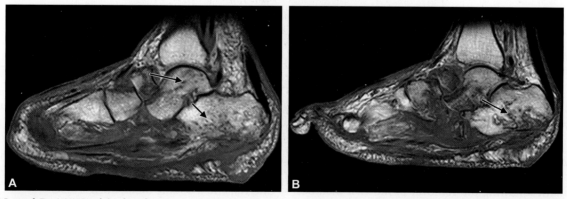

Figs. 10A and B: (A) MRI of the foot for a patient with Charcot's foot revealing the involvement of the talus and calcaneum with islands of edema within the bone (shown with the arrows).

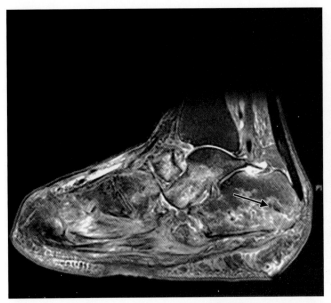

Fig. 11: T2 weighted MRI image of the foot of the same patient showing involvement of the calcaneus (Edema within the bone is shown with arrow).

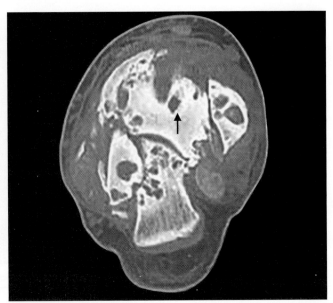

Fig. 12: CT scan of the foot showing edematous infiltrates in the bones of the foot (shown with arrow).

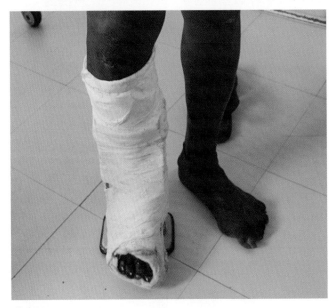

Fig. 13: Total contact cast on the right leg.

weight bearing (PWB) with assistive devices (e.g. crutches, walkers).

2. Post Acute Phase

Management following the removal of the cast includes life-long protection of the involved extremity. Patient education and professional foot care on a regular basis are integral aspects of life-long foot protection. After cast removal, patients should wear a brace to protect the foot. Many types of braces may be used, including a patellar tendon-bearing brace, accommodative footwear with a modified AFO, a Charcot restraint orthotic walker (CROW), and a double metal upright AFO.

Custom footwear includes extra depth shoes with rigid soles and a plastic or metal shank. If ulcers are present, a rocker-bottom sole can be used. Also, Plastazote inserts can be used for insensate feet. This regime may be eliminated after 6–24 months, based upon clinical and radiographic findings. Continued use of custom footwear in the post-acute phase for foot protection and support is essential.

The total process of healing typically takes 1–2 years. Preventing further injury, noting temperature changes, checking feet every day, reporting trauma, and receiving professional foot care are also important steps of treatment.

Custom footwear includes extra depth shoes with rigid soles and a plastic or metal shank. If ulcers are present, a rocker-bottom sole can be also used.

Ankle-Foot Orthosis (Figs. 14 to 17)

Ankle-foot orthosis (AFO) is also known as fixed ankle brace (FAB). It helps to completely immobilize the foot and ankle in cases of instability at the subtalar or ankle joints. It is prescribed after surgically stabilizing the above instabilities and also after resolution of an acute Charcot's foot, to protect these joints. It functions by restricting all the joint movements in such feet, thereby reducing stress and protecting the joints. A moulded

insole can be given to support the deformity and equalize the plantar pressures.

Patellar Tendon-bearing Orthosis (Figs. 18A and B)

When there is permanent destruction of joints in the foot, extensive scarring of the plantar surface and a shortened foot becomes insufficient to support the body weight during standing and walking. Such feet require a patella-tendon bearing (PTB) orthosis.

This is similar to the AFO/FAB, explained above, the only difference being that the AFO/FAB comes to the level of the calf, whereas in the PTB it extends all the way up to the knee joint. A shelf is made below the patella tendon to bear most of the body weight while the foot bears minimal weight. This is used generally in patients with Charcot's foot who need off-loading and need to continue ambulation.

Surgical Therapy

Surgery is warranted in less than 15% of cases. Surgery is performed when a deformity places the extremity at risk for ulceration and when the extremity cannot be protected

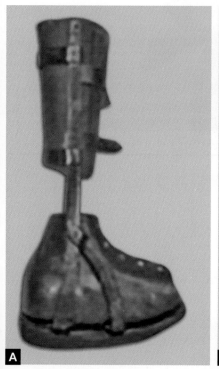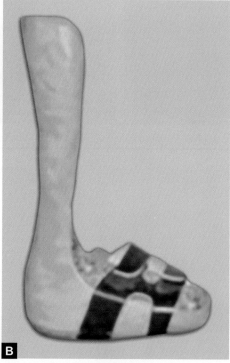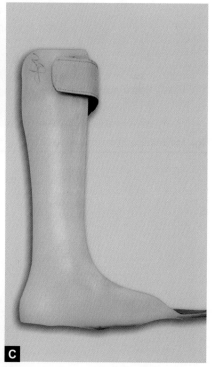

Figs. 14A to C: Three different types of AFOs/FABs are depicted in the subsequent pictures on the right side. (A) conventional orthosis. (B) AFO made of mouldable plastic sheets; (C) AFO made of a resin material, which is bi-valved at calf level. AFO/FAB comprises of orthosis, which extends from the heel to calf level, moulded insole with rigid rocker outer-sole.

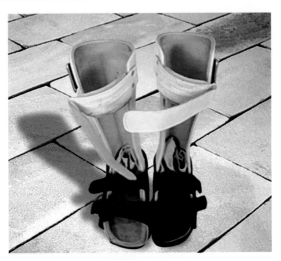

Fig. 15: Ankle-foot orthosis modified with an insole.

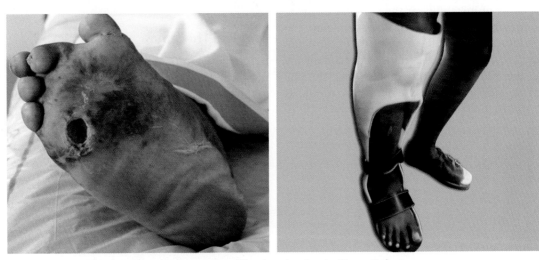

Fig. 16: Modified Patellar tendon-bearing orthosis given for off-loading the ulcer in Charcot's foot.

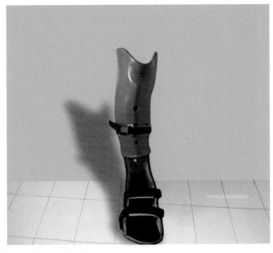

Fig. 17: Modified ankle-foot orthosis with patellar-tendon brace.

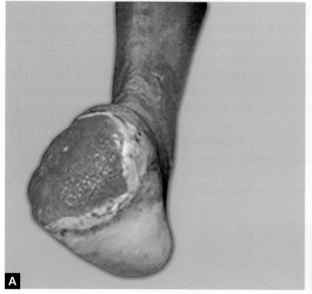 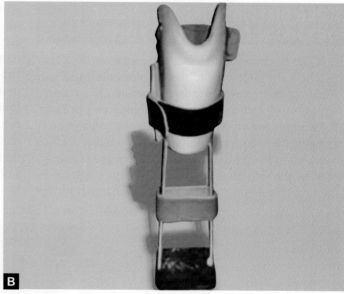

Figs. 18A and B: Patellar tendon-bearing Böhler-iron orthosis, given for complete off loading of the foot for ulcers or amputation wounds in the weight bearing areas.

safely by accommodative footwear. The goal of reconstruction is to create a stable plantigrade foot, that can be protected appropriately in accommodative footwear and that can support ambulation. Surgery is indicated for malaligned, unstable, or nonreducible fractures or dislocations, as well as when nonsurgical means fail.

Medical Therapy

For reduction of inflammation and osteoporosis, use of oral Alendronate 70 mg once a week for 3 months or intravenous Pamidronate 60 mg once in three months is recommended for patients with acute charcot's foot.

OTHER DIFFERENTIAL DIAGNOSIS FOR CHRONIC CHARCOT'S FOOT

One of the important differential diagnosis for the Charcot's foot in the tropical countries is Mycetoma, especially in endemic countries like India. Mycetoma is a chronic subcutaneous infection caused by actinomycetes or fungi. This infection results in a granulomatous inflammatory response in the deep dermis and subcutaneous tissue, which can extend to the underlying bone. Mycetoma is characterized by the formation of grains containing aggregates of the causative organisms that may be discharged onto the skin surface through multiple sinuses. Mycetoma caused by microaerophilic actinomycetes is termed actinomycetoma, and mycetoma caused by true fungi is called eumycetoma. The earliest sign of mycetoma is a painless subcutaneous swelling. The causal agent can be stained better in biopsy samples with gram stain (actinomycetoma) or gomori methenamine silver or periodic acid-Schiff stains (eumycetoma). In the treatment of mycetoma, dapsone and trimethoprim and sulfamethoxazole in double strength should be attempted first and may need to be combined with surgery, especially for eumycetoma lesions in the extremities (Figs. 1 and 2).

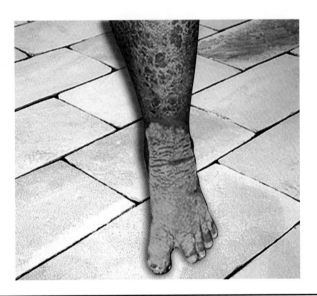

Fig. 1: Mycetoma foot.

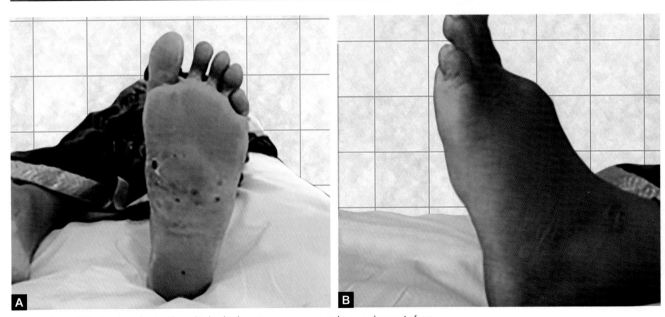

Figs. 2A and B: Madura foot with multiple discharging sinuses mimicking a charcot's foot.

CASE 25

A 52-year-old male, a chronic smoker, known to have diabetes for past 5 years presented with rest pain and blackening of right foot for past 3 months. On examination, his bilateral lower limb pulses were absent. There was also distinct blackening of the toes on the right foot. The blackened area had a boggy feel on touch (Fig. 1).

The ankle-brachial pressure index was calculated and was found to be 0 on the right and on the left, it was 0.2.

WHAT IS THE DIAGNOSIS?

The angiography showed juxta-renal aortic occlusion and confirmed the diagnosis Peripheral Artery Occlusive Disease (Fig. 2).

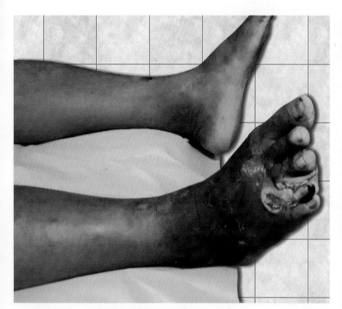

Fig. 1: Clinical picture of the patient.

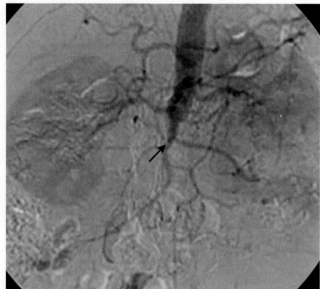

Fig. 2: Angiography of the abdominal vessels showing an arterial occlusion (shown with arrow).

CASE 26

A 60-year-old male, chronic smoker, known to have diabetes for the past 10 years presented with non-healing ulcer in the left second web space for past 3 months (Fig. 1).

On examination, there was no warmth or pus discharge from the wound. The peripheral pulses on the left foot were absent.

Ankle brachial pressure index on the right was 0.5, and on the left was 0.32.

WHAT IS THE DIAGNOSIS?

The angiography showed occlusion of common femoral artery and confirmed the diagnosis of Peripheral Artery Occlusive Disease (Figs. 2A and B).

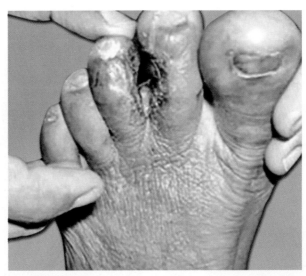

Fig. 1: Non-healing ulcer in the second web space.

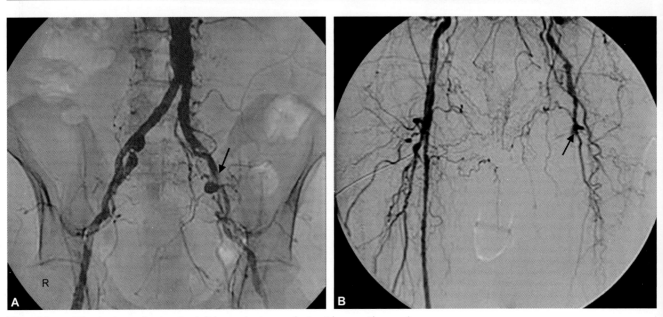

Figs. 2A and B: Angiography showing left femoral artery occlusion (shown with arrow).

CASE 27

Mr. S, a 64-year-old gentleman, diagnosed to have diabetes nellitus 4 years ago, presented to the foot clinic with complaints of ulcers over the tips of his toes, which occurred 3 months ago and have not yet healed. Two years ago, he developed acute black discoloration of his left 3rd toe, for which he underwent an amputation at a peripheral hospital (Figs. 1 and 2). He was not further evaluated at that time.

For the past 3 years, he complains of pain upon walking a brief, specific distance, which relieved by rest. These symptoms had been progressive. The pain was in his calves, but not in his thighs, nor buttocks. He did not have associated angina or its' equivalents. He smokes tobacco and has a history of 10 "pack years". His ankle brachial pressure in the right leg was 0.6 and in the left leg was 0.4. Toe pressure in the right was – 60 mm Hg and in the left was 45 mm Hg.

WHAT IS THE DIAGNOSIS?

Angiography was done and confirmed bilateral peripheral arterial occlusion.

He was advised medical management in the form of antiplatelet therapy and observation. His foot wear modification involved a scoop within the inner sole at the point of contact of the ulcers with the footwear to offload pressure over the same. No debridement was advised in view of Peripheral arterial occlusive disease.

DISCUSSION

Prevalence of diabetic peripheral artery occlusive disease (PAOD) in India varies between 6 and 16 percent. Peripheral arterial occlusive disease is four times more prevalent in patients with diabetes than in nondiabetics with early large vessel involvement coupled with distal symmetrical neuropathy. The arterial occlusion typically involves the infrapopliteal arteries but spares the dorsalis pedis artery.

Smoking, hypertension and hyperlipidemia commonly contribute to the increased prevalence of peripheral arterial occlusive disease in diabetics. For every 1 percent increase in hemoglobin A1C there is a corresponding 26 percent increased risk of PAD.

The presence of lower extremity ischemia is suggested by a combination of clinical signs and symptoms plus abnormal results on noninvasive vascular tests. Signs and symptoms may include claudication, pain occurring in the arch or forefoot at rest or during the night, absent popliteal or posterior tibial pulses, thinned or shiny skin,

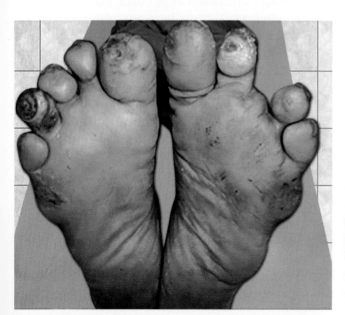

Fig. 1: Peripheral arterial occlusive disease (PAOD) related trophic ulcers.

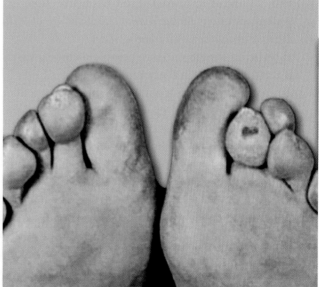

Fig. 2: Feet with peripheral artery disease.

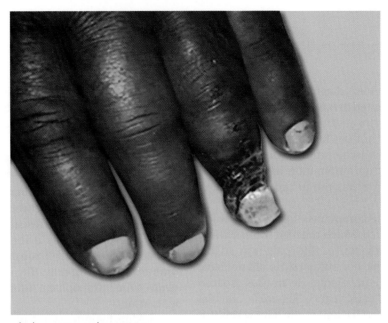

Fig. 3: Gangrene of the upper limb seen in another patient.

and absence of hair on the lower leg and foot, thickened nails, redness of the affected area when the legs are dependent. In patients with uncontrolled hyperglycemia the gangrene can also occur in the upper limbs, though it is rare (Fig. 3). The need for a major amputation is five to ten times higher patient with diabetes than those without diabetes.

Osteomyelitis increases the risk for the need of amputation by 23-fold as compared to soft-tissue infection.

Recommendations by the diabetic foot society of India for vascular evaluation and treatment are:

- All diabetics should undergo complete clinical vascular evaluation once in every 6 months.
- ABI should be done as a part of the initial examination to differentiate arterial claudication from neurogenic or venous claudication.
- All patients with PAD should have baseline lab studies which include lipid profile, ECG. The abnormalities should be addressed and treated.
- Duplex scan (Doppler ultrasound) is recommended as the first imaging modality in patients with claudication, ulcer or gangrene. The scan should be performed by an experienced sonologist as it is operator dependant.

- Angiogram (DSA, CTA, and MRA) should be done only after a judicious clinical evaluation.
- All patients with intermittent claudication should be placed on a (supervised) exercise program, lifestyle modification, control of risk factors and appropriate pharmacotherapy.
- Patients, who after adequate medical therapy develop disabling claudication or rest pain, need to be treated early and aggressively by a vascular surgeon. This includes patients with ABI of less than 0.5 and/or toe pressure and/or transcutaneous oxygen measurement (TcPO2) of less than 40.
- The "watch and wait" policy in India after debridement of an ischemic lesion often results in increased morbidity, mortality and cost to the patient.
- Do not amputate—if you can help it.

Diabetes Maintenance Therapy for Vascular Disease Prevention includes,

- Glycemic control
- Blood pressure control
- Blood lipid control
- Antiplatelet therapy
- Miscellaneous treatment
  - Smoking cessation
  - Foot care program

CASE 28

Mr. TKV is a gentleman with diabetes of 15 years duration. He presented with complaints of an infected fissure,

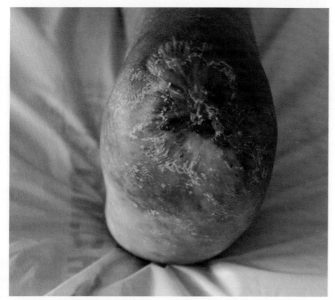

Fig. 1: Stump with ulcer.

which was initially treated with oral antibiotics, and he improved. Subsequently, the depth had increased giving rise to an ulcer, and 4 weeks later was associated with slough and foul smelling ooze. He was subsequently admitted and underwent surgical debridement. His past history was significant for a trans-metatarsal amputation 8 months ago in the right foot, secondary to wet gangrene after a thorn prick in the fore foot (Fig. 1). The stump has healed well and he was using crutches as an offloading measure for the right foot.

In view of his past history, the present ulcer would have been difficult to offload with a patellar tendon brace, therefore offloading his foot using crutches was the best option.

DISCUSSION

Foot wear modification following an amputation

1. *Stump of Trans-metatarsal amputation*: "elephant hoof" footwear can be used to prevent callosities at the stump, the front straps of this footwear should not be in constant contact with each other (Fig. 2).
2. *Below knee amputation*: An appropriate prosthesis must be used for (Fig. 3)

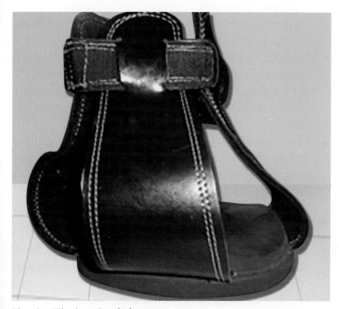

Fig. 2: "Elephant hoof" footwear.

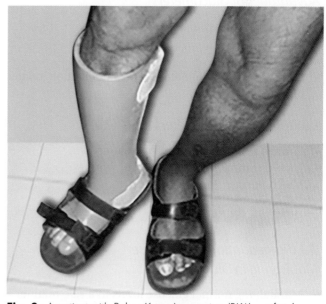

Fig. 3: A patient with Below Knee Amputation (BKA), artificial prosthesis.

GADGETS IN DIABETES

Diabetes self-care technology has come a long way. At present there are numerous options available to make living with diabetes easier than it was a few years ago. They include:

- Blood glucose monitoring devices
- Insulin delivering devices
- Gadgets of convenience that help with activities of daily living.

A. Blood Glucose Monitoring Devices

Self-management of diabetes has proven to improve glycemic control, quality of life and delay onset of complications in an individual with diabetes. A very important aspect of self-management is monitoring blood glucose values regularly with various options available, e.g.

- Glucometer
- Continuous glucose monitoring systems (CGMS)
- Others advanced devices, e.g. glucophone

Glucometer (Fig.1)

There are a variety of glucometers available which work using different principles and technologies, e.g.
a. Reflectance photometry—based on the principle of colorimetry
b. Biosensor technology—based on electrochemistry.

Advantages of Glucometers

- Convenience/easy to use
- Precision
- Affordability
- Overcomes color blindness and illumination related problems

Limitations of Glucometers

- Limited analytical measurement interval
- Lack of compatibility with control samples
- Matrix effects
- Temperature effects causing false results
- Higher costs of consumables

Recommendations for Glucose Monitoring in Diabetes

- Maintaining normal glucose levels in a safe manner is encouraged amongst individuals with diabetes.
- Use of calibration and control solutions assures accuracy of results.

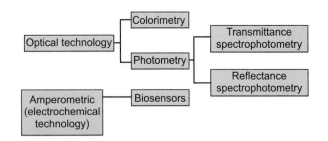

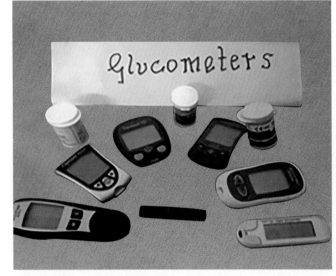

Fig. 1: Various types of glucometers.

- Ensure that the instrument is calibrated to whole blood or plasma glucose.
- The user should maintain proper use of the device and interpret it's results as advised.
- Health professionals should assess the performance of the patient's glucometer and the ability of the patient to use the data at regular intervals by comparative measurement of blood glucose using a method of higher reliability.
- When using enzyme impregnated strips for glucose measurement it is imperative that the strips are properly stored airtight in the screw cap container provided until use for maximum shelf life

When to Check Glucose?

- It is best measured once before Breakfast, 2 hours after Breakfast, and 2 hours after Lunch, 2 hours after Dinner, at least 1 or 2 times a week.
- In case of gestational diabetes mellitus, blood glucose levels are measured once before breakfast (fasting), 1 hour after breakfast, 1 hour after lunch, 1 hour after dinner at least 2–3 times in a week.

- To confirm hypoglycemia.
- During acute phase of illness, to prevent hyperglycemia.

Barriers to SMBG (Self Monitoring of Blood Glucose)

Many individuals find that incorporating monitoring into their daily routines may be troublesome. Whether it's a child with type 1 diabetes that goes to school, afraid that their friends will discover diabetes or a employer who is apprehensive of an employee discovering his diabetes is a stigma in the society at present. It is important to counsel these individuals and break the barriers to manage their diabetes well. Patient education plays a key role in emphasizing this and encouraging maintenance of an SMBG diary.

Record Keeping

It is not only of convenience, but is crucial in patient care. As a subject maintaining this record, they may, by themselves discover a pattern and mend their meal timings etc. based on their records. As a practitioner it helps in adjusting treatment and further empowering the individual with diabetes about how to deal with small doubts that come up on a daily basis. It should consist of

- Blood Glucose levels
- Meal timings, content and quantity
- Time and date
- Insulin dose adjustments
- Special events affecting glycemic control [e.g. illness, parties, exercise etc...]
- Hypoglycemic episodes and description of severity and measures taken to correct the same.

Continuous Glucose Monitoring System (CGMS) (Figs. 2A to C)

CGMS is a device which is available commercially. It allows continuous monitoring of glucose levels and provides glucose as long it is attached to the subject.

The device consists of a sensor that inserted into the subcutaneous layer of the skin over the anterior abdominal wall and measures interstitial fluid glucose. The glucose penetrates the semi-permeable membrane of the sensor reacts with glucose oxidase in the sensor to produce electrons that thence produces an input signal. This signal is translated to a glucose value.

Whereas glucometer readings obtained by finger pricks are at best single, "snapshots", providing readings at selected times over a time period, continuous glucose monitoring enables tracking of blood glucose levels on a continuous basis over several hours without multiple pricks. This would enhance our awareness of excursions in glucose readings, particularly during nocturnal hours, when hypoglycemia may be recognized. It is designed to continuously and automatically monitor glucose values in subcutaneous tissue fluid within a range of 40-400 mg/dl. Up to 2 weeks of glucose data can be stored in the monitor's memory and then transferred to a personal computer for analysis.

This device is a helpful tool in management of brittle diabetes and hypoglycemia unawareness.

Recommendations of use of CGMS:

- While stabilizing individuals on continuous Subcutaneous insulin infusion (insulin Pump)
- Evaluation of Brittle diabetes mellitus
- It is a guide for future management of patients.

Limitations

- It is an expensive device
- Glucose levels are not reported in "real time".

Warnings/Precautions

Infection, inflammation or bleeding at the glucose sensor insertion site is a possible risk of glucose sensing. Glucose sensor should be removed if redness, pain, tenderness or swelling develops at the insertion site.

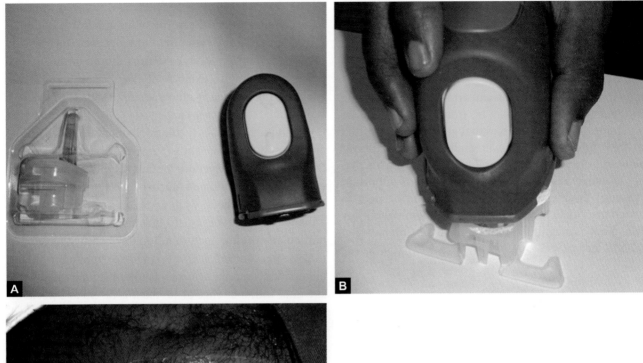

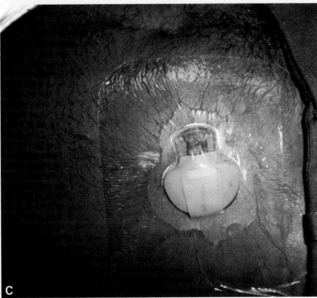

Figs. 2A to C: (A) CGM sensor (B) The application device enclosing the sensor. (C) The CGM device attached to a sensor whose probe is in the subcutaneous space of the anterior abdomen wall.

CASE 29

Mr. N is known to have Type 1 diabetes mellitus for the past 6 years, being very stringent with his glycemic control, he frequently suffered from severe hypoglycemic episodes without preceding symptoms of hypoglycemia (Fig. 1). He was admitted one morning for an episode of convulsions followed by a fall, resulting in a fracture of his right humerus which needed a surgical fixation. In retrospect, he remembers having had nightmares almost every night for the past week, and skipping his night time snacks as his fasting values were in the higher range. He was also increasing the dose of basal insulin. Suspecting that he was experiencing early morning hypoglycemia, he was subjected to a CGM (Continuous Glucose Monitoring) study, which revealed the following graph.

WHAT IS THE DIAGNOSIS?

A typical Somogyi phenomenon: Hypoglycemia in the early morning hours, but upon waking up in the morning, his fasting blood sugars were elevated, owing to correction of hypoglycemia by counter regulatory hormones.

DISCUSSION

The fact that he had no manifestation of autonomic symptoms (palpitations, sweating, headache and hunger) or neuroglycopenic symptoms. Mr. N was diagnosed to have hypoglycemia associated autonomic failure (HAAF) (Figs. 1 and 2). His glycemic targets were relaxed, and he was re-educated on the importance of regular monitoring, adjustment of insulin doses and especially the importance of a regular meal and snack pattern- seeing that even in the afternoon hours he would have hypoglycaemia pre lunch- during which time also, he was completely asymptomatic. The dawn phenomenon, an opposite of somogyi effect, is an early-morning (usually between 2 a.m. and 8 a.m.) hyperglycemia due to the inadequate insulin or increased calorie intake at bedtime (Fig. 3).

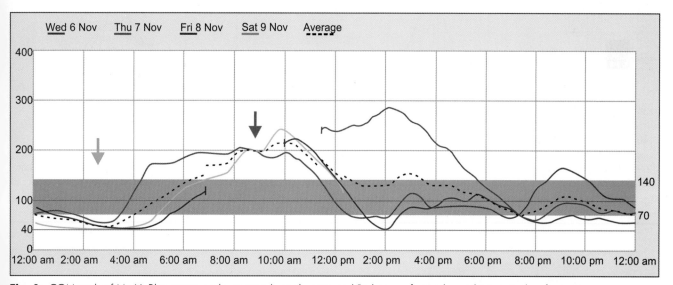

Fig. 1: CGM study of Mr. N, Blue arrow: early morning hypoglycemia and Red arrow: fasting hyperglycemia in the afternoon.

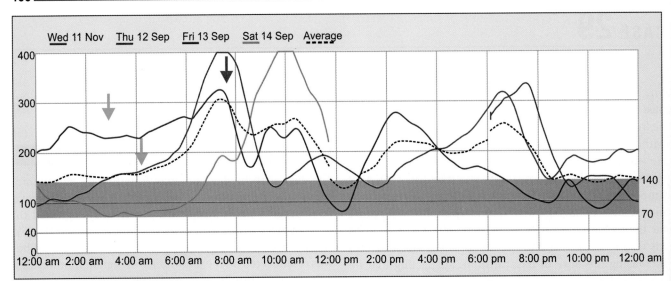

Fig. 2: A 43-year-old Mrs S known to have type 1 diabetes mellitus for the past 20 years was admitted for persistent poor glycemic control. Her CGMS curve showed a hyperglycemia starting from early morning (blue arrow: early morning hyperglycemia, red arrow: fasting hyperglycemia) suggestive of a Dawn phenomenon.

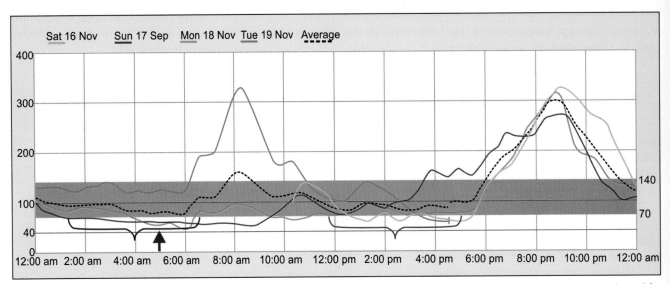

Fig. 3: A 27-year-old newly-married Mrs K, a known diabetic since 2006, presently admitted with 7 weeks pregnancy. She was admitted for recurrent asymptomatic episodes of hypoglycemia at night (shown with arrow) which were asymptomatic.

INSULIN DELIVERING DEVICES

The array of insulin delivery devices has gone from a simple insulin syringe to an insulin pen and now the readily available insulin pump device. The use of each one is greatly dependent upon ease of use, costs for maintenance etc.

1. *Syringes (Fig. 1)*: A 40 IU insulin syringe for use with a 40 IU/mL insulin vial and 100 IU insulin syringe for use with a 100 IU/mL insulin vial.
2. *Insulin Pen Device (Figs. 2A to E):* There are two types of pens.
   a. The disposable pens may be discarded after the cartridge gets drained. Can be dialled up to 80 units.

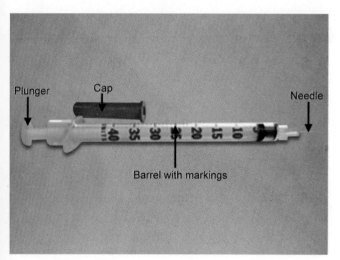

Fig. 1: Insulin syringe.

b. The reusable pen has a pre-filled insulin cartridge that can be replaced with another cartridge when the insulin has been used. This is intended for long term/permanent insulin therapy. The cartridges and needles have to be changed from time to time. Can be dialed up to around 60-70 units. One cartridge contains 3 mL/300 IU of insulin. With the reusable pen, the patient inserts an insulin cartridge into the pens delivery chamber. This allows greater flexibility for some patients (i.e. changing types of insulin without having to buy another pen when prescription changes) and it may be more economical than using pre-filled pens.

Insulin Administration with a Pen Device

- The pen should be turned through 180° angle for mixing the insulin
- The pen should be primed before each use
- Each needle can be used till it is painless (5–6 times). Needles should not be wiped or sterilized.
- Needles should be disposed in a plastic/metal container.
- Clean the site with a spirit swab.
- After dialing the dose, Insulin should be administered in the same way as by the syringe method.
- The dose window should be visible. The button should be pressed till the dial comes back to "Zero".
- After administration the pen should be held in place for a count of 10 for better absorption and to prevent loss of the dose through the injection site.
- Pen cartridges should be stored in the refrigerator door including the one being used.
- Needle should be removed after each use.

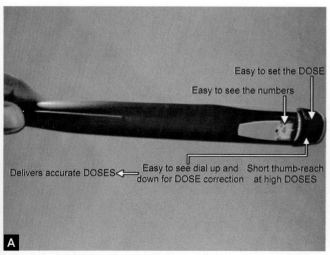

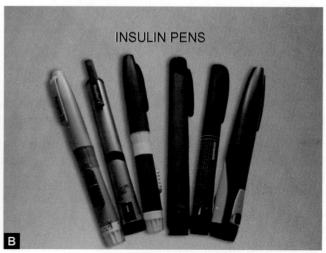

Figs. 2A and B: Insulin pen; types and parts.

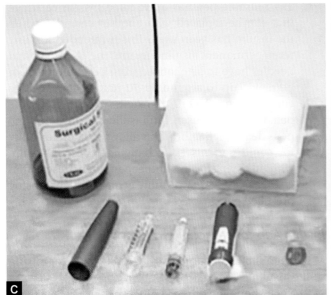

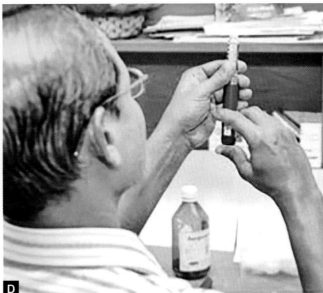

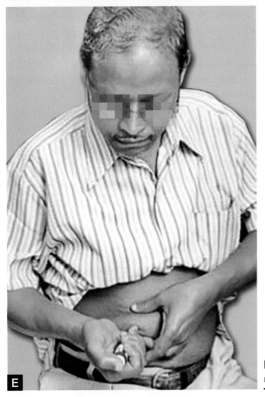

Figs. 2C to E: Steps during administration of insulin using insulin pen; make sure all required items are ready; prime the insulin pen; pinch and administered.

- Anterior abdominal wall is the best site for insulin administration.

Advantages of Insulin Pen Devices over Conventional Insulin Syringes:

- Dial on the pen devices have a magnifying glass for aiding those who are visually impaired

- More convenient insulin delivery.
- More accurate dosing.
- Less pain because smaller gauge needles are used.
- Better quality of life.
- Easier compliance with insulin regimen.
- Simpler for specific populations to use (e.g. elderly, children, adolescents and pregnant women).
- Improved social acceptability, especially at school.

- More flexibility because of disposable or reusable options. Insulin pen devices are unique in that they combine the insulin containers and the syringe in a single unit.

Who Benefits from Pen Devices?

- Patients with erratic eating habits may benefit. However, people who take regular or Lispro insulin before meals or snacks and NPH at bed time usually need two pens, one for each type of insulin. Also, patients who take mixture of two kinds of insulin in one syringe (e.g. Regular/Lispro and NPH or lente other than 30/70 premixed insulin) would need to use two pens and two injections for each dose. This is less desirable than the single-syringe injection of mixed insulin.
- Children often have more positive feelings about the pens compared to conventional syringes because of less pain.
- Treatment of women with pre-gestational and gestational diabetes requiring pharmacologic therapy. The convenience, flexibility and ease of use with insulin pen can simplify treatment and reduce therapy related stress for pregnant women during an already stressful time.
- In older patients with vision problems, air bubbles that are drawn into the syringe may go unnoticed leading to variations in insulin delivery from day to day. Not only do insulin pens improve dosing accuracy and compliance but they also may be easier for patients with compromised fine-motor coordination.

Continuous Subcutaneous Insulin Infusion (CSII, Figs. 3A to C)

It was first introduced in 1978. The pump is small, light weight and has a large, backlit liquid crystal display (LCD). It stores approximately 90 days worth of data in memory. The theoretical advantage of pump therapy is its ability to mimic physiological insulin release in patients with insulin deficiency, when compared to multiple daily insulin injection therapy. They are small more efficacious, easier to use and weigh around 400 g. The pump contains an insulin-filled cartridge connected to a catheter that is inserted into the subcutaneous tissue. It continuously delivers pre-determined basal rates to meet non-prandial insulin requirements. It also infuses a bolus to cover mealtime or snack time insulin requirements.

The system consists of a pump, reservoir syringe and infusion set. The reservoir volume is 3 mL/300 IU and has to be disposed after each use. The infusion set also has to be changed every 2–3 days, to maximize the benefits of pump therapy.

Basal Insulin

This is continuous infusion of small amounts of rapidly acting insulin over 24 hours. This aims to match endogenous hepatic glucose production and generally comprises 40–50% of total daily insulin dose. The rate of infusion can be individually programmed throughout the day, increasing during times of relative insulin resistance and decreasing during periods of activity. A properly set basal rate keeps the blood glucose levels stabilized in the absence of food.

- Higher basal rates for less activity periods
- Lower basal rates for more active periods

Bolus Insulin

These are patient-activated doses given with meals to correct hyperglycemic crisis. Some recent pump models incorporate bolus dose calculator technology. The dose calculator is programmed with both the individual patient's insulin requirements per gram of carbohydrate (insulin: carbohydrate ratio) and their insulin sensitivity factor (used to calculate correction bolus doses) Mealtime doses are calculated based on current and target blood glucose levels and the carbohydrate content of the meal.

Benefits of CSII:

- Closer to normal blood glucose levels throughout the day—within the target range.
- Fewer erratic swings in blood glucose and thus a decreased risk of hypoglycemia more appropriate matching of insulin to food intake
- Improved chances for a long, healthy life.
- Increased flexibility in coping with daily living.
- Improved targeting of the "dawn phenomenon".

Risks of CSII:

- Diabetic Ketoacidosis: Since there is no subcutaneous depot of long-acting insulin with CSII, if the flow of the short-acting insulin is interrupted, diabetic ketoacidosis can develop more rapidly and frequently with CSII. The interruption may be intentional allowing patient to participate in certain activities or unintentional, caused by catheter occlusion, dis-insertion, battery failure, depletion of insulin supply and other causes such as patient error and inadequate training.

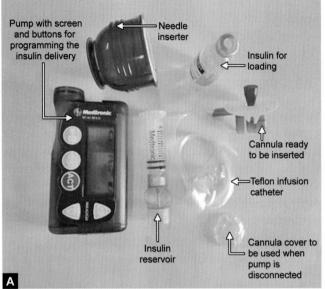

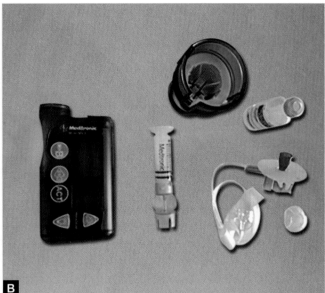

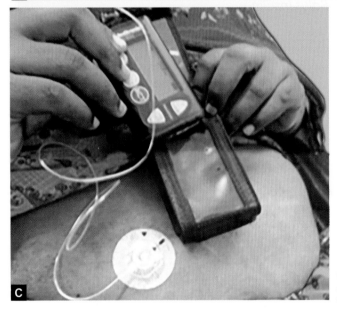

Figs. 3A to C: (A and B) Insulin pump and its parts; (C) Insulin pump on a patient.

Patients should be trained to check their blood glucose at least 4 times a day.

- *Hypoglycemia:* Generally occurs less frequently with CSII than with MDI, mainly due to unintentional insulin delivery or "Pump runaway". Frequent SMBG allow early recognition of hypo glycaemia.
- *Catheter Site Infection and Contact Dermatitis:* Most common complication associated with CSII is infection at the infusion site. Occasional cases of contact dermatitis attributed to the components of the infusion site and tapes have been described. Change of catheter site every 2–3 days minimizes the risk of developing skin infections.
- *Weight Gain:* Weight gain is a common adverse effect of impaired glycemic control. Exercise and dose attention to caloric intake can result in weight maintenance and if necessary, weight reduction.

MULTIPLE CHOICE QUESTIONS

1. All of the following are true regarding immunoendo-crinopathy, *EXCEPT:*
   A. *AIRE* gene mediates peripheral antigen presentation in thymus
   B. Autoantibodies against TNF-α and TNF omega are seen in most patients of APS- 11
   C. FOX P3 mutations present with Type 1 DM, enteropathy and immune dysregulation
   D. Wolframs syndrome is associated with non-autoimmune destruction of pancreatic beta cells

2. A 38-year-old lady with type 2 diabetes mellitus, weighing 100 kg, asks you about treatment options but is afraid of using medication for the treatment of diabetes. Which *one* of the following is the MOST effective method of achieving significant weight loss in patients with diabetes mellitus without using oral antidiabetic medications?
   A. Diets emphasizing fewer calories.
   B. Increased physical activity.
   C. Diets emphasizing a reduction in saturated fats.
   D. Bariatric surgery.

3. In neonatal diabetes, which of the following statements are true?
   A. Patients diagnosed before 6 months are very unlikely to have type 1 diabetes and genetic causes for neonatal diabetes should be looked for
   B. Patients with KCNJ11 (Kir6.2) mutations are extremely sensitive to sulfonylureas and require lower doses than used in type 2 diabetes
   C. Neurologic features in patients with KCNJ11 (Kir6.2) mutations are normally the result of brain injury occurring when patients have severe diabetic ketoacidosis
   D. Approximately 10% of patients who have transient neonatal diabetes will be diabetic after 30 years of age.

4. A patient with diabetes has a callosity on the right foot which is located on the 1st metatarsal head and recurs after removal. Examination of the foot shows mild clawing and she has a monofilament sensation perception of 10 g. After removal again, which of the following methods would you use to prevent a recurrence:
   A. Total Contact Cast.
   B. Patellar tendon baring brace
   C. Microcellular rubber foot wear without a broad toe box and a back strap
   D. Footwear with a Metatarsal bar

5. In the urgent care clinic, you are evaluating a 47-year-old woman with poorly controlled diabetes who has a chief complaint of "sinusitis." She does not have a history of atopy. She first noticed a headache 2 days ago and now feels very congested in her upper nasal passages. She has hyperesthesia over her nasal bridge as well and is inquiring about antibiotics to treat her infection. She has a bloody nasal discharge with occasional black specks. On examination, the sinuses are full and tender. She has a temperature of 38.3°C. Oral examination shows a black eschar on the roof of her mouth surrounded by discolored hyperemic areas on the palate. What is the most appropriate intervention at this time?
   A. Ciprofloxacin and quarantine for possible anthrax
   B. ENT consultation if no improvement with oral antibiotics
   C. Immediate biopsy of the involved areas and lipid amphotericin
   D. Immediate biopsy of the lesion and voriconazole

6. A 70-year-old man has below knee amputation following progressive wet gangrene. He is obese and has osteoarthroses. The stump ulcer is about 4 cm in size. He wishes to have a prosthesis on a long term basis following healing of the ulcer. Which of the following forms of therapy would you use for now?
   A. Patellar Tendon Bearing brace.
   B. Silver sulphadiazine dressing.
   C. Walker.
   D. MCR foot wear with meta tarsal bar

7. A 30-year-old man presented with polyuria and polydipsia, abdominal pain and weight loss of 10% of his body weight, and is normotensive. He has been married for 3 years and is infertile.
   His urine ketones were negative. His blood sugars were 420 mg/dL. C-peptides were 3.0 ng/dL. GAD Antibodies are negative. Urine microscopy shows numerous WBCs and the culture grows E coli. A CT scan done to rule out pyelonephritis shows a normal pancreas, liver and bilateral renal cysts with normal sized kidneys.
   Your most likely diagnosis is:
   A. MODY 1
   B. MODY3
   C. MODY5
   D. MODY7

8. A 40-year-old gentleman with diabetes presents pain in the medial aspect of his foot and which is persistent. Examination shows edema and tenderness of the medial aspect of the foot. His monofilament testing reveals non-perception of a 10 g monofilament and Biothesiometry of 35 mV. A plain X-ray reveals features of Charcot's type 2 arthropathy, by the Mrdjenovic classification. He is otherwise physically fit with a BMI of 22 kg/m², and can walk 6 km a day, but for the pain in his foot, and feels well otherwise and his glucose levels on Glimepiride and metformin are equivalent to a HbA1c of 6.7%. The most suitable form of therapy would be:
   A. A moulded insole with a rigid rocker, with a shore value of less than 16 and more than 8 for the insole.
   B. A clog with the cutout of the outer-sole on the medial aspect below the first metatarsal head and an insole with a shore value of less than 16 and more than 8.
   C. Ankle-foot Orthosis with a boot and an insole with a shore value of more than 8 and less than 16.
   D. Standard microcellular foot-wear with a back-strap and a insole with a shore value of less than 16 and more than 8.

9. A 50-year-old man has diabetes for 10 years duration and he is on maximum dosage of oral hypoglycemic agents with which he has been compliant with. He is currently on Metformin, Pioglitazone, Voglibose, Linagliptin and Glimepiride. He did not want to take insulin till this point. On examination his BMI is 21 kg/m² and he does not have complications of diabetes. Self Monitored sugars on 5 days of the week, shows an average of 250 mg/dL and HbA1c is 9.0%. He is willing for a single daily add on drug to the current medications. Cost is not an issue, essentially it should be effective. Which one would you choose?
   A. Degludec
   B. Glargine
   C. Gliclazide-XL
   D. Liraglutide

10. A 40-year-old gentleman has been on monotherapy for his diabetes for 6 months. He is experiencing recurrent urinary tract infections, which his doctor is ascribing to pharmacological therapy. Which one is the most likely cause?
    A. Sitagliptin
    B. Glucokinase inhibitors
    C. Dapagliflozin
    D. Albiglutide

11. A 50-year-old lady is on metformin therapy for diabetes for 4 years. She is very cautious with pharmacotherapy and has heard that adding on other oral drugs can cause hypoglycemia, some of which may pose a risk for pancreatic tumors.

    Though not proven, some cause abdominal distension, some cause edema and some cause urinary tract infections. Which oral drug then would you use as an add on which do not have any of the adverse effects that have been mentioned?
    A. Sitagliptin
    B. Liraglutide
    C. Acarbose
    D. Bromocriptine

12. A 28-year-old gentleman presented with hypertension, diabetes and cardiac failure. He had weight loss of 20 kg and subsequently his bone marrow showed evidence of histoplasmosis. He was advised to take the following medication for 2 years after initial stabilization:
    A. Itraconazole
    B. Ketoconazole
    C. Voriconazole
    D. Metronidazole

13. A 50-year-old gentleman with diabetes and on chronic corticosteroid therapy for SLE, presents with cough with expectoration. There are gram positive filamentous organisms in his sputum. After stabilization he is given a 6 week course of oral medications and is well after that. What has he been given?
    A. Cotrimoxazole
    B. Voriconazole
    C. Fluconazole
    D. Ampicillin

14. A 40-year-old gentleman has difficult to control diabetes requiring 200 units of insulin per day. Which of the following infections would he possibly have?
    A. Hepatitis A
    B. Hepatitis B
    C. Hepatitis C
    D. Hepatitis E

15. For the anti-hyperglycemic agent Metformin, select *one* primary mechanism of action largely associated with it.
    A. Reduces gluconeogenesis in the liver.
    B. Stimulates post-prandial insulin secretion.
    C. Delays the absorption of carbohydrates in the gut.
    D. Enhances insulin sensitivity in the peripheral tissues.

16. A 50-year-old woman with type 2 diabetes mellitus is seen in the office with a blood pressure of 150/90 mm Hg and the lipid profile shown below. She has a normal amount of albumin in her urine and normal renal function.

Total Cholesterol –215 mg/dL

Triglycerides –120 mg/dL

HDL-C 51 mg/dL

LDL-C 140 mg/dL

If her doctor elects to start her on medication for her blood pressure, which *one* of the following classes of antihypertensive agents would be BEST to reduce her chance of progression to microalbuminuria?
   A. Alpha blockers
   B. Diuretics
   C. ACE inhibitors
   D. Beta blockers

17. She is reluctant to take a statin. Which *one* of the following statements is INCORRECT regarding statins and the prevention of CVD?
   A. Statins have been shown to reduce the chances of a CV event in individuals that have no known CVD (primary prevention).
   B. All the large published studies which evaluated statins' ability to prevent all-cause mortality have shown a benefit.
   C. Statins have been shown to reduce the chances of a second CV event in individuals that have known CVD (secondary prevention).
   D. Statins have been shown to reduce the chances of having a CV event irrespective of LDL levels L

18. After taking a statin, she develops muscle aches and pains. Her Creatine phosphokinase (CPK) levels are now: 800 IU. On stopping statins, the drug that would be useful, purely for treating the elevated cholesterol would be:
   A. Fenofibrate
   B. Nicotinic acid
   C. Ezetimibe
   D. Gemfibrozil

19. A 70-year-old gentleman with diabetes for 11years presents with fever and chills for 4 days. Urine microscopy shows multiple white blood cells in the analysis. A urine culture is performed and reveals Extended spectrum beta lactamase (ESBL) organisms present in high titers. What would you do next:
   A. Start Meropenem
   B. Start Amoxicillin
   C. Start Gentamicin
   D. Start Nitrofurantoin

20. The fever persists after three days. An ultrasonogram is performed which shows edema of the right kidney and gas in the perinephric space. What is the most likely organism as a cause?
   A. E. Coli
   B. Klebsiella
   C. Clostridium
   D. Peptostreptococcus

21. Following a urological procedure, the fever persists, and the patient has a unilateral nephrectomy. The infection spreads to the opposite side and the opposite side is nephrectomised as well. The patient is started on hemodialysis. After that, the fever subsides. Functionally he is well, and leads an independent life, he would like to spend much of his time at home, without frequent hospital visits. What would you give as an option for this patient for long term renal replacement therapy?
   A. Hemodialysis
   B. Cadaver based renal transplantation
   C. Live related renal transplantation
   D. Continuous ambulatory peritoneal dialysis

22. A 31-year-old, economically challenged farmer presents with abdominal pain and diarrhea for 12 years. He is on premixed insulin for diabetes for 5 years, the HbA1c is 9.5% and his BMI is 18 kg/m². He has frequent hypoglycemic attacks early morning and also post meal. The 72 stool fat measurement is 34 g. The CT scan shows duct dilatation in the pancreas and large pancreatic calculi within the ducts.

The most likely problem that he has is:
   A. Cystic fibrosis gene mutation.
   B. Serine kinase 4 mutation
   C. SPINK-1 mutation
   D. Alcoholic pancreatitis

23. For better control of blood sugars, you put him on three meals and three snacks, give him pancreatic enzyme supplements. Which of the following insulin regimens would you prefer?
   A. Aspart insulin thrice a day with a pen and glargine at bedtime
   B. Soluble insulin with a syringe thrice a day and NPH at bedtime.
   C. Degludec insulin once a day and Humalog thrice a day.
   D. Try out Glimepiride with metformin and top up with Acarbose if still uncontrolled

24. You are located in a tertiary care center and he comes to you annually for a follow-up. Your protocol would include:

A. DOTATATE scan and Ca 19-9 once a year
B. CT Abdomen and CEA once year
C. DOTATATE scan and CEA once a year
D. Ultrasound abdomen and Ca-19.9 once a year.

25. A 26-year-old nurse is applying for a job. She is found to have fasting plasma glucose of 130 mg/dL, her postprandial sugars are normal. She is otherwise well, with a normal blood pressure, a BMI of 21kg/m², no features of insulin resistance and has no dysmorphic features. She has no ketones in her urine. Her GAD auto-antibodies are negative, C-peptides are 3.0 ng/dl and she has a normal ultrasound of the abdomen. Her father had diabetes diagnosed at the age of 31 and her grand-father at the age of 44. Her only brother had a urinary tract infection and was diagnosed at the age of 29 years to have diabetes.

Going by the textbook, she is most likely to have:
A. MODY1
B. MODY2
C. MODY3
D. MODY4

CHAPTER 3

Aggressive Adrenal
(Disorders of the Adrenal Gland)

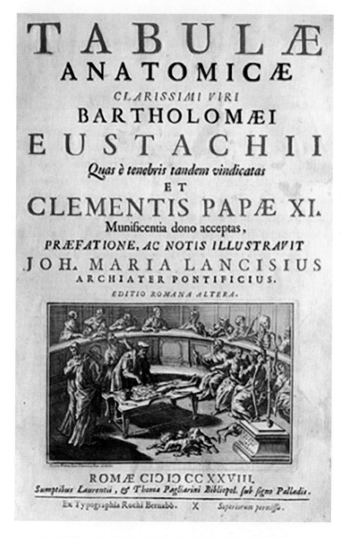

Batholemeus Eustachius (1520–1574), in his book:
"Tabulae Anatomicae Bartholomei Eustachi quas a tenebris tandem vindicatas" Which are
Anatomical Illustrations of Bartholomeo Eustachi rescued from obscurity) first explained
"Glandulae renibus incubentis" or "glands lying on the kidneys...."

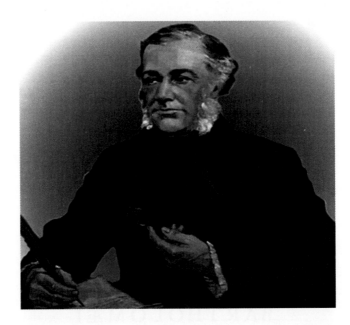

Thomas Addison (2 April 1793–29 June 1860) was a renowned 19th-century English physician and scientist. He is traditionally regarded as one of the "great men" of Guy's Hospital in London.

Among other pathologies he discovered Addison's disease and Addisonian anemia (pernicious anemia).

Dr Thomas Addison described adrenal insufficiency in the year 1849, in the era where other endocrine functions had yet to be explained in detail which he described from the autopsies he performed. At the time, there was no cure for adrenal insufficiency. Addison also noticed that 70–90% of patients with adrenal insufficiency had tuberculosis as well.

CASE 1

A 28-year-old lady presented with history of fever, weight loss and cough for the past since 6 months. On examination she had skin lesions over the face, palmar creases and the oral mucosa (Figs. 1 and 2). There were episodes of abdominal pain and features suggestive of proximal myopathy. There was no history of vomiting, jaundice or diarrhea. Chest X-ray (Fig. 3) was done and the images are displayed below.

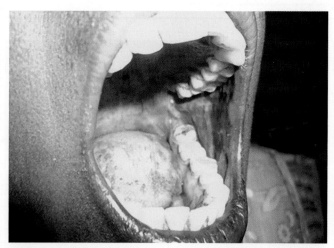

Fig. 1: Mucosal hyperpigmentation.

WHAT IS THE DIAGNOSIS?

Her investigations revealed a low serum sodium with high potassium levels. The serum cortisol levels were undetectable with elevated Adrenocorticotropic harmone (ACTH) levels (1250 pg/mL). In view of hyperpigmentation with low blood pressure and a low serum sodium level, primary adrenal insufficiency was diagnosed. She was given parenteral hydrocortisone.

Chest X-ray revealed a bilateral nodular and branching pattern involving the upper zones (Fig. 3). Subsequently she underwent a CT scan of the thorax and abdomen which confirmed the presence of nodular opacities involving the upper lobes of the lung bilaterally (Fig. 4).

A CT abdomen showed bilateral supra renal masses (Figs. 5A and B). Subsequently the patient underwent a CT guided adrenal FNA biopsy which showed a granulomatous reaction with epithelioid histiocytes, lymphocytes and multinucleate giant cells. (Fig. 6). The biopsies of the skin lesions and the bone marrow have grown Histoplasma capsulatum. Subsequently, she was started on liposomal Amphotericin which was later changed to Itraconazole.

She was shifted to oral prednisolone and in due course of time fludrocortisone was added. Her sodium

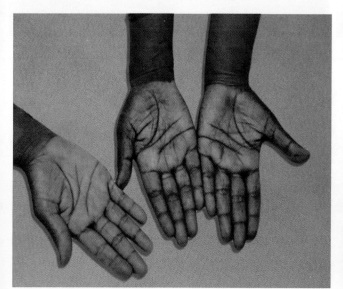

Fig. 2: Hyperpigmentation of the palmar creases on comparing her sister's palms on the left side.

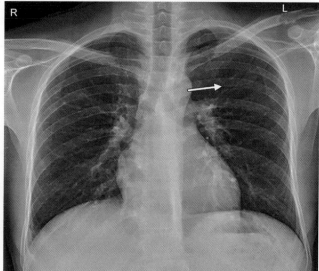

Fig. 3: Nodular branching pattern involving the upper zone.

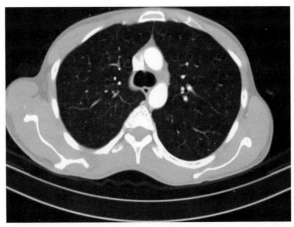

Fig. 4: CT Thorax showing nodular opacities involving the upper lobes of the lung.

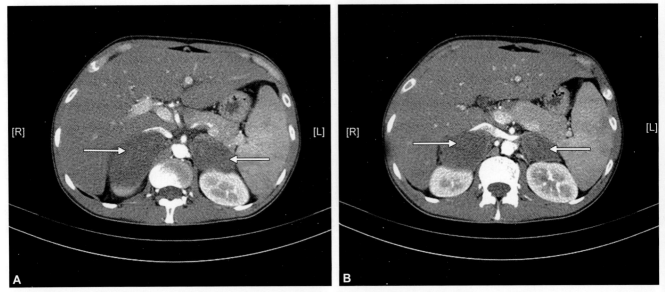

Figs. 5A and B: CT Abdomen with Bilateral adrenal masses (shown with the arrows).

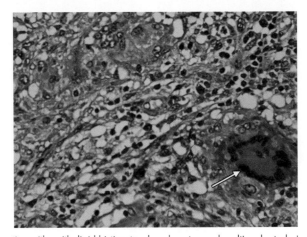

Fig. 6: Illustrating a granulomatous reaction with epithelioid histiocytes, lymphocytes and multinucleated giant cells (shown with arrow) (H&E × 200).

levels normalised on starting oral fludrocortisone. She responded well to the treatment and gained a body weight of 10 kg over the last one year. At present she is on regular follow up.

DISCUSSION

Disseminated histoplasmosis occurs in one in every 2000 patients with acute infection. It is usually seen in patients with altered immunity and at extremes of age however progressive illness can be seen in acute stages of infection before cellular immunity evolves. Histoplasma capsulatum is a dimorphic fungus which develops from microconidia that are inhaled into the lungs. It induces three types of tissue responses, including diffuse histoplasmosis, focal histoplasmosis and tuberculoid granulomas.

Fungal culture remains the gold standard for the diagnosis, being positive in 75% of cases of Disseminated Histoplasmosis.[1]

Treatment includes Intravenous Liposomal Amphotericin B (3–5 mg/kg/day) for 3 weeks followed by Oral Itraconazole 200 mg twice daily long term.[2]

REFERENCES

1. Vyas S, Kalra N, Das PJ, et al. Adrenal histoplasmosis: An unusual cause of adrenomegaly. Indian J Nephrol. 2011;21(4):283–5.
2. Subramanian S, Abraham OC, Rupali P, et al. Disseminated histoplasmosis. J Assoc Physicians India. 2005;53:185–9.

CASE 2

A 36-year-old gentleman presented with 4-months history of ulcer over the tongue. The ulcer had slowly increased in size and was associated with pain, odynophagia and discomfort in speech. There was no history of associated trauma, intake of alcohol, smoking or chewing tobacco. He has a grocery shop and was not involved in farming or working in caves. On examination a 2 × 2 cm ulcer with elevated margins was seen at the posterior aspect of the tongue (Fig. 1). On palpation the ulcer was tender and indurated. Images of the ulcer are displayed below.

WHAT IS THE DIAGNOSIS ?

The patient was thoroughly investigated. His hemogram, chest X-ray and HIV serology were normal. Biopsy of the

ulcer revealed a characteristic "sunflowers in bloom" appearance of macroconidia of Histoplasma capsulatum and the microconidia were also seen (Fig. 2). Subsequently he was started on Tab. Itraconazole 200 mg thrice daily for 3 days followed by twice daily for 12 months.

He also had bilateral adrenal enlargement (Fig. 3) for which a CT guided FNAC was done which showed dimorphic capsulated fungi suggestive of histoplasmosis (Fig. 2).

DISCUSSION

Histoplasmosis or Cave's disease or Darling's disease was discovered in 1905 by Darling while working in the Canal Zone in Panama. Although localized oral lesions

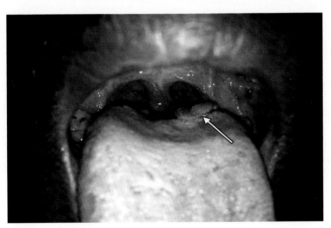

Fig. 1: An elevated ulcer in the posterior aspect of the tongue.

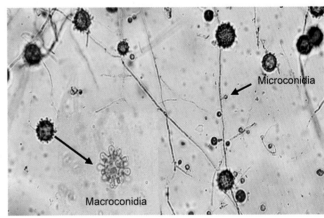

Fig. 2: Lactophenol cotton blue preparation (400 ×) showing macro and microconidia of the Histoplasma capsulatum.

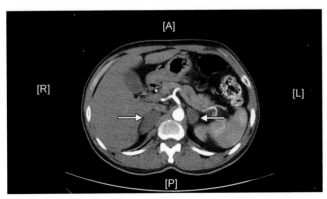

Fig. 3: CT abdomen with contrast showing bilateral adrenal enlargement (shown with the arrows).

without any systemic involvement are uncommon, the presence of mucocutaneous lesions should always be considered as a manifestation of disseminated disease.[1] Goodwin et al. stated that the most characteristic lesion in chronic disseminated histoplasmosis is an oropharyngeal ulcer and is seen in up to 70% of cases.[2]

REFERENCES

1. Dunlap CL, Barnes WG. Oral histoplasmosis. J Mo Dent Assoc. 1969;49(7):26–9.
2. Goodwin RA, Shapiro JL, Thurman GH, et al. Disseminated histoplasmosis: clinical and pathologic correlations. Medicine (Baltimore). 1980; 59(1):1–33.

CASE **3**

A 28-year-old gentleman from Bangladesh presented with history of intermittent fever, weight loss and cough with expectoration for the past 6 months. On examination he had multiple papular lesions with crust over the face (Figs. 1A to C). A CT abdomen that was done in his hometown showed bilateral adrenal gland enlargement (Figs. 2A and B). He was empirically started on anti-tubercular therapy (ATT) by his family physician with no clinical improvement. His biopsy showed a necrotic focus with a few small spherical structures resembling histoplasma (Figs. 3A and B). A silver methenamine and PAS diastase staining from the adrenal biopsy also showed a similar finding (Fig. 4).

WHAT IS THE DIAGNOSIS?

This patient had biochemical features suggestive of hypocortisolemia and was diagnosed to have Histoplasmosis of the face and the adrenal gland. He was given prednisolone with fludrocortisone and itraconzole.

DISCUSSION

In India, the Gangetic state of West Bengal is the site of the most frequent infections, with 9.4 percent of the population testing positive.[1] Histoplasma capsulatum was isolated from the local soil proving endemicity to West Bengal. The fungus seems to grow best in soils having a high nitrogen content, especially those enriched with bird manure or bat droppings.

The normal reservoir for Histoplasma is droppings of birds and bats and moist soil, particularly beneath trees. The mode of infection is by the inhalation of the dimorphic soil fungus. The organisms reach alveolar spaces where it multiplies in mononuclear phagocytes and is not

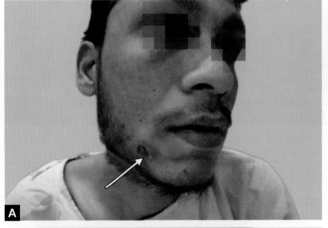

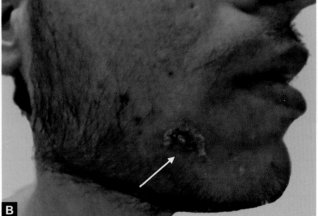

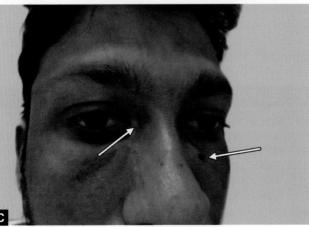

Figs. 1A to C: Plaques with crusts over the face (shown with the arrows).

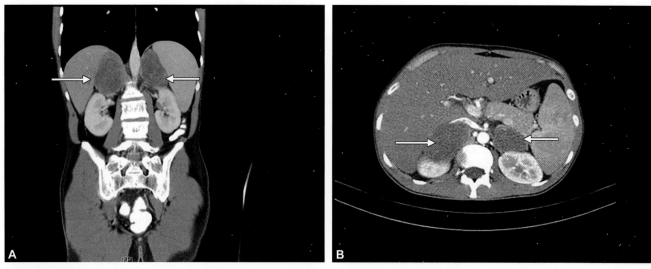

Figs. 2A and B: CT abdomen showing bilateral enlarged adrenal glands (shown with the arrows).

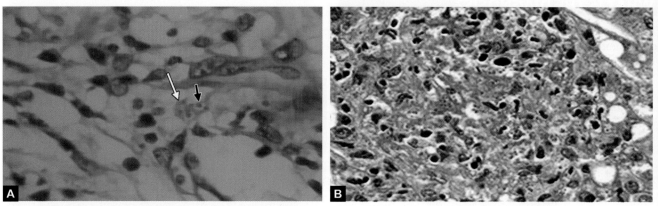

Figs. 3A and B: Histopathological specimen from the adrenal gland showing a necrotic focus (shown with white arrow) with few small spherical structures (shown with black arrow) (Periodic acid Schiff with diastase × 400).

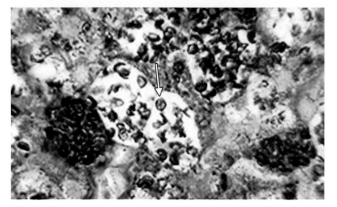

Fig. 4: Silver methenamine staining of the adrenal gland biopsy tissue showing spherical microorganisms (shown with arrow) and necrotic tissue.

contagious. The Culture usually shows a tan-white-brown wooly mold at 25–30° C on Sabouraud dextrose agar. In microscopy the Organisms will have delicate, septate hyphae, 1–2 microns thick, with large rough-walled macro–conidia 5–15 microns. The organism reverts to yeast form at 37° C on sheep blood agar.[2]

REFERENCES

1. Sanyal, Maya, Thammayya. A. Histoplasma capsulatum in the soil of Gangetic plain in India. Indian J Med Res. 1975; 63(7):1020-8.
2. Ajello L, Hay RJ, 1997. Medical Mycology Vol 4 Topley & Wilson's Microbiology and Infectious Infections. 1997 9th Edition, Arnold London.

CASE 4

A 48-year-old lady with no previous significant co-morbidities presented with the history of abdominal pain and vomiting for one month. She also noticed hyperpigmentation of the face and the palmar creases and also unintentional weight loss of about 10 kg over 1 year duration. She did not give any history of kochs in the past or an exposure to tuberculosis. She was hypotensive with a BP of 80/60 mm Hg, when presented to the emergency department. Her clinical image and CT abdomen were shown in the Figures 1 and 2 respectively.

WHAT IS THE DIAGNOSIS?

Further investigations revealed a low serum sodium level with high potassium levels and acidosis suggesting corticosteroid as well as mineralocorticoid deficiency. She had undetectable serum cortisol levels with high plasma ACTH levels (1250 pg/mL). The CT abdomen image revealed bilateral adrenal enlargement with calcification within the adrenal glands (Fig. 2). The CT guided biopsy of the adrenal gland revealed granulomas composed of epithelioid histiocytes, lymphocytes, few plasma cells and Langhans' type of multinucleate giant cells suggestive of tuberculosis.

She was started on oral prednisolone and fludrocortisone was added later. She was also treated with anti-tubercular treatment for one year. At present, she is on follow up in our Endocrine clinic and on prednisolone and fludrocortisone.

DISCUSSION

Thomas Addison described cases of adrenal insufficiency more than 150 years ago where in his initial series found more than 50% of patients had tuberculosis (6/11).[1]

Though autoimmune disorders became the most common cause of adrenal insufficiency in developed countries, hematogenous spread of pulmonary tuberculosis, continues to be a cause of adrenal insufficiency in developing countries. The diagnosis of adrenal tuberculosis, especially with enlargement of adrenal glands, can be difficult with differentials like histoplasmosis, adrenal hemorrhage due to infections or APLA need to be ruled out.

Dissemination of M. tuberculosis may occur at the time of primary pulmonary infection or later from re-infection or reactivation of previous infection.

Enlargement of both adrenal glands may occur in nearly (90%) patients with tuberculous adrenal insufficiency. Bilateral adrenal enlargement is the typical finding and

this may include a central necrotic area of low attenuation and a peripheral enhancing rim in CT Imaging. In the phase of healing, the enlargement of tuberculous adrenals may partially or completely resolve, with or without calcification or atrophy. However the glucocorticoids and mineralocorticoid replacements have to be continued on a long term basis.[2]

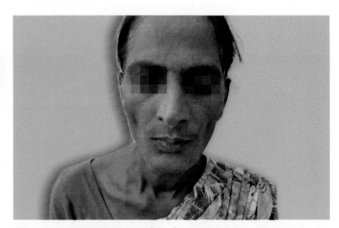

Fig. 1: Hyperpigmentation of the face.

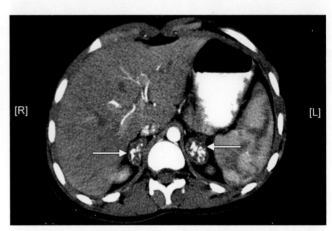

Fig. 2: CT abdomen showing bilateral adrenal enlargement and calcification within the adrenal glands (shown with the arrows).

REFERENCES

1. T. Addison, On the Constitutional and Local Effects of Disease of the Suprarenal Capsules, Warren & Son, London, UK, 1855.
2. Al-Mamari A, Balkhair A, Gujjar A, et al. A Case of Disseminated Tuberculosis with Adrenal Insufficiency. Sultan QaboosUniv Med J. 2009;9(3):324-7.

CASE 5

A 40-year-old female presented with complaints of abdominal pain over a week. She was initially evaluated by gastroenterologists for abdominal pain. As a part of evaluation and routine physical examination, hemogram, renal and liver function tests were done and were normal. A CT abdomen was done which revealed a left adrenal mass which was heterogeneously enhancing with multiple cystic areas and an intervening solid compartment (Figs. 1A to D).

WHAT IS THE DIAGNOSIS?

On endocrine assessment she had a history of intermittent headache and palpitations for the past 4 years. She was on treatment for hypertension and diabetes for the past 4 years. There was no history of menstrual irregularities, easy bruisability of the skin, fractures or hirsutism. Her 24-hour urinary metanephrine levels were elevated and she had normal suppressible serum cortisol levels following a 1 mg over night dexamethasone suppression test.

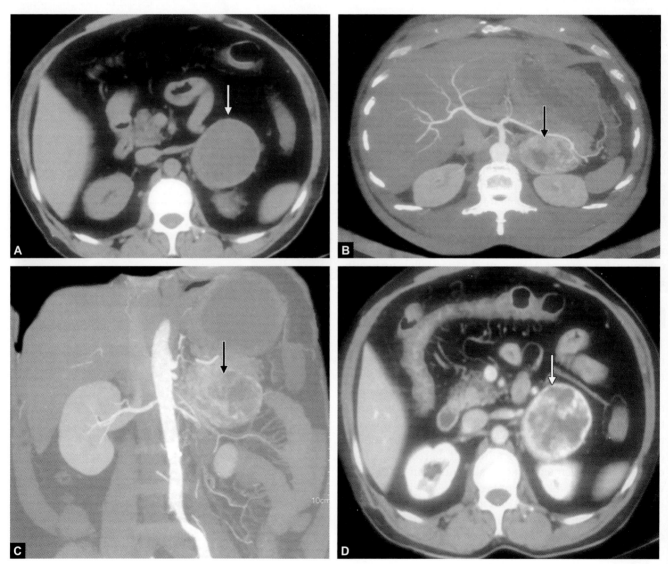

Figs. 1A to D: Heterogeneously enhancing left adrenal mass with multiple cystic and an intervening solid compartment (shown with arrow).

A differential diagnosis of left adrenal adenoma or a pheochromocytoma was made.

After preoperative treatment with alpha adrenergic blockade and beta blockers she underwent laparoscopic adrenalectomy and the histopathology report was positive for a pheochromocytoma.

DISCUSSION

An adrenal mass may be detected in about 5% of patients imaged for a non-adrenal pathology. Increased reliance on diagnostic imaging, a progressively aging population and improved precision of these investigations are the reasons for an increased frequency of detection of incidentalomas. Adrenal incidentalomas are mostly benign but they have the potential to become malignant with high mortality rates. In 85% of cases these lesions are non-functioning benign adenomas. Size appears to be the single most important predictor of malignancy, lesions less than 4 cm in size below 10 HU (Hounsfield) washout, more than 50% on non-contrast CT scan are adenomas and are unlikely to be malignant and can be treated conservatively, where as in lesions more than 5 cm in size surgical intervention with removal of the lesion becomes necessary as there is an increased risk of malignancy. For masses that appear to be benign (<10 HU; washout, >50%), small (<4 cm), and completely non-functioning, imaging and biochemical re-evaluation at 1–2 year is appropriate. To avoid unnecessary radiation exposure and to cut down the health care costs some authors have proposed that no further testing of small non-functioning incidentalomas is required.[1,2]

REFERENCES

1. Lynnette K. Nieman. Approach to the Patient with an Adrenal Incidentaloma. J Clin EndocrinolMetab. 2010; 95(9):4106-13.
2. Kapoor A, Morris T, Rebello R. Guidelines for the management of the incidentally discovered adrenal mass. Can Urol Assoc J. 2011;5(4):241-7.

CASE 6

A 37-year-old lady was diagnosed to have hypertension 17 years ago at the age of 20 and presented with 2 episodes of features suggestive of proximal muscle weakness. She did not have palpitations, easy skin bruisability or hirsutism. On examination she had elevated blood pressure and had no clinical evidence of muscle weakness. The abdominal image is shown in Figure 1.

WHAT IS THE DIAGNOSIS?

On thorough investigation she was found to have borderline hypernatremia (144 meq) with significant hypokalemia (1.8 mq) associated with suppressed plasma renin and elevated serum aldosterone. She also had features suggestive of hypertensive retinopathy and left ventricular hypertrophy on ECHO and ECG. CT abdomen revealed a well-defined hypodense lipid rich lesion arising from the left adrenal gland, that measured about 18 × 16 mm (shown with arrow).

Preoperatively, she was started on potassium sparing diuretics and potassium supplements. She underwent left adrenalectomy and the histopathology report of the surgical specimen was suggestive of an adrenal adenoma. Postoperatively her serum potassium normalised and on discharge her blood pressure was under control without antihypertensives.

DISCUSSION

Conn's syndrome is a state of primary hyperaldosteronism producing adrenal adenoma and was first described in 1955 by Jerome W Conn an American endocrinologist. Aldosterone producing adrenal adenomas constitutes about 35% of all cases of Primary Aldosteronism. Adrenal adenomas are considered to be second most common cause of primary hyperaldosteronism after adrenal hyperplasia. An Aldosterone:Renin ratio more than 30 is considered indicative of primary hyperaldosteronism. The usual presenting features include muscle cramps, weakness, headache, polydypsia, polyuria etc. Fine cut

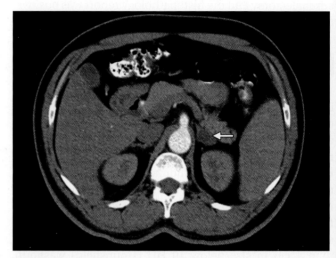

Fig. 1: CT scan abdomen showing a lipid rich adenoma on the lateral limb of the left adrenal gland (shown with arrow).

CT scanning of the adrenal region is the investigation of choice as it provides an excellent visualisation of adrenal morphology.

Surgical intervention is indicated in patients with a confirmed mineralocorticoid excess and a unilateral lesion and in patients with confirmed lateralisation as documented by adrenal venous sampling (AVS) procedure. Laparoscopic adrenalectomy is the usual preferred method of surgery. Patients who are not surgical candidates and in whom a bilateral hyperplasia of the adrenal, as detected by CT scanning or AVS procedures are treated with spironolactone or eplerenone.[1,2]

REFERENCES

1. Funder JW, Carey RM, Fardella C, et al. Case detection, diagnosis, and treatment of patients with primary aldosteronism: an endocrine society clinical practice guideline. J Clin Endocrinol Metab. 2008;93(9):3266–81.
2. Gupta V. Mineralocorticoid hypertension. Indian J Endocrinol Metab. 2011;15(Suppl4):S298–312

CASE 7

A 64-year-old male presented with diffuse abdominal distension, a feeling of heaviness in the abdomen and loss of appetite for one year duration. He did not have any history of proximal muscle weakness, easy skin bruisability, hematuria, hypertension or pigmentation of the skin over the abdomen. On examination his blood pressure was 150/90 mm Hg and there was 6 × 6 cm globular mass in the in the left upper quadrant. A CT scan of the abdomen was done and the images are displayed below.

WHAT IS THE DIAGNOSIS?

The CT abdomen showed a 14 × 11 cm large well circumscribed fat attenuation lesion in the left adrenal gland with features suggestive of an adrenal myelolipoma (Figs. 1A and B). The biochemical evaluation was negative for an-ACTH independent cushings syndrome. His 24-hour urinary metanephrines and normetanephrines were not elevated. Serum dehydroepiandrosterone sulfate (DHEAS) was also within normal limits. He had open surgical excision of the lesion.

DISCUSSION

Adrenal myelolipomas are benign tumor like lesions composed of mature adipose tissue and hematopoietic elements in various proportions. Both the myeloid and lipomatous elements have a monoclonal origin which supports the hypothesis that myelolipomas are neoplastic lesions. Adrenal cortical cells are able to differentiate and may reversibly change into fat or blood forming cells. Myelolipomas are found unexpectedly at autopsy in 0.08–0.4% of the cases.[1] They most commonly occur in the adrenal glands and constitute 3% of all adrenal tumors.The gross cut surface has varying colors from red to yellow to mahagony brown. They are usually asymptomatic but have been reported to present with symptoms such as flank pain from tumor bulk, necrosis and spontaneous retroperitoneal hemorrhage. The CT scan of the adrenal gland is the most sensitive diagnostic modality. Surgical excision is recommended for large tumors because of associated spontaneous bleeding, Symptomatic tumors, growing tumors and tumors greater than 10 cm should be excised.[2]

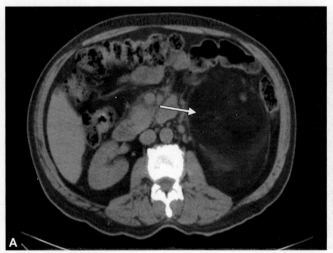 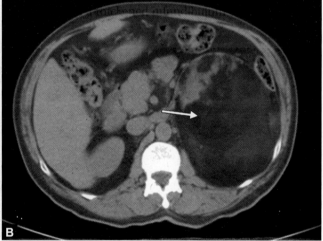

Figs. 1A and B: CT abdomen showing a well-circumscribed mass with a large component of fat and also soft tissue density in the left suprarenal region (shown with arrow).

REFERENCES

1. Nabi J, Rafiq D, Authoy FN, et al. Incidental Detection of Adrenal Myelolipoma: A Case Report and Review of Literature. Case Rep Urol. 2013;20;2013:e789481.

2. Al Harthi B, Riaz MM, Al Khalaf AH, et al. Adrenal myelolipoma a rare benign tumor managed laparoscopically: Report of two cases. J Minimal Access Surg. 2009;5(4):118–20.

CASE 8

A 22-year-old lady presented with paroxysms of palpitations, headache and sweating of 2 months duration. Historically, 2 months back she was told to have high blood pressure but was not on any treatment. There were no history suggestive of proximal muscle weakness, hyperpigmentation or hirsutism. Her clinical examination was unremarkable except for an elevated blood pressure. A CT abdomen was done and images are shown in Figures 1A and B.

WHAT IS THE DIAGNOSIS?

Her 24-hour serum metanephrine was markedly elevated. Subsequent CT abdomen showed an intensely enhancing well defined lesions in the right and the left adrenal glands. The Meta Iodo Benzyl Guanidine (MIBG) scan (Figs. 2A and B) showed an abnormal tracer accumulation in both supra renal regions suggestive of functioning neuroendocrine tumors essentially—bilateral pheochromocytomas. She

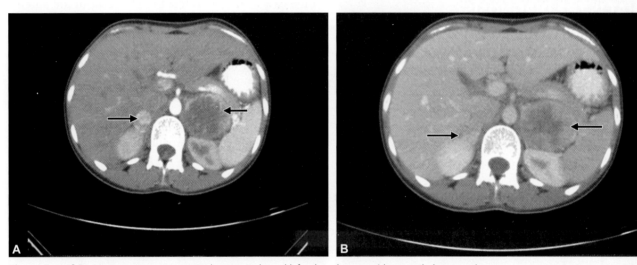

Figs. 1A and B: Heterogeneous contrast enhancing right and left adrenal masses (shown with the arrows).

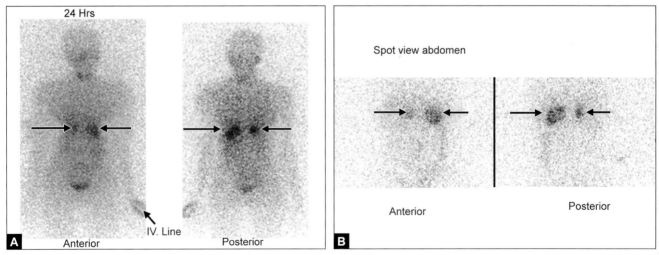

Figs. 2A and B: Meta Iodo Benzyl Guanidine (MIBG) scan showing an increased tracer uptake in the right and left supra renal regions (shown the arrows).

was started on alpha adrenergic blocking agents and was planned for surgical excision of the tumors.

DISCUSSION

The term "Pheochromocytoma" reflects the black colored staining caused by oxidation of intracellular catecholamines when exposed to dichromatic salts. In Greek *phaios* means dark and *chroma* means color. Pheochromocytomas are catecholamine producing tumors of the medulla of the adrenal glands originating in the chromaffin cells and the sympathetic ganglia. Tumors may arise sporadically or as a part of MEN type 2 or several other pheochromocytoma associated syndromes. The diagnosis of pheochromocytoma provides a correctable cause of elevated blood pressure levels. The clinical presentation ranges from adrenal incidentaloma to a patient with hypertensive crisis with cardiovascular and cerebrovascular complications.[1] The prevalence of pheochromocytoma ranges from 0.1% to 0.6%. Pheochromocytomas traditionally have been taught to be tumors that follow the rule of tens which states that 10% are bilateral, 10% are extra adrenal, 10% are malignant, 10% are benign sporadic pheochromocytomas which are detected as adrenal incidentalomas, 10% occur in children, 10% are familial and 10% recur after surgical removal. However about 25% of the patients have an inherited mutations including germ line mutations in the *RET, VHL, NF1, SDHB, SDHC, SDHD,* or *SDHAF2* genes.[2] The definitive treatment of choice is surgical resection.

REFERENCES

1. Chen H, Sippel RS, Pacak K. The NANETS Consensus Guideline for the Diagnosis and Management of Neuroendocrine Tumors: Pheochromocytoma, Paraganglioma & Medullary Thyroid Cancer. Pancreas. 2010;39(6):775–83.
2. Fishbein L, Nathanson KL. Pheochromocytoma and Paraganglioma: Understanding the Complexities of the Genetic Background. Cancer Genet. 2012;2005(1-2):1–11.

CASE 9

A 59-year-old gentleman presented with pain on the left side of the abdomen with paroxysms of palpitations, headache and sweating. He had recent onset of hypertension, for which he was on treatment. He did not have history of muscle weakness or hyper pigmentation. He underwent CT (Fig. 1) and MRI abdomen (Fig. 2), images are displayed below.

WHAT IS THE DIAGNOSIS?

The CT abdomen showed an intensely enhancing large right adrenal mass with central necrosis. His urinary 24-hour metanephrine and normetanephrine levels were elevated and the Meta Iodo Benzyl Guanidine (MIBG) scan showed an increased uptake in the region of the right adrenal gland suggestive of a pheochromocytoma (Fig. 3). He was started on alpha blocking agents and was planned for surgical excision of the tumor. He underwent left adrenalectomy and the histopathology report showed zellenballen appearance suggestive of a pheochromocytoma (Fig. 4).

DISCUSSION

Felix Frankel in 1886 first described a patient with pheochromocytoma. The term pheochromocytoma was first coined by Ludwig Pick, a pathologist in 1912.[1] Pheo-

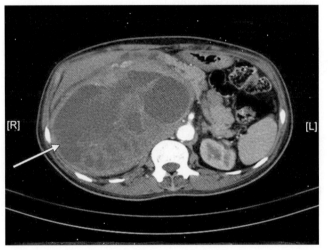

Fig. 1: CT abdomen showing a contrast enhancing 15.7 x 15.4 x 16.2 cm well defined, lesion predominantly cystic with multiple septations and peripherally located solid components which show heterogeneous enhancement (shown with arrow).

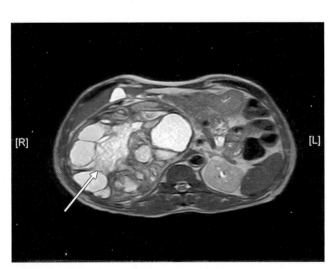

Fig. 2: MRI abdomen showing a hyperintense mass with patchy areas of restricted diffusion in T2 weighted image (shown with arrow).

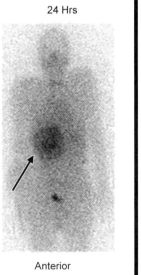
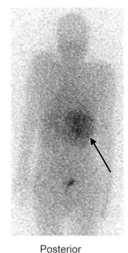

24 Hrs

Anterior   Posterior

Fig. 3: MIBG showing an increased tracer uptake in the right suprarenal region (shown with arrow).

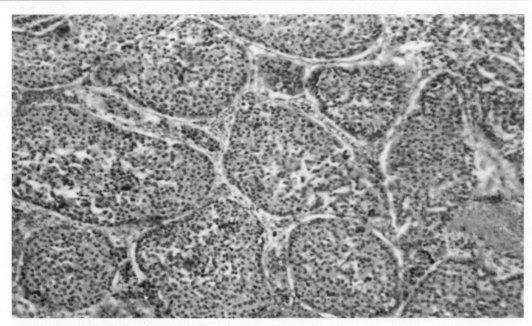

Fig. 4: Histopathology showing Zellballen appearance from the right suprarenal mass.

chromocytoma has been termed "the great masquerade" due to its variable presentation. About 5% of the adrenal incidentalomas are proved to be pheochromocytomas. Both CT and MRI are similar in sensitivity in detecting pheochromocytomas and CT with contrast should be the initial diagnostic mode of choice.[2] Pheochromocytomas can be localised by using radioactive tracers like I 131 or I 123-meta iodo benzyl guanidine (MIBG) due to the selective uptake by these tumors.

REFERENCES

1. Messerli FH, Michalewicz L. Clinical and experimental pheochromocytoma. JAMA. 1997;2;278(1):78–9.
2. Chen H, Sippel RS, Pacak K. The NANETS Consensus Guideline for the Diagnosis and Management of Neuroendocrine Tumors: Pheochromocytoma, Paraganglioma & Medullary Thyroid Cancer. Pancreas. 2010;39(6): 775-83.

CASE 10

A 29-year-old lady presented with history of low back pain for more than 6 months' duration with radiation to both the lower limbs. A computed tomography (CT) scan of the lower back showed an irregular lytic lesion involving the first and second segments of the sacrum (Figs. 1A and B). She was found to be hypertensive for which she underwent a surgery of the abdomen. After her referral to the endocrinology department, I 131 meta iodo benzyl guanidine (MIBG) scintigraphy was performed—the 72-hour post-MIBG images are shown in Figure 2.

WHAT IS THE DIAGNOSIS?

An initial differential diagnosis of a giant-cell tumor or a metastasis from an unknown primary tumor was considered, however the biopsy finding from the lumbar spinal mass showed features suggestive of pheochromocytoma (Fig. 3). The patient had surgery to treat an extra-adrenal pheochromocytoma (located in the organ of Zuckerkandl at the bifurcation of the aorta) before 12 years, when she presented with hypertension and a palpable abdominal mass. She was under regular follow up only for the first 3 years postoperatively. She had been asymptomatic and normotensive over the next 9 years until the present episode of lower back pain occured. She was treated with an ablative dose of 105 mCi of I 131 MIBG followed by external beam radiotherapy for local pain and α-adrenergic receptor blockade.

DISCUSSION

Paragangliomas are found where there is chromaffin-tissue, along the paraaortic sympathetic chain, within the organ of Zuckerkandl (at the origin Inferior Mesenteric Artery), in the wall of urinary bladder and along the sympathetic chains of the neck or mediastinum. Familial paragangliomas are caused by *SDHB* mutations. Malignancy occurs in 2.6–26% of individuals with pheochromocytomas. Paragangliomas of the retroperitoneum have a much higher reported rate of malignancy. The common sites of metastasis are bone, liver, and lungs.[1] Malignant Pheochromocytomas may recur early or late in the clinical course of the illness, the latest reported occurrence is more than 20 years after initial surgery.[2] Therapy for malignant pheochromocytoma and paraganglioma includes local excision, I 131 MIBG, and external beam radiotherapy. In patients with rapidly progressing malignancy, chemotherapy should be used as a first line of treatment.

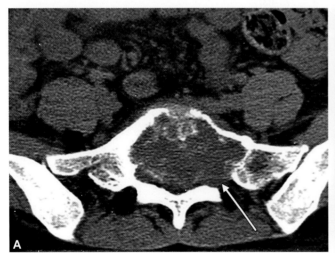
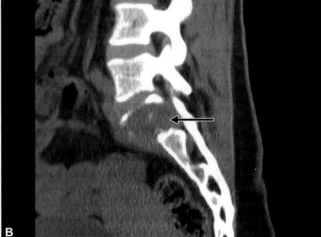

Figs. 1A and B: CT scan showing destruction of the neural foramina and involvement of the pedicle of the L5 vertebra (shown with arrow).

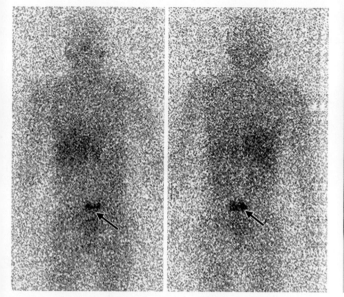

Fig. 2: MIBG scintigraphy showing an intense uptake in the same region as the lytic lesion seen in computed tomography (shown with arrow).

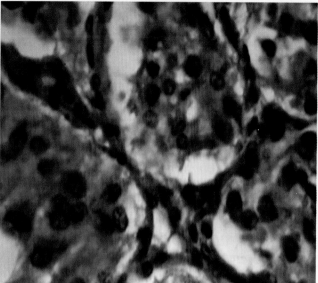

Fig. 3: Histopathology specimen showing high power view of the zellballen appearance from the tumor site.

REFERENCES

1. Fishbein L, Nathanson KL. Pheochromocytoma and Paraganglioma: Understanding the Complexities of the Genetic Background. Cancer Genet. 2012;205(1-2):1–11.

2. Baez JC, Jagannathan JP, Krajewski K, et al. Pheochromocytoma and paraganglioma: imaging characteristics. Cancer Imaging. 2012;7;12(1):153–62.

CASE 11

A 51-year-old gentleman presented with intermittent abdominal pain, paroxysms of headache, palpitations and sweating for 2 months. On examination he had features of marfanoid habitus and elevated blood pressure. His neck examination revealed a diffuse goitre. He underwent a computed tomography (CT) abdomen as a part of the evaluation of his abdominal pain (Figs. 1A and B).

WHAT IS THE DIAGNOSIS?

Computed tomography (CT) Abdomen showed a well defined heterogeneously enhancing lesion arising from the right adrenal gland. His 24-hour urine metanephrine and normetanephrine levels were elevated. A MIBG scan showed an increase in uptake by the adrenal tumor in the right adrenal region (Figs. 2A and B).

On evaluation for a syndromic association of pheochromocytoma, the patient had a palpable thyroid nodule with elevated calcitonin level. Subsequently he underwent. Fine needle aspiration cytology (FNAC) of the thyroid nodule and cytological report of which was suggestive of medullary carcinoma of thyroid. Hence, this patient was diagnosed to have MEN-2B where pheochromocytoma with medullary carcinoma of thyroid, marfanoid habitus and mucosal neuroma all coincide. Patient was started on alpha blocking agents followed by beta adrenergic blockage and planned for both right adrenalectomy and thyroidectomy.

DISCUSSION

Multiple endocrine neoplasia type 2B is an autosomal dominant disorder caused by mutations in RET (Re-arranged during Transfection) proto-oncogene, which encodes for a tyrosine kinase. MEN type 2B represents 5% of all MEN 2 cases. It includes Medullary thyroid cancer, pheochromocytoma (usually bilateral), mucosal neuromas, marfanoid habitus, thickened corneal nerve and intestinal ganglioneuromas. Mucosal neuromas and marfanoid habitus are the most distinctive features and are recognisable in childhood. Medullary thyroid cancer is seen in all patients with MEN 2 but pheochromocytoma occurs in only about 50% of these patients. Prophylactic thyroidectomy has been performed in many carriers of RET mutations and pheochromocytoma should be excluded before considering the surgery in patients with medullary carcinoma thyroid. Family education is important in the management of MEN 2. Death from medullary carcinoma of the thyroid can be prevented by early thyroidectomy. The identification of the RET (Re-arranged during Transfection) protooncogene mutations and with the application

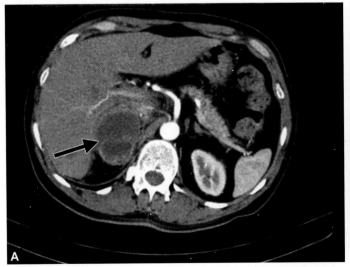 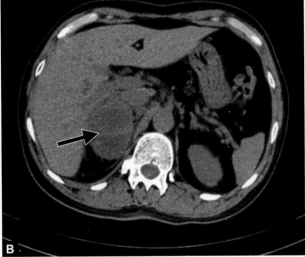

Figs. 1A and B: CT Abdomen showing a heterogeneous mass in the right suprarenal region (shown with arrow).

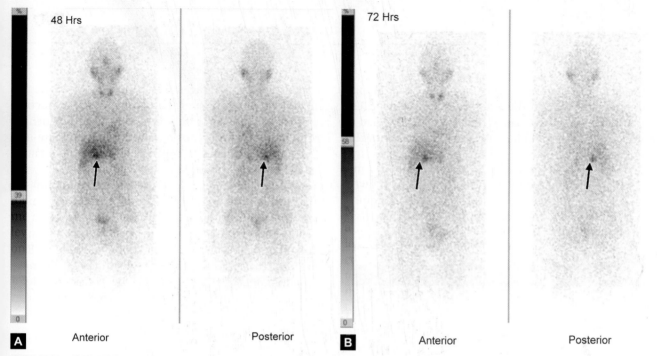

Figs. 2A and B: MIBG at (A) 48 hours and (B) 72 hours showing an increased tracer uptake in the right suprarenal area (shown with arrow).

of DNA based molecular diagnostic techniques has simplified the screening process.[1] The RET proto-oncogene analysis can be performed in patients with suspected MEN 2B to detect codon 883, 918, 923 mutations.[2] Annual screening for pheochromocytomas in patients with germline RET mutation should be performed by measuring 24-hour urine catecholamines and metanephrines.

REFERENCES

1. Finny P, Jacob JJ, Thomas N, et al. Medullary thyroid carcinoma: a 20-year experience from a centre in South India. ANZ J Surg. 2007;77(3):130–4.
2. Mahesh D, Nehru A, Seshadri M, et al. RET mutations in a large Indian family with medullary thyroid carcinoma. Indian J Endocrinol Metab. 2014;18(4):516

CASE 12

A 28-year-old lady presented with headache, palpitations and abdominal pain to the emergency department. On examination she was anxious, diaphoretic. She had a Pulse rate 180/min with Blood pressure: 240/160 mm Hg. Her physical examination revealed a Scar from old thyroid surgery (at age 8- probable total thyroidectomy) and mucosal neuroma of the tongue (Fig. 1). Fundus showed Grade III hypertensive changes. Computed tomography (CT) image showed bilateral well defined adrenal mass with central necrosis (Fig. 2).

WHAT IS THE DIAGNOSIS?

Multiple endocrine neoplasia type 2B/Mucosal neuromata with endocrine tumors/Multiple endocrine neoplasia type 3 also known as Wagenmann Froboese syndrome is a genetic disease comprising of marfanoid habitus, mucosal neuromas, medullary carcinoma of thyroid, pheochromocytoma and craniosynostosis. Variations in the Re-arranged during Transfection (RET) proto-oncogene cause MEN 2B.[1]

DNA testing is now the preferred method of establishing a diagnosis of MEN 2B, and is thought to be almost 100% sensitive and specific. Approximately 95% of all individuals with the MEN 2B phenotype have a single point mutation in the tyrosine kinase domain of RET at codon 918 in exon 16, which substitutes a threonine for methionine.[2] MEN 2B should be considered in a patient with medullary carcinoma thyroid where it can be confirmed by simple serum calcitonin evaluation.

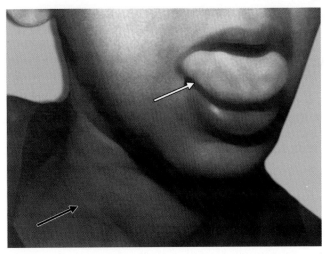

Fig. 1: Post thyroidectomy scar in the neck (shown with black arrow) and mucosal neuroma of the tongue (shown with white arrow).

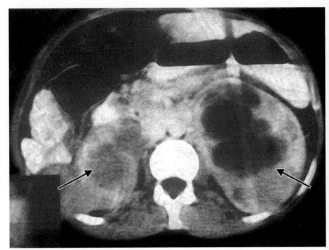

Fig. 2: CT image showing bilateral contrast enhancing adrenal masses with central necrosis (shown with the arrows).

REFERENCES

1. Mahesh DM, Nehru AG, Seshadri MS, et al. RET mutations in a large indian family with medullary thyroid carcinoma. Indian J Endocrinol Metab. 2014;18(4):516–20.

2. Pai R, Ebenazer A, Paul MJ, et al. Mutations seen among patients with pheochromocytoma and paraganglioma at a referral center from India. Horm Metab Res Horm stoffwechselforschung Horm Metab. 2014;30.

CASE 13

A 44-year-old gentleman presented with history of Grade 2 Hypertension for 2 years duration and a recent onset diabetes mellitus. He felt that he had become more nervous for the past one year. Historically, he had a history of fracture of his right neck of femur after a trivial fall.

WHAT IS THE DIAGNOSIS?

His fundoscopy revealed grade 4 hypertensive retinopathy with electrocardiography (ECG) showing left ventricular hypertrophy. His serum calcium level was high (11 mg%)

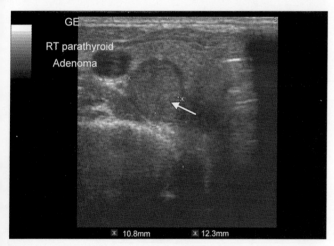

Fig. 1: Ultrasonography of the neck showing a right parathyroid adenoma (shown with arrow).

and phosphate was low with phosphaturia (TMPO4/GFR <1.5%). His parathormone levels were inappropriately high for the serum calcium level. The ultrasound neck and the Sestamibi-Parathyroid scintigraphy were concordant for a right inferior parathyroid adenoma (Figs. 1 and 2). A 24-hour urinary VMA —16 mg and 12 mg on 2 occasions (normal <7 mg/24 hrs) were found to be elevated. Subsequently the CT Abdomen revealed a 3.1 × 1.4 cm right adrenal mass and a 5 × 3.7 cm left adrenal mass. The functional imaging in the form of MIBG scan revealed uptake of both the adrenal glands (Fig. 3).

Initially he underwent bilateral adrenalectomy after adequate preoperative preparation. After one year, he was subjected to a right parathyroidectomy. Intra operatively he was found to have a bulky right lobe of thyroid and in view of the same, he had a right hemi thyroidectomy. The biopsy was reported to be a parathyroid adenoma with medullary thyroid carcinoma, following which he underwent a completion thyroidectomy with central neck dissection. So the final diagnosis was MEN 2A (Medullary thyroid carcinoma + parathyroid adenoma + pheochromocytoma). He was asymptomatic on subsequent follow-up visits. The Genetic analysis revealed a RET mutation in the codon 634 (Fig. 4).

DISCUSSION

Multiple endocrine neoplasia type 2 (MEN 2) is classified into three subtypes: MEN 2A, FMTC (familial medullary

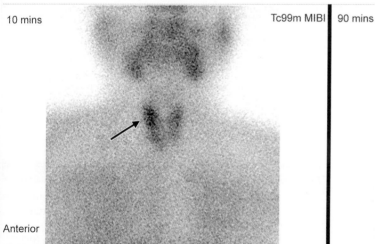

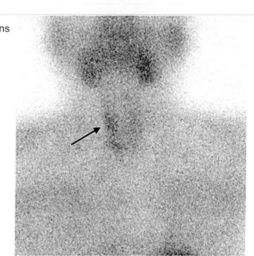

Fig. 2: Sestamibi scan showing an increased tracer uptake after 90 minutes in the right superior parathyroid region suggesting a parathyroid adenoma (shown with arrow).

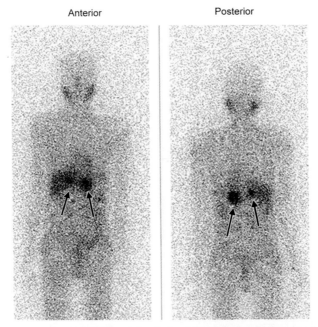

Fig. 3: MIBG scan at 72 hours showing an abnormal tracer uptakes in the right and left suprarenal region (shown with the arrows).

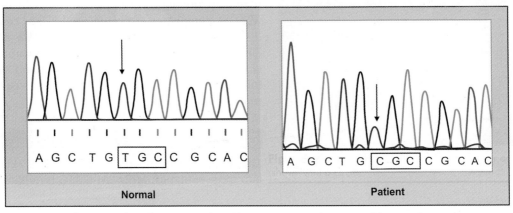

Fig. 4: RET mutation in codon 634, where thymine is replaced by cytosine on a phenogram (shown with arrow).

thyroid carcinoma), and MEN 2B. All the three subtypes involve high risk for development of medullary carcinoma of the thyroid (MTC); MEN 2A and MEN 2B have an increased risk for pheochromocytoma; MEN 2A has an increased risk for parathyroid adenoma or hyperplasia. The mucosal neuromas of the lips and tongue, distinctive facies with enlarged lips, ganglioneuromatosis of the gastrointestinal tract, and an asthenic "marfanoid" body habitus are the additional features in MEN 2B. MTC typically occurs in early childhood in MEN 2B, early adulthood in MEN 2A, and middle age in FMTC.

Re-arranged during Transfection (RET) is the only gene in which mutations are known to cause MEN type 2. Molecular genetic testing of RET identifies disease-causing mutations in 98% of individuals with MEN 2A, more than 98% of individuals with MEN 2B, and in about 95% of families with FMTC. The major disease-causing mutations are non-conservative substitutions located in one of six cysteine codons 609, 611, 618, and 620 in exon 10 and codons 630 and 634 in exon 11.[1,2]

REFERENCES

1. Mahesh DM, Nehru AG, Seshadri MS, et al. RET mutations in a large Indian family with medullary thyroid carcinoma. Indian J Endocrinol Metab. 2014;18(4):516–20.
2. Takahashi M, Asai N, Iwashita T, et al. Molecular mechanisms of development of multiple endocrine neoplasia 2 by RET mutations. J Intern Med.1998;243:509–13.

CASE **14**

A 27-year-old male presented with right loin pain and two episodes of painless hematuria. On examination he was found to have hypertension and a palpable mass in the right lumbar region. Computed tomographic scans of the abdomen were performed to evaluate the mass

(Figs. 1 and 2). His magnetic resonance imaging (MRI) Brain showed a contrast enhancing lesion in the cerebellum.

WHAT IS THE DIAGNOSIS?

This patient had high levels of urinary catecholamine products. In view of the right pheochromocytoma, bilateral renal masses, pancreatic cysts and cerebellar hemangioblastoma, this patient was diagnosed to have a fully expressed index case of V*on Hippel-Lindau (VHL) disease.*

DISCUSSION

Von Hippel-Lindau (VHL) disease is an autosomal dominant neoplastic syndrome caused by a germline mutation in the *VHL* gene. These mutations lead to the development of several benign or malignant tumors, and cysts in many organ systems.[1] The susceptible organs are the adrenals, kidneys, pancreas, central nervous system (CNS), retina, and reproductive adnexal organs. Von Hippel-Lindau disease is not very rare and has very high penetrance of around 90% by 65 years of age.

Fig. 1: CT abdomen showing a mass in the region of the right adrenal gland (shown with black arrow), with multiple renal cysts/masses (shown with white arrow).

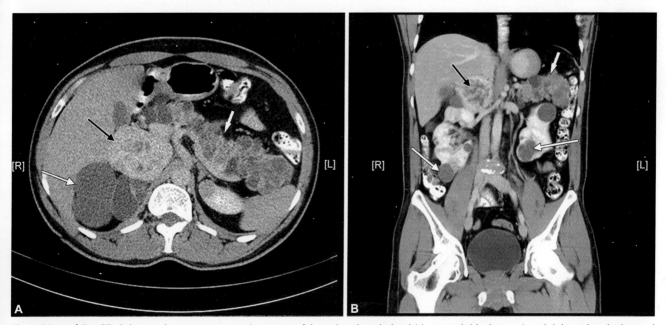

Figs. 2A and B: CT abdomen showing a mass in the region of the right adrenal gland (shown with black arrow), with bilateral multiple renal cysts/masses (shown with white arrow) and multiple cysts in the pancreas (shown with broad white arrow).

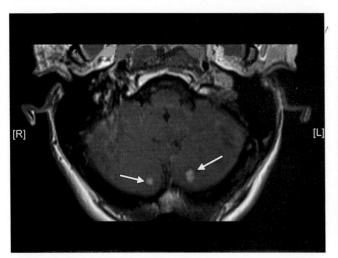

Fig. 3: MRI Post-gadolinium showing cerebellar hemangiomas (shown with the arrows).

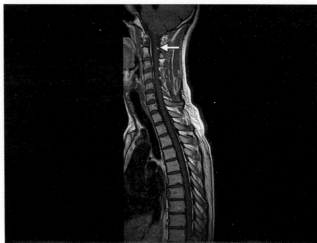

Fig. 4 MRI spine showing a hemangioma at the C2 vertebra level (shown with arrow).

The diagnosis of VHL disease is mainly based on the clinical criteria.

The common tumors found in the CNS are cerebellar, spinal cord, brainstem, nerve root and supratentorial hemangioblastomas, as well as retinal hemangioblastomas (Figs. 3 and 4). Specific presentation patterns have emerged, which have helped with the screening and counseling of individuals. Type 1 patients rarely have pheochromocytomas but can develop all other tumor types. Type 2 patients are at high risk of developing pheochromocytomas (often bilateral) but are either at low risk for RCC (type 2A) or high risk for RCC (type 2B). Type 2C patients have familial pheochromocytoma alone, with no other tumors.[2] A multi-specialty approach is needed for the optimal assessment and treatment of these patients. Comprehensive serial screening of the family members and regular follow-up are essential for proper care.

REFERENCES

1. John AM, C GPD, Ebenazer A, et al. p.Arg82 Leu von Hippel-Lindau (*VHL*) Gene Mutation among Three Members of a Family with Familial Bilateral Pheochromocytoma in India: Molecular Analysis and In Silico Characterization. PLoS ONE. 2013;23;8(4):e61908.
2. Jacob JJ, Paul TV. A man with painless hematuria and hypertension. Hong Kong Med. 2007;13(2): 162–3.

CASE 15

A 7-year-old boy presented with progressive difficulty in walking, and drooling of saliva for the last 8 months. He was noticed to have progressive hyperpigmentation for the last 8 months (Fig. 1). He was aphasic for the past 2 months along with decreased memory. He had normal perinatal history with normal milestones. He was irritable with hyperpigmentation of the lips, fingers and toes. He had a generalized increase in tone with brisk deep tendon reflexes with bilateral Babinski signs being positive.

WHAT IS THE DIAGNOSIS?

His investigations revealed an elevated plasma adrenocorticotropic hormone (ACTH) level (971 pg/mL) with an 8 am Cortisol in the normal range. His post Synacthen stimulation test with 250 mcg did not reveal a positive response suggesting subclinical Addisons disease. His Serum lactic acid, ammonia and blood arylsulphatase were normal. His visual evoked potential (VEP) showed right optic nerve dysfunction. The MRI Brain is showed below (Figs. 2 and 3).

DISCUSSION

X-linked adrenoleukodystrophy (X-ALD) is the most common peroxisomal disorder. The disease is caused by mutations in the *ABCD1* gene that encodes the peroxisomal membrane protein ALDP which is involved in the transmembrane transport of very long-chain fatty acids (VLCFA-more than 22 carbons).[1] A defect in ALDP results in elevated levels of VLCFA in plasma and tissues. The clinical spectrum in males with X-ALD ranges from an isolated adrenocortical insufficiency and slowly progressive myelopathy to devastating cerebral demyelination. X-ALD is a metabolic disorder characterized by impaired peroxisomal beta-oxidation of VLCFA, which is reduced to about 30% of control levels.[1,2] Consequently, there is an accumulation of VLCFA in plasma and all tissues, including the white mater of the brain, the spinal cord and the adrenal cortex.

Adrenocortical insufficiency (or even an Addisonian crisis) can be the presenting symptom of X-ALD in boys and men, years or even decades before the onset of neurological symptoms. X-ALD is a frequent cause of Addison's disease in boys and adult males when the auto-antibodies are absent. It is therefore important to

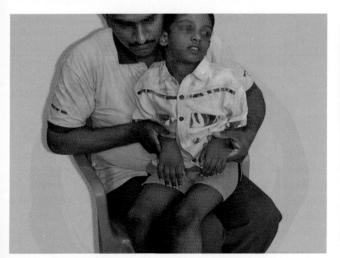

Fig. 1: Clinical image of the boy with hyperpigmentation.

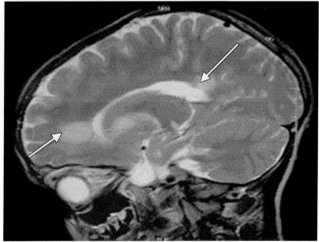

Fig. 2: AT 2 Weighted sagittal view of the MRI Brain showing areas of demyelination in the periventricular region, highlighted with arrow marks. Demyelination is also noted in the bilateral frontal white mater.

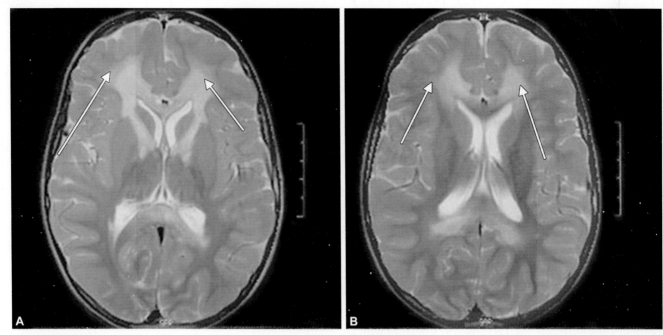

Figs. 3A and B: T2 Weighted MRI Brain showing areas of demyelination in the periventricular region and also in the bilateral frontal white mater (shown with the arrows).

consider X-ALD in any boy or adult male presenting with Addison's disease. Adrenocortical insufficiency initially affects the glucocorticoid axis later on involving the mineralocorticoid function. Allogeneic bone marrow transplant remains the only therapeutic intervention that can arrest the progression of cerebral demyelination. Certain dietary products like rapeseed oil or mustard seed oil that are rich in erucic acid (C22:1) can result in the lowering of carbon 26 levels.[2] Presently, prenatal testing to prevent unnecessary new cases of this devastating disease is available.

REFERENCES

1. Engelen M, van der Kooi AJ, Kemp S, et al.: X-linked adrenomyeloneuropathy due to a novel mis-sense mutation in the ABCD1 start codon presenting as demyelinatingneuropathy. J Peripher Nerv Syst. 2011,16:353–5.
2. Engelen M, Kemp S, de VisserM, et al.-The BT.X-linked adrenoleukodystrophy (X-ALD): clinical presentation and guidelines for diagnosis, follow-up and management. Orphanet J Rare Dis. 2012;13;7:51.

CASE 16

A 44-year-old lady presented with acute onset left sided abdominal pain associated with nausea, vomiting palpitation and high BP (180/100 mm Hg). She had repeated episodes with similar attacks during her hospital stay over two days with hypotension. All her investigations were within normal limits except for high activated partial thromboplastin time (APTT) levels (67.3 seconds). Her serum cortisol levels on admission were normal. However, in view of the vomiting and low serum sodium the serum cortisol was repeated which was suppressed with a blunted response to intravenous synacthen. Pre-synacthen ACTH level was 675 pg/dL (normal upto 46 pg/dL). She did not give a history of recurrent miscarriage. Computed tomography (CT) abdomen done on the first and the third day of admission are given in Figures 1 and 2.

WHAT IS THE DIAGNOSIS?

Further investigations revealed a high Anticardiolipin Antibodies—30 GPL Units (upto 25 GPL Units) with moderate lupus Anticoagulant, (LAC) being positive. The diagnosis was a bilateral adrenal Hemorrhagic infarct and the etiology was due to an autoimmune anti-phospholipid syndrome. The Hypoadrenalism was evidenced by biochemically low cortisol with a blunted response to ACTH stimulation with High plasma ACTH level and positive anti-lupus and anti-cardiolipin antibodies. Generally the markers of connective tissue disorders and procoagulant factor (protein-S, C) will be negative. The treatment includes Glucocorticoid and Mineralocorticoid replacement with Optimal anti-coagulant therapy to keep an INR (between) 2.5 to 3.5.

DISCUSSION

Overt Addison's disease is reported in only 0.4% of patients with ascertained APLA syndrome. Usually 80% of cases are due to autoimmune adrenalitis with infections due to tuberculosis and histoplasmosis accounting for about 15% of patients. Hypoadrenalism in APS is probably related to adrenal vein thrombosis and a consequent hemorrhagic infarction. The proposed mechanism is a rich arterial supply, but a limited venous drainage by a single vein. This transition from artery to the capillary system is so sharp that it forms a kind of functional vascular dam. Such patients should be advised long term steroid and fludrocortisone replacement with hydrocortisone injection protocol during the situations of stress.[1,2]

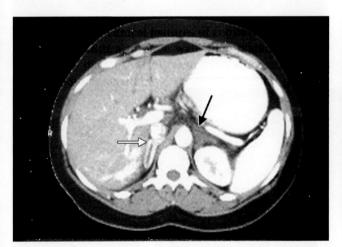

Fig. 1: Day 1 CT scan of the abdomen showing an enlarged left adrenal gland (shown with black arrow) and a normal sized right adrenal gland (shown with white arrow).

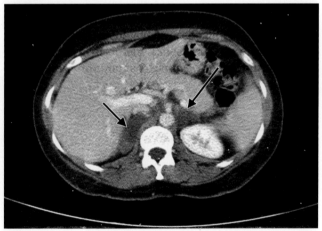

Fig. 2: A repeat CT abdomen on the third day showing bilateral enlarged adrenal glands (shown with the arrows).

REFERENCES

1. Presotto F, Fornasini F, Betterle C, et al. Acute adrenal failure as the heralding symptom of primary anti-phospholipid syndrome: Report of a case and review of the literature. Eur J Endocrinol. 2005;153:507–14.

2. Betterle C, Dal Pra C, Mantero F, et al. Autoimmune adrenal insufficiency and autoimmune polyendocrine syndromes: Autoantibodies, autoantigens, and their applicability in diagnosis and disease prediction. Endocr Rev. 2002;23: 327–64

CASE 17

A 28-year-old lady from Bangladesh presented with fever, polyarthritis and weight loss over 8 months. She gave birth to a child at home 15 days prior to the onset of symptoms with no perinatal complications. She also gave history of loss of appetite with weight loss of 25 kgs over 9 months. On examination she was emaciated with generalised lymphadenopathy, hepatosplenomegaly and polyarthritis involving both the large and small joints. She did not have an elevated blood pressure or features of myopathy, hirsutism or hyper pigmentation. She underwent sequential chest imaging (Figs. 1 to 5) which is shown below.

Her blood culture for bacteria, tuberculosis and fungal culture was negative. Beta-HCG and gynecological evaluation for gestational trophoblastic disease was negative. Her blood pressure levels are in the normal range with normal 24-hour urine metanephrines and normetanephrines values. Subsequently she underwent MIBG and DOTANAC scan to assess the uptake of the lesions (Fig. 5).

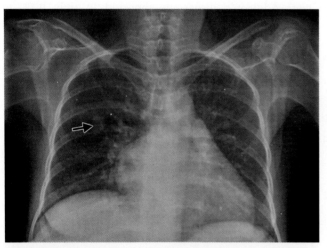

Fig. 1: Chest X-ray with a cannon ball lesion (shown with arrow).

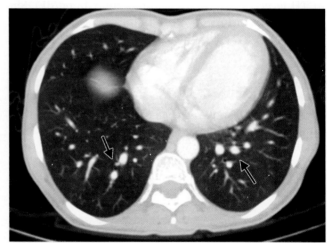

Fig. 2: CT thorax showing multiple nodular lesions (shown with the arrows).

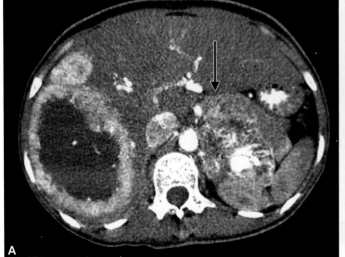

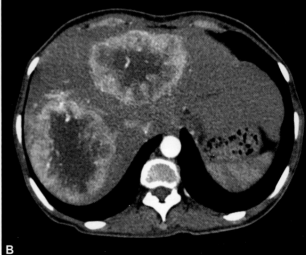

Figs. 3A and B: CT abdomen showing a large vascular lesion in the left adrenal gland (shown with arrow) and similar multiple lesions with central necrosis seen in both the lobes of liver.

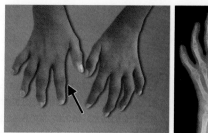
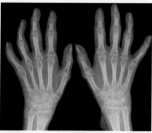

Fig. 4: Dactylitis (shown with arrow) and X-ray of the hand and wrist with periarticular osteopenia involving proximal and distal interphalengeal joints suggestive of arthritis.

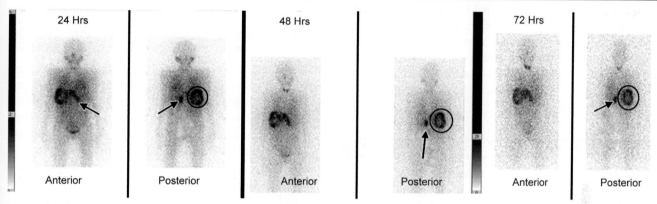

Fig. 5: MIBG scan at 24, 48 and 72 hours showing an abnormal tracer uptake in the left suprarenal region (shown with arrow) and a large area of circumferential tracer activity noted in the liver with central photopenia (shown with circle).

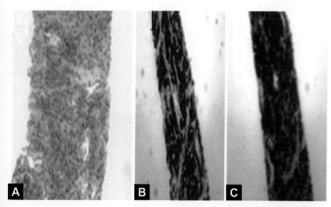

Figs. 6A to C: (A) Hematoxylin and Eosin x 200 showing a nested arrangement of tumor cells (zellballen appearance). Immuno histo-chemistry x 100 positive for (B) synaptophysin and (C) chromogranin.

Due to the highly vascular nature of the tumor, biopsy of the adrenal tumor was not done, instead a biopsy of the liver lesions was done and histopathology of it showed a well differentiated neuroendocrine tumor with chromogranin and synaptophysin positivity, which are markers of neuroendocrine tumor with MIB1 Index of 15–20% suggesting intermediate proliferation index (Figs. 6A to C). In view of multiple lung and liver metastases she was considered for a MIBG ablation and Octreotide injection therapy.

DISCUSSION

Paraneoplastic polyarthritis is a well-described entity, but it is seen in association with certain cancers, mainly adenocarcinoma, but is also seen in solid tumors like ovarian, lung, gastric, colon, breast, and laryngeal neoplasms. Paraneoplastic polyarthritis is predominantly a diagnosis of exclusion. Most of the etiologies of polyarthritis can be diagnosed based on the mode of presentation, patterns of articular involvement, associated systemic symptoms, radiological presentation, inflammatory markers, and auto-antibodies.[1] The pathogenesis of paraneoplastic polyarthritis has not been fully understood. However certain unknown circulating immune complexes and platelet activating factors have been postulated to cause sterile inflammatory response in the synovium leading to polyarthritis.[2]

REFERENCES

1. Zupancic M, Annamalai A, Brenneman J, Migratory Polyarthritis as a Paraneoplastic Syndrome. J Gen Intern Med. 2008;23(12):2136–9.
2. Shetty s, Hephzibah J, Borah B, et al. Paraneoplastic arthritis in association with metastatic neuroendocrine tumor of the addrenal gland. Australas med J. 2014;7(8): 345-9.

CASE **18**

ADRENOCORTICAL CARCINOMA

A 36-year-old lady presented with amenorrhea, hirsutism and acne on the face along with palpitations and head ache for 2 years. On examination she had cushingoid features along with virilisation (Figs. 1 and 2). There was mild clitoromegaly. Her Modified ferriman-gallwey score revealed a score of 16/36. She was also found to be hypertensive. Blood investigations showed increased serum cortisol, dehydroepiandrosterone sulfate (DHEAS) and testosterone with hypokalemia. Plasma ACTH was found to be suppressed. She had abdominal imaging done, which is displayed.

WHAT IS THE DIAGNOSIS?

On abdominal imaging there was a mass with heterogenous echotexture in the right adrenal gland. She was diagnosed to have having high blood glucose levels requiring insulin for glycemic control. Her blood pressure was controlled with increasing doses of spironolactone, prazosin, nebivolol and ramipril. Subsequently a whole body DOTATATE PET-CT was done (Figs. 3 and 4).

Whole body PET-CT showed metabolically active linear focus in right sacrum, with no corresponding lesion in CT scan. Differentials considered were Insufficiency fracture and metastasis and was planned to follow-up after the surgical management is over. After optimization of BP, she underwent right open adrenalectomy and biopsy of specimen was suggestive of Adrenocortical carcinoma with capsular and lymphovascular invasion with modified weiss score of 7 (Fig. 5).

DISCUSSION

Adrenocortical carcinoma is a rare malignancy with incidence of 1–2 cases per million population. Most commonly used histopathological classification in grading the tumors is the Weiss score which takes mitotic rate > 5/HPF as high nuclear grade, typical mitosis, < 25% clear cells, diffuse architecture and presence of necrosis, invasion of venous system, sinusoidal structures and capsule.[1] Surgical excision of the tumor is the treatment of choice. Adjuvant chemotherapy with mitotane should be considered in patients with high risk of recurrence as determined by the tumor size of > 8 cm, vascular and capsular invasion and Ki67 proliferation index ≥ 10%. Single metastases can be treated with surgery or radiofrequency ablation. Inoperable tumor can be treated with mitotane. Chemotherapy with the Berutti regimen (containing cisplatin, etoposide, doxorubicin and mitotane) should be considered if the

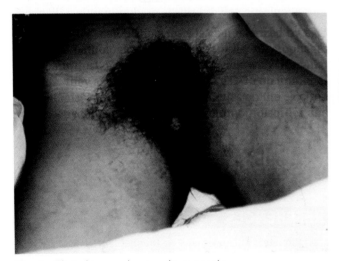

Fig. 1: Clinical image showing clitoromegaly.

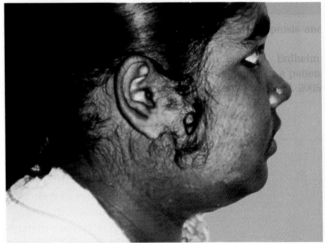

Fig. 2: Hirsutism.

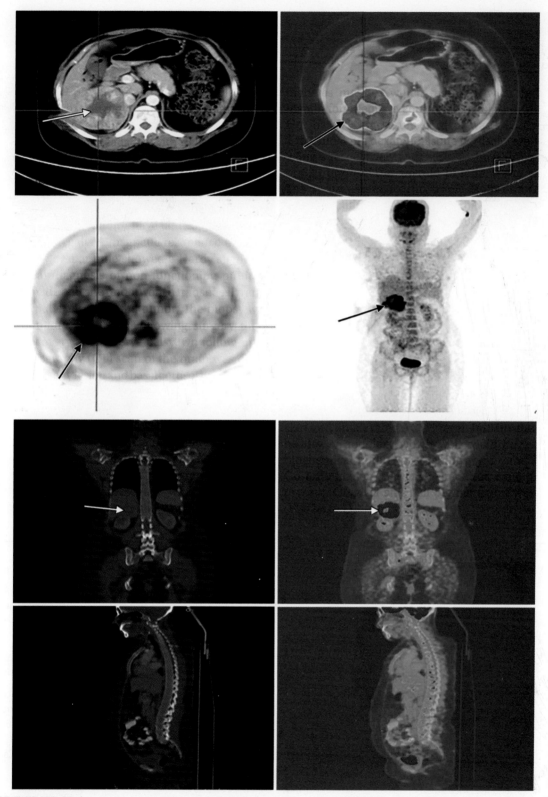

Fig. 3: DOTATATE PET CT showing an increased tracer uptake in the right suprarenal area (shown with arrow).

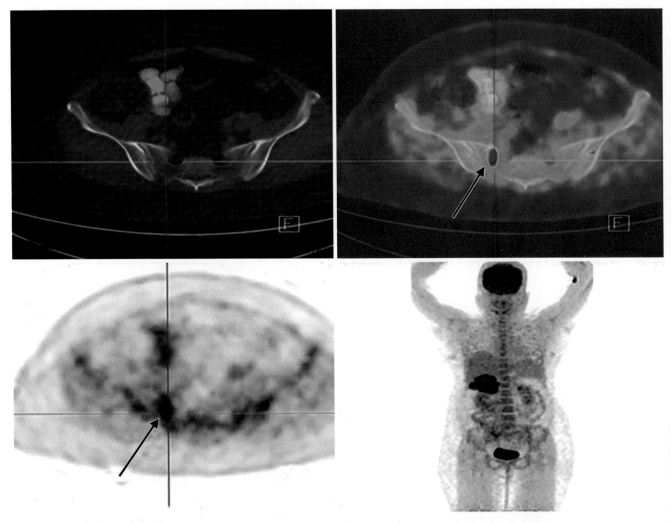

Fig. 4: DOTATATE PET CT showing an abnormal tracer uptake in the right sacral bone (shown with arrow).

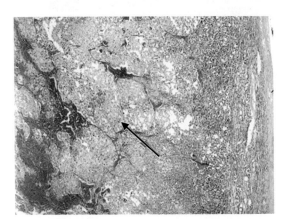

Fig. 5: Histopathological specimen with poorly cohesive cell clusters in necrotic background with vacuolated cytoplasm (shown with arrow).

tumor recurs or progresses during mitotane treatment.[2] The overall survival rate is 30–40%. Tumor suppressor gene *TP53* mutations are found in 25% of sporadic cases of adrenocorical carcinoma.

REFERENCES

1. Wang C, Sun Y, Wu H, et al. Distinguishing adrenal cortical carcinomas and adenomas: a study of clinicopathological features and biomarkers. Histopathology. 2014;64(4):567-76.
2. Fassnacht M, Terzolo M, Allolio B, et al. Combination Chemotherapy in Advanced Adrenocortical Carcinoma. N Engl J Med. 2012; 2;366 (23):2189-97.

CASE 19

A 28-year-old woman presented with a history of recurrent episodes of chest pain with profuse sweating and palpitations for 4 years, five such episodes occurred during micturition or soon after micturition. She also had an episode of hematuria. Her admission blood pressure was 140/90 mm Hg. After micturition her pulse rate increased to 120/min and the blood pressure increased to 160/110 mm Hg. A fundus examination revealed grade 2 hypertensive retinopathy changes.

WHAT IS THE DIAGNOSIS?

All her investigations were within normal limits except for the 24-hour urinary Vanillyl Mandelic Acid (VMA) levels which were elevated at 8 mg and 11 mg (normal <7 mg/24 hours). An ultrasound abdomen followed by MRI pelvis and MIBG scan were done. (Figs. 1 to 3).

A cystoscopy under general anesthesia revealed a 3 × 3 cm extra mucosal mass arising from the right lateral bladder wall, above the right ureteric orifice. She was adequately hydrated with oral fluids, oral salt and alpha blockade followed by beta blockade pre-operatively for a duration of 2 weeks. There was no fluctuation of blood pressure during surgery. Histopathology of the tumor confirmed the diagnosis of pheochromocytoma arising from the bladder wall (Figs. 4 and 5). On follow-up, her urinary metanephrine levels have normalized and she remained asymptomatic.

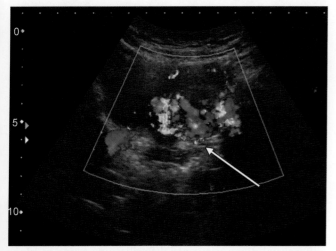

Fig. 1: Ultrasound Abdomen revealing an intravesical mass extending into the perivesical space (shown with arrow).

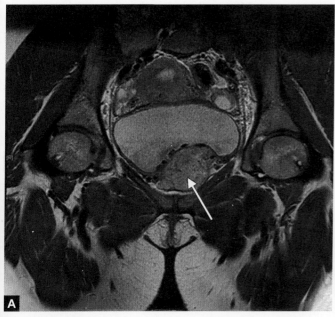

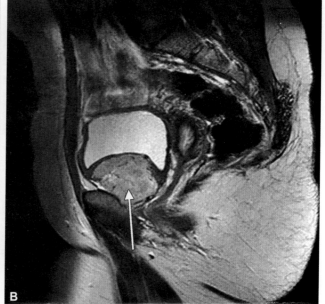

Figs. 2A and B: MRI pelvis with a 3 × 4 × 4 cm submucosal mass in the inferolateral wall of the urinary bladder (shown with arrow).

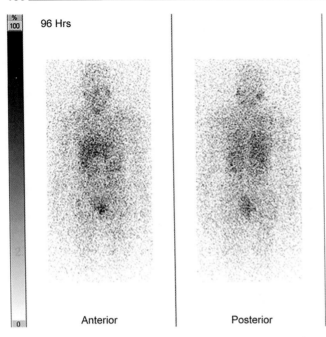

96 Hrs

Anterior   Posterior

Fig. 3: MIBG (Meta-Iodo-Benzyl-Guanidine) scan showing no abnormal tracer uptake even after 96 hours.

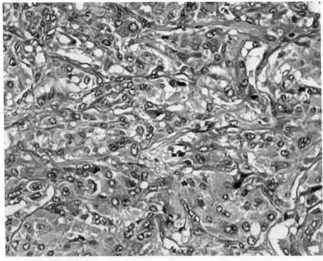

Fig. 4: Histopathological examination with typical 'zell-ballen' arrangement of tumor cells, separated by a delicate network of capillary sized blood vessels.

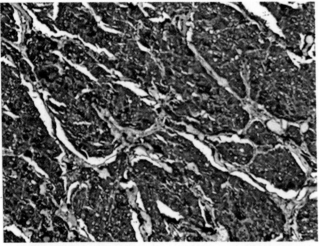

Fig. 5: Histopathological image with the tumor cells positive for Chromogranin A.

DISCUSSION

Pheochromocytoma of the urinary bladder is a rare tumor. Such tumors arise from the chromaffin tissues associated with sympathetic nerves located within the bladder wall. They are hormonally active and cause symptoms including palpitations, sweating, headache and hypertension (paroxysmal/sustained). The classical presentation is micturition syncope.[1] One of the important differential diagnosis is atrial fibrillation. A rise in blood pressure can be demonstrated immediately following micturition. The other uncommon precipitating factors include abdominal palpation, defecation and sexual intercourse. Most vesical pheochromocytomas are intramural as the sympathetic plexus is scattered between all the layers of the bladder wall. At cystoscopy these tumors may appear granulated and lobulated with or without ulceration.[2] Transurethral resection is not recommended as it will not remove the entire tumor. Open surgery is required to completely resect these tumors. Laparoscopic tumor resection has also been attempted.

REFERENCES

1. Rajaratnam S, Seshadri MS, Gopalakrishnan G, et al. Pheochromocytoma of the urinary bladder. J Assoc Physicians India 1999;Vol 47: 246-7.
2. Kapoor N, Seshadri M, Thomas N, et al. Pheochromocytomas of the vesical and paravesical region. BJUI [Internet]. 2012;8 [cited 2014 Nov 18].

CASE **20**

A 27-year-old male presented with history of palpitations, sweating, weight loss, periorbital headache and off and on vomiting for 1½ years. He was also found to have elevated blood pressure values requiring an ICU stay. He was started on antihypertensive agents. Clinically he did not have any features suggestive of adrenal hypersecretion. His biochemical reports were normal for urinary metanephrines/normetanephrines, DHEAS and workup for Cushings syndrome was negative. He subsequently underwent a contrast enhancing-CT abdomen, which showed a right side adrenal mass (Fig. 1).

WHAT IS THE DIAGNOSIS?

He underwent MIBG scan which showed normal physiological uptakes (Fig. 2). In the background of the clinical picture and investigation reports, he was suspected to have a pheochromocytoma most likely and was prepared for surgery with adequate α-blockade for more than 2 weeks followed by β-blockers. In view of his nature and size of the mass, and keeping in mind the history of hypertensive crisis in the past, he underwent right adrenalectomy.

Surgical specimen biopsy was consistent with right sided pheochromocytoma.

DISCUSSION

Certain patients can have both normal urinary catecholamine excretion and a normal MIBG scan. The normal catecholamine in the blood/urine may be due to necrosis of the tumor or dopamine secreting tumor. These are the most specific tests for the diagnosis of pheochromocytoma/paraganglioma. PETCT imaging is considered as the "gold standard" in localization of adrenal and extra adrenal pheochromocytomas.[1] MIBG has a functional imaging where in 15% can have a negative scan. Therefore in patients who are suspected to have a pheochromocytoma but have a negative MIBG scan should be subjected to FDG-PET scanning for localization of extra adrenal pheochromocytoma and metastasis.[2]

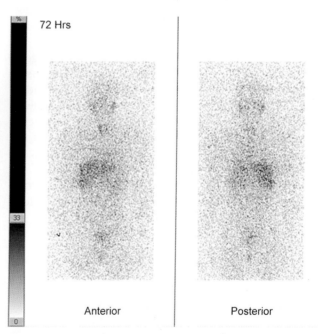

Fig. 2: MIBG with normal tracer uptakes in the liver, submandibular gland and urinary bladder.

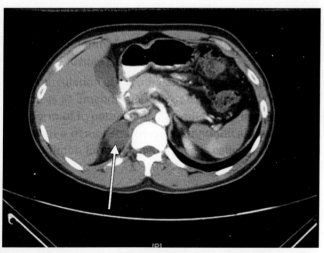

Fig. 1: CT abdomen showing a lesion in the right adrenal gland region which is same as that of the gall bladder density (shown with arrow).

REFERENCES

1. Chen H, Sippel RS, Pacak K. The NANETS Consensus Guideline for the Diagnosis and Management of Neuroendocrine Tumors: Pheochromocytoma, Paraganglioma& Medullary Thyroid Cancer. Pancreas. 2010;39(6):775–83.

2. Boedeker CC. Paragangliomas and paraganglioma syndromes. GMS Curr Top Otorhinolaryngol Head Neck Surg [Internet]. 2012;26 [cited 2014 Oct 26];10.

CASE **21**

A 31-year-old male presented with complaints of weakness and fatigue for 4 months associated with episodic vomiting, headache, palpitations, sweating and giddiness. On examination he had elevated blood pressure levels. He had no features suggestive of hyperpigmentation, easy bruisability or proximal muscle weakness. He had family history of his brother and sister with bilateral carotid body tumors. His 24-hour urinary catecholamine levels were elevated. Subsequently CT abdomen revealed a heterogenous mass in the right supra renal region (Fig. 1).

WHAT IS THE DIAGNOSIS?

He was initiated on alpha blocking agents and subsequently underwent open excision right adrenal pheochromocytoma and two paragangliomas in the organ of zuckerkandl region. The histopathology report was suggestive of pheochromocytoma. Postoperatively he was off alpha blocking agents and was alright for 10 days after which he started developing giddiness and palpitations for which he was evaluated and found to have no recurrence of pheochromocytomas.

His blood pressure normalised after the initial surgery. After 1 year of the surgery he had similar symptoms of paroxysms. For which he was re-evaluated and found to have elevated urinary metanephrine levels. A MRI showed a large well defined hyperintense gadolinium enhancing masses occupying the carotid space in both sides of the neck with long lesions and increased vascularity (Figs. 2A to F)

He later under went surgical excision of bilateral carotid body tumors at two different settings and histopathology report was suggestive of carotid body paraganglioma. He was evaluated for the presence of any mutations and was found to be positive for SDH-D mutation suggestive of Familial Pheochromocytoma.

He was asymptomatic for a duration of five months after which he had a recurrence of paroxysms. A DOTATATE PET CT showed a Functioning neuroendocrine tumor—bilaterally in the carotid space—and on the right side of the neck (Fig. 3).

Ultrasound neck showed a well defined hypoechoic vascular lesion in the posterior to inferior pole of right lobe of thyroid measuring 13 × 9.5 mm. A whole body "DOTATATE PET" study was done to rule out new lesions. His MIBG scan was negative for a functioning neuroendocrine tumor. One of the reasons for the negative uptake could be due to a "dopamine" secreting neuroendocrine tumor, however there is no hard evidence to back up this.

In view of the inoperable nature of the tumors in the neck and the fluctuating blood pressure, it was decided to proceed with radio nucleotide (Lutetium) based therapy.

DISCUSSION

The *paraganglioma syndromes* have been classified based on the genetic analysis of the families with history of head and neck paragangliomas. Subunits of the enzyme succinate dehydrogenase (SDH) an important component of Kreb's cycle is encoded by susceptible genes. The SDH enzyme complex is made up of several subunits (SDHA, SDHB, SDHC, SDHD, and SDH assembly factor 2) and is integral in linking the tricarboxylic acid (TCA) cycle to the process of oxidative phosphorylation within mitochondria. Specifically, SDHB is a known tumor

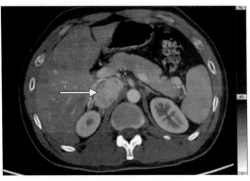
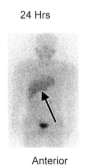
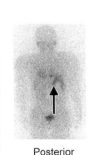
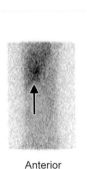
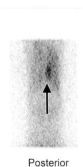

24 Hrs

Anterior   Posterior   Anterior   Posterior

Fig. 1: CT abdomen showing a right supra renal mass (shown with white arrow) with a concordant increased tracer uptake in the MIBG scan (shown with black arrow).

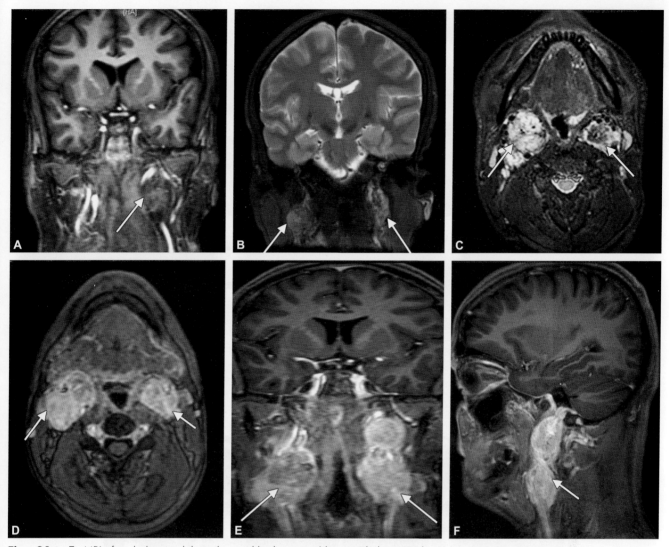

Figs. 2A to F: MRI of neck showing bilateral carotid body tumors (shown with the arrows).

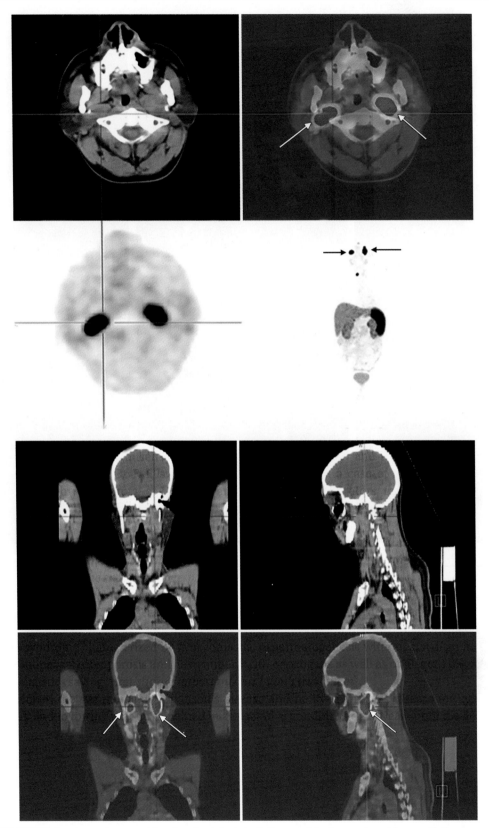

Fig. 3: DOTATATE PET CT showing an increased functional uptake in both the carotid artery regions (shown with the arrows).

suppressor gene which functions to prevent the accumulation of toxic metabolites during the TCA cycle.[1] Mutations of SDHA do not predispose to paraganglioma tumors instead cause Leigh's disease which is characterised by progressive loss of mental and movement abilities and results in death within a couple of years usually due to respiratory failure. Transmission of disease in carriers of SDHB, SDHC and SDHAF2 is by autosomal dominant but in SDHD involved families only the progeny of affected fathers develop the tumors if they inherit the mutation. PGL1 is the most common type of paraganglioma syndromes and about one third of the patients with PGL4

develop metastases.[2] Routine genetic counseling and testing are recommended in the family of patients with paraganglioma.

REFERENCES

1. Pai R, Manipadam MT, Singh P, et al. Usefulness of Succinate dehydrogenase B (SDHB) immunohistochemistry in guiding mutational screening among patients with pheochromocytoma-paraganglioma syndromes. APMIS 2014; 122(11):1130–5.
2. Kapoor N, Pai R, Ebenazer A, et al. Familial carotid body tumors in patients with SDHD mutations: a case series. Endocr Pract. 2012;18(5):e106–10.

MULTIPLE CHOICE QUESTIONS

1. A 27-year-old gentleman is brought with recurrent weakness of all four limbs. On examination his blood pressure was 190/130 mm Hg.
   A. Additional history and examination may reveal all *EXCEPT*:
   B. Grade 2 motor power
   C. Grade 3 hypertensive changes
   D. List of antihypertensive drugs being taken
   E. Mucocutaneous neuromas on the tongue

2. His laboratory evaluation showed serum sodium 144 meq/L (Normal 135–144 meq/L), serum potassium 2 meq/L (Normal 3.5–5 meq/L) and serum bicarbonate 30 meq/L. Further tests required in this patient include all *EXCEPT*:
   A. Tc 99m Renal scintigraphy
   B. Renal arterial doppler
   C. Plasma Aldosterone levels
   D. Plasma renin activity

3. Which imaging modality is required for this patient
   A. Ultrasound abdomen   B. PET scan
   C. CT scan   D. MIBG scan

4. A 19-year-old unmarried female presented with history of irregular cycle since 2 years and history of secondary amenorrhea for 2 months. She had no prior history of galactorroea or visual complains. She had history of intermittent intake of oral contraceptive pill for irregular cycle. On examination her BMI is 28.5 kg/m², FGS score of 12/36 but had no features of virilization. Hormonal investigations showed prolactin of 23 ng/mL (Normal < 20 ng/mL) and TSH – 2.3 µIU/mL. All of the following clinical condition can be associated with menstrual irregularities and hirsutism *EXPECT*:
   A. Polycystic ovarian syndrome
   B. Idiopathic hirsutism
   C. Hyperprolactinemia
   D. Nonclassical adrenal hyperplasia

5. Which of the following statement is *Not True* about hirsutism and amenorrhea.
   A. Prolactin and TSH should be performed in all patients
   B. CT adrenal and ovary indicated if DHEAS level is > 8 µg/mL
   C. Basal 17-hydroxyprogesterone in follicular-phase of < 2 ng/mL effectively rules out Non – classical CAH
   D. Hilus tumor of ovary is most frequent in 2nd to 3rd decades

6. Hirsutism during pregnancy seen in all *EXCEPT*:
   A. Fetal congenital adrenal hyperplasia
   B. Hyperreactio luteinalis
   C. Aromatase deficiency in fetus
   D. Luteoma of pregnancy

7. A 58-year-old lady presents with history of swelling of bilateral lower limb and abdomen in addition swelling, enlarged pulsatile neck veins since 3 months. She also complained of intermittent episodes of flushing since 2 years. There was no history of hypertension and diabetes 1. What is the most likely associated neuroendocrine tumor?
   A. ACTH secreting pituitarytumor
   B. Carcinoid tumor   C. Conns adenoma
   D. Acromegaly

8. Thirty-five days infant reared as a female child born of non-consanguineous marriage presented with vomiting since 10 days, loose motions and refusal of feeds since 2 days and anuria since 12 hours. She was a full term normal delivery without any antenatal or post-natal complications with a birth weight of 3.5 kg. She was exclusively breastfed and 3 of her elder siblings are normal. On examination, she was hypothermic and malnourished (Weight = 2.5 kg, < 5th centile), (Height = 53 cm, 25th centile)] with grade 3 dehydration. Her blood pressure was 60 mm of Hg (systolic). She had ambiguous genitalia in form of clitoromegaly with rugosity of fused labia majora and hyper-pigmentation of external genitalia. Bilateral testes were not palpable. Other systemic examination was normal. The most likely enzyme deficiency is:
   A. Lipoid adrenal hyperplasia
   B. 3 beta HSD – type 2 deficiency
   C. 21 – α hydroxylase deficiency
   D. 17 – α hydroxylase deficiency

9. Biochemical changes seen in the above said condition are all *EXCEPT*:
   A. Hypoglycemia   B. Hyponatremia
   C. Hyperkalemia   D. Raised plasma renin activity

10. Treatment and monitoring of this condition include all *EXCEPT*:
    A. Hydrocortisone at a dose is preferred in childhood at a dose of 10–15 mg/m² per day
    B. Fludrocortisone dose requirement per µg/m² increases in adolescence and adulthood
    C. In untreated nonclassical CAH final height not compromised without treatment
    E. Testicular adrenal rest tumor in male can regress with glucocorticoid suppression.

CHAPTER 4

Pituitary Passions

(Pituitary, Hypothalamus and Pineal Gland)

EIGHT — THE SYRACUSE HERALD: SUNDAY MORNING, AUGUST 18, 1918. — Magazine Section

New and Interesting Facts from Science and Life

Has SCIENCE at LAST LOCATED the SEAT of LOVE?

"PITUITARY BODY" Now SAID to RULE and DIRECT the AFFECTIONS

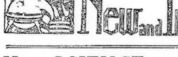

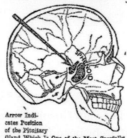

Arrow Indicates Position of the Pituitary Gland Which Is One of the Most Carefully Protected Organs of the Human Body.

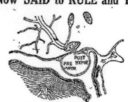

Detailed Sectional View of the Pituitary Gland and Its Surrounding Tissues.

An article on Pituitary Gland published in "THE SYRACUSE HERALD-NEW YORK" Magazine section on August 18th 1918.

HAROLD LEEMING SHEEHAN

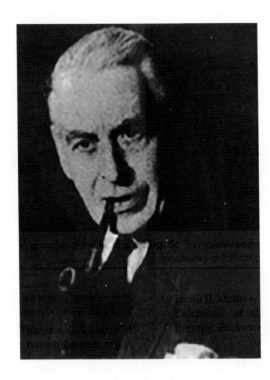

Professor **Harold Leeming Sheehan**, who was George Holt Chair, Professor of Pathology at Liverpool University from 1946 to 1965, was born in Carlisle in 1900. He graduated in Medicine from Manchester University in 1921 and several years later became demonstrator and subsequently was a lecturer in pathology at the same university. In 1935, he became the Director of Research at the Royal Maternity Hospital, Glasgow in 1935. In 1939 he joined the Territorial Army served in the Royal Army Medical Corps, thereby becoming the deputy director of pathology at the allied forces' headquartering Italy. He was elected to be the chair of pathology in Liverpool.

He built up a prestigious department, covering the pathological services for the local hospitals and gaining an international reputation for research in 1946. His first contribution was a description of chloroform causing liver damage that were used as an anesthetic agent in pregnant women, a condition that became known in France as "Maladie de Sheehan,". His highly important discovery was the postpartum haemorrhage (PPH)and necrosis of the pituitary and the clinical symptoms and signs of PPH. In Liverpool he wrote his classic paper on postpartum hypopituitarism, a condition now generally known as Sheehan's syndrome. At the age of 82, his last book, Postpartum Hypopituitarism, was written in collaboration with Dr JC Davis and was published in the year 1982.

CASE 1

A 32-year-old, lady presented with recurrent episodes of headache over a period of 6 months. She was not on any specific medication. The rest of her history was unremarkable.

On examination, she had bilateral papilledema. Visual field examination revealed an enlargement of the blind spot. Her height was 155 cm and she weighed 115 kg. A Computed Tomography (CT) scan of the brain was done and revealed no hydrocephalus. An area of the brain is demonstrated below on a CT scan (Fig. 1).

WHICH OF THE FOLLOWING IS TRUE?

1. She requires urgent transsphenoidal surgery.
2. Serum prolactin may be elevated.
3. An association with heavy smoking has been described in this condition.
4. The prevalence of this CT finding in the general population is around 1/1000.
5. Diabetes insipidus may complicate the natural history of this disorder.

The primary empty sella syndrome is a condition that is associated with the extension of the subarachnoid space through an incompetent diaphragmatocele into the sellaturcica in a patient who has not had previous pituitary surgery or radiation. In fact some radiologists believe that when it occurs in a partial form, it need not be reported as it is well within the realms of normal radiological anatomy.[1]

DISCUSSION

The incidence of the partial empty sella may be as high as 1–2% of the general population. However, the complete empty sella though often benign, needs to be viewed critically. It is associated with a greater frequency of pseudotumor cerebri (benign intracranial hypertension).[2] Pseudotumor cerebri may in fact be the cause of empty sella due to raised intracranial pressure. Both these conditions have a lot in common. They have a similar clinical profile in that there is an increased female predominance

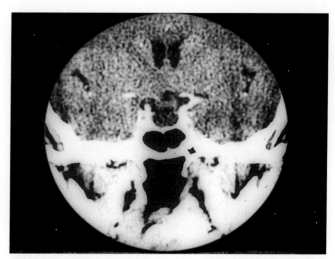

Fig. 1: Computed tomography (CT) scan of the brain.

(4:1), headache as a primary symptom of presentation (80%) and endocrine related symptoms (20%). Visual field defects are seen in a small but significant proportion of patients with the empty sella (16%). Hypopituitarism is often associated with the empty sella syndrome in those who have an enlarged sella turcica (4), the most common hormonal deficit being that of growth hormone followed by the gonadal axis and later on the vital pituitary-adrenal axis and culminating with the pituitary-thyroid axis.

Subjects who are detected with the complete empty sella syndrome should therefore have their visual fields screened along with a hormonal profile. Hyperprolactinemia due to stalk compression may be seen in a significant number. Follow-up on an annual basis is also necessary since a proportion of patients may develop further herniation of the optic chasm into the sella leading to worsening of vision.[1,2]

REFERENCES

1. Elster AD. Modern imaging of the pituitary. Radiology. 1993;187(1):1-14.
2. Foley KM, Posner JB. Does pseudotumorcerebri cause the empty sella syndrome? Neurology. 1975;25(6):565-9.

CASE 2

A 54-year-old lady, a mother of 5 children, was admitted with history of weight loss over past 1.5 years. She was apparently well 2 years before when she was bitten by a snake of an unidentified species. She did not seek medical attention then but a few days later she was admitted with history of vomiting and giddiness, elsewhere. She also had edema of legs at the time of presentation. She was diagnosed to have hypothyroidism and hyponatremia, initially. She gives a history of vomiting and giddiness on and off. On examination, her blood pressure was 150/90 mm Hg in the supine position and 128/80 mm Hg on standing. Rest of her vital signs were normal. The thyroid gland was not palpable. Her skin was dry and thin. Systemic examination was grossly normal.

Her investigations revealed Thyroid-Stimulating Hormone (TSH) of 3 μIU/mL (0.3–4.5), free thyroxine -0.4 ng/dL (0.8–2) and Luteinizing Hormone (LH) 4.74 mIU/mL, Follicle-Stimulating Hormone (FSH) - 8.73 mIU/mL. Her serum Prolactin (HPRL) was 9.49 ng/mL and 8 am serum Cortisol of 1.07μg/mL (5–15).

An Magnetic Resonance Imaging (MRI) of pituitary was done and is shown below (Figs. 1A to F).

WHAT IS YOUR IMPRESSION?

This lady has significant postural fall in blood pressure with hyponatremia and an inappropriately low serum cortisol level suggestive of Adrenocorticotropic Hormone (ACTH) deficiency. Also she had low free thyroxine levels with simultaneously inappropriately low serum TSH level suggesting a central hypothyroidism. Even though she attained menopause 7 years before, her serum FSH was also inappropriately low for her postmenopausal status. So the combined biochemical evaluation showed features suggestive of panhypopituitarism. Subsequently the MRI pituitary revealed an empty sella, with rest of the brain being normal.

She was then started on parenteral glucocorticoids after which her serum sodium level normalized and was subsequently changed over to oral corticosteroids with oral thyroxine supplements. In patients with hypocortisolemia and hypothyroidism, the glucocortoids should be supplemented initially followed by oral thyroxine. The reason for the initial glucocorticoid therapy is to avoid a hypocortisolemic crisis as thyroxine increases the metabolic clearance rate

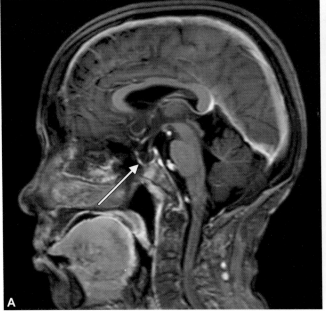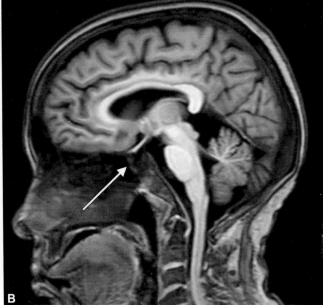

Figs. 1A and B

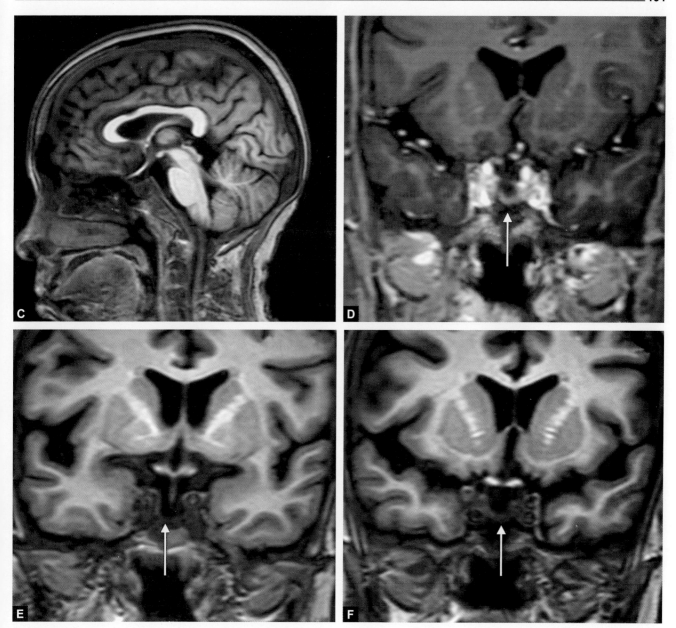

Figs. 1A to F: Magnetic resonance imaging (MRI) pituitary.

of cortisol. If thyroxine is started prior to the glucocorticoids there is a possibility of aggravation in hypocortisolemic symptoms.

DISCUSSION

A viper bite can release procoagulant molecules leading to a disseminated intravascular coagulation like state which may cause abnormal thrombosis and/or bleeding in diverse organs; this mechanism when acts in the pituitary may develop an acute or a chronic hypopituitarism or even diabetes insipidus.[1] An empty sella may be classified as primary when this occurs in people who have not received pituitary radiation or pituitary surgery, whereas an empty sella discovered following surgical procedures is classified as a secondary empty sella. In view of the increased intracranial pressure and traction over the optic chiasma caused by the post surgical adhesions, visual field defects are also known to occur and often require treatment. Cerebrospinal fluid (CSF) rhinorrhea can occur presenting as a non-traumatic and persistent nasal discharge. A long standing increase in the intrasellar pressure can also lead to pituitary dysfunction, which, if present needs to be corrected with appropriate hormone replacement therapy.[2]

REFERENCES

1. Uberoi HS, Achuthan AC, Kasthuri AS, et al. Hypopituitarism following snake bite. J Assoc Physicians India 1991; 39:579-80.
2. Garg M, Brar K, Pandit A, et al. Clinical spectrum of hypopituitarism in India: A single center experience. Indian J Endocrinol Metab. 2012;16(5):803.

CASE 3

Mrs S, is a 56-year-old lady, known to have hypothyroidism and has been on thyroxine for the same since the past 10 years. She was seen by many doctors and was continued on the same treatment which she had stopped prior to coming here. She was a postmenopausal lady for the past 2 years (Fig. 1). She had a past history of postpartum hemorrhage during her last child birth. She was then seen by a diligent physician who noticed a reduction in the axillary and pubic hair and asked for a Serum Cortisol (8 am) and Prolactin and ordered for a Magnetic Resonance Imaging (MRI) of the pituitary, in view of a probable Panhypopituitarism.

WHAT IS THE DIAGNOSIS?

On investigation, she was found to have a serum Prolactin (HPRL): 2.79 ng/mL, 8 am Serum Cortisol: 1.94 µg%, TSH: 0.018 µIU/mL with T4- Total Thyroxine – 2.5 µg/mL, FTc-0.56 ng/mL, FSH-4 mIU/ml. The investigations revealed an inappropriately low FSH for her postmenopausal status.

An MRI of the brain was done and revealed the following.

The MRI pituitary revealed an empty sella (shown with the arrows) with rest of the brain normal (Figs. 2A to E). She was diagnosed with an empty sella syndrome and panhypopituitarism due to Sheehan's syndrome. She was

then treated with replacement doses of thyroxine with initial parenteral corticosteroid therapy and later continued on oral corticosteroids.

DISCUSSION

Sheehan's syndrome occurs as a result of ischemic pituitary necrosis due to massive postpartum hemorrhage.

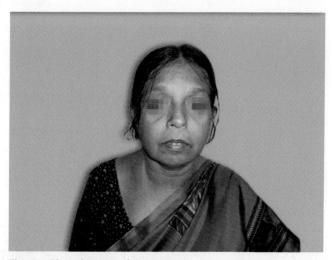

Fig. 1: Clinical picture of the patient.

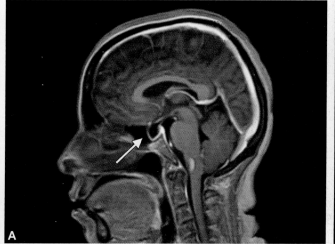

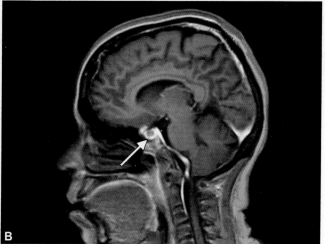

Figs. 2A and B

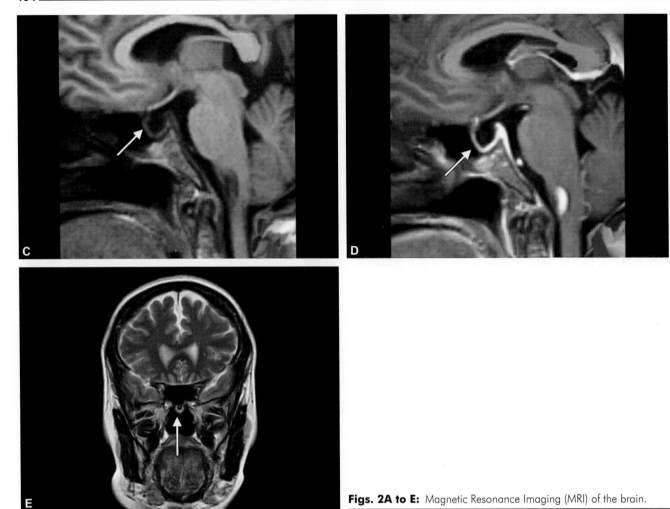

Figs. 2A to E: Magnetic Resonance Imaging (MRI) of the brain.

It may rarely be seen without massive bleeding or even after a normal delivery. With advances of obstetric care, Sheehan's syndrome has become uncommon except for certain developing countries.[1] The pathogenesis that have been suggested in Sheehan's' syndrome are a small sella size, disseminated intravascular coagulation and auto-immunity following a severe postpartum hemorrhage. These patients need to be taught about the hydrocortisone stress protocol to avoid a relative hypocorticolemic state during the stressful events.[2]

REFERENCES

1. Keleştimur F. Sheehan's syndrome. Pituitary. 2003;6(4):181–8.
2. Garg M, Brar K, PanditA, et al. Clinical spectrum of hypo-pituitarism in India: A single centre experience. Indian J Endocrinol Metab. 2012;16(5):803.

CASE 4

A 22-year-old student, Mr P suffered an extensive traumatic brain injury after a road traffic accident. He was admitted, investigated and underwent a left temporoparietal craniotomy and evacuation of subacute extradural hematoma and necrotized brain tissue. Subsequently, 2 years later he noticed a decrease in frequency of shaving and progressive weight gain. More, recently he was experiencing fatigue during the day. He occasionally had bouts of vomiting too.

WHAT IS THE DIAGNOSIS?

He was then evaluated here for rehabilitation and on investigation he was found to have hypothyroidism. On further evaluation he was found to have deficiency of all the anterior pituitary hormonal axes.

A repeat Magnetic Resonance Imaging (MRI) brain was done which revealed an empty sella (Fig. 1, shown with arrow).

From history and clinical evaluation he was thus diagnosed to have post-traumatic panhypopituitarism and was advised prednisolone, thyroxine and testosterone replacement.

DISCUSSION

Traumatic brain injury (TBI) is one of the main causes of death and disability in young adults. Post-traumatic hypopituitarism (PTHP) was thought to be a rare occurrence. However recent clinical evidence has demonstrated that TBI may frequently cause hypothalamic-pituitary dysfunction thereby hampering the recovery in a patient with TBI. The infundibular hypothalamic pituitary structure is particularly very fragile due to its peculiar anatomical and vascular structure. Cerebral damage due to TBI resulting from trauma can be classified into 2 types, primary which occurs during the insult and secondary which is at any point of time after the event. Similarly the pituitary dysfunction following a traumatic events can be classified as: (a) functional alterations during the acute phase post

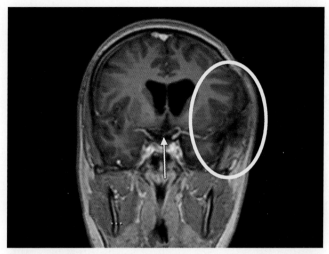

Fig. 1: Magnetic resonance image (MRI) of the brain showing severe traumatic brain injury (shown with a circle).

injury, which result in a temporary increase or decrease in blood pituitary hormone concentrations; (b) alterations in the pituitary hormonal secretion that may occur at any time after the initial insult resulting in a permanent hypopituitarism caused either at the pituitary and/or hypothalamic level. The pituitary gland responds to acute traumatic events with two types of secretory patterns: (1) Adrenocorticotropin (ACTH), prolactin (PRL) and growth hormone (GH) levels increase, (2) while luteinizing hormone (LH), follicle-stimulating hormone (FSH) and thyrotrophin (TSH) levels may either decrease or remain unchanged, associated with a decreased activity of their target organs.[1,2]

REFERENCES

1. Bondanelli M, Ambrosio MR, Zatelli MC, et al. Hypopituitarism after traumatic brain injury. Eur J Endocrinol. 2005;1;152(5):679–91.
2. Zheng P, He B, Tong W. Dynamic pituitary hormones change after traumatic brain injury. Neurol India. 2014;62(3):280.

CASE 5

A 28-year-old, lady presented with a history of oligomenorrhea for 6 years with (cycles once in 3–4 months) amenorrhoea for 1 year prior to the present event. She also complained of headache and vomiting over 2 days with left eye ptosis (Fig. 1). She was married for 4 years with primary infertility. Examination revealed normal genitalia with

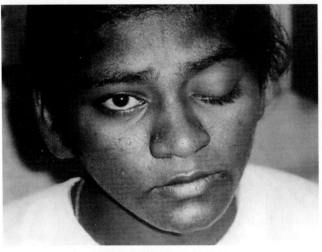

Fig. 1: Clinical picture of the patient.

no galactorrhea. Nervous system examination was normal except for a left third nerve palsy. The hormonal evaluation revealed the following: Follicle-Stimulating Hormone (FSH): 1.2 mIU/mL (4–12), Luteinizing Hormone (LH): 1.4 mIU/mL (4–12), Prolactin: 800 ng/mL (<25 ng/mL), FT4: 0.56, T4: 2.1, Thyroid Stimulating Hormone (TSH): 4.2 mIU/mL. Serum 8 am Cortisol: 25 mcg/dL. Magnetic Resonance Imaging (MRI) brain images are demonstrated in the Figures 2A and B.

WHAT IS THE DIAGNOSIS?

The patient was started on thyroxine 100 mcg/day and triiodothyronine 25 mcg three times a day. She also underwent transsphenoidal decompression of pituitary adenoma after three days of thyroxine and triiodothyronine therapy. The visual fields improved by 80% in a week and the left 3rd nerve palsy resolved in 4 weeks.

The histopathology is shown in the Figures 3A and B, where it revealed a hemorrhagic necrosis with no identification of the specific cell types of the pituitary with numerous red blood cells interspersed with in the tissue of a pituitary macroadenoma. Figure 4 shows the histopathology of pituitary adenoma without apoplexy for comparison.

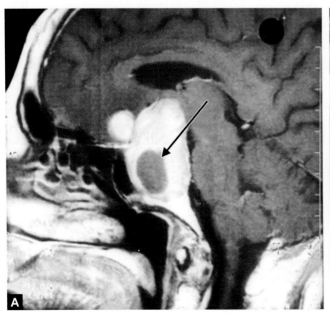

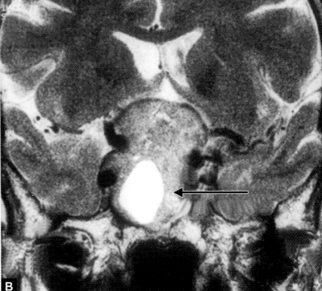

Figs. 2A and B: MRI of the pituitary showing a large suprasellar with apoplexy (shown with arrow).

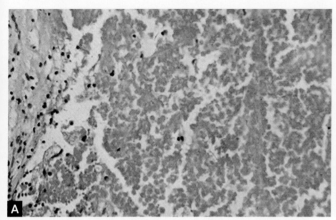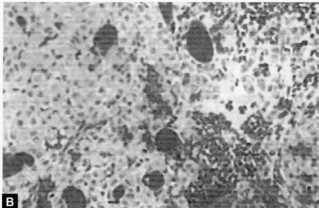

Figs. 3A and B: Pituitary adenoma with apoplexy.

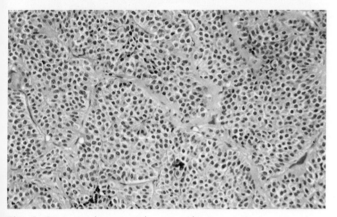

Fig. 4: Pituitary adenoma without apoplexy.

So this patient has had an episode of pituitary apoplexy that precipitated an acute episode of left third nerve palsy as evidenced by the ptosis. The diagnosis is that of a probable macroprolactinoma with an apoplexy.

DISCUSSION

The normal pituitary consists of a mixture of different cell types encased in a reticulin meshwork but the pituitary adenoma is characterized by a monomorphic expansion of one cell type with lack of reticulin network among neoplastic cells. The growth pattern can be diffuse, trabecular pseudoacinar or pseudopapillary.

Emergency surgery is indicated in this setting owing to the presence of progressive deterioration of visual fields.

Apoplexy can be a devastating complication in patients who have an underlying pituitary macroadenoma and can be sudden in onset.[1] Some of the complications that occur with apoplexy may be irreversible or fatal such as hypothalamic dysfunction due to suprasellar enlargement, third ventricular hemorrhage and hemiplegia due to compression of the middle cerebral or carotid arteries.

Hypopituitarism that occurs secondary to apoplexy has a greater likelihood of being permanent,[2] since the normal gland undergo ischemic necrosis in part and partly due to a high proportion of hypothalamic-releasing hormone deficiency. This adds on to the long term morbidity and mortality. Apoplexy may also be precipitated by numerous factors, like anticoagulants both oral and heparin, and with age and intercurrent illness where these agents are likely to be used increasingly. Apoplexy is liable to be induced by provocative testing with LHRH agonists in particular.

The differential diagnosis includes basilar artery occlusion, sub-arachnoid hemorrhage due to ruptured intracranial aneurysm, hypertensive encephalopathy, cavernous sinus thrombosis, intra-cerebral hematoma, encephalitis, retrobulbar neuritis, temporal arteritis, and ophthalmologic migraine.[1,2]

REFERENCES

1. Ranabir S, Baruah MP. Pituitary apoplexy.Indian J Endocrinol Metab. 2011;15(Suppl3):S188–96.
2. Rogg JM, Tung GA, Anderson G, et al. Pituitary Apoplexy: Early Detection with Diffusion-Weighted MR Imaging. Am J Neuroradiol. 2002;1;23(7):1240–5.

CASE 6

A 45-year-old man, with no known co-morbidities presented with history of acute onset, complete ptosis of right eye over 2 days (Fig. 1). He also had associated headache with the symptom of ptosis. There was no history of seizures, vomiting or loss of consciousness. An Magnetic Resonance Imaging (MRI) of the pituitary was done 2 months prior showed a pituitary macroadenoma (Fig. 2, shown with a circle).

WHAT IS THE DIAGNOSIS?

The repeat MRI of pituitary identified a pituitary macroadenoma with apoplexy (Fig. 3, shown with arrow). The hormonal evaluation showed hypocortisolemia and central

hypothyroidism for which he was replaced with prednisolone and thyroxine respectively. As he did not have visual compromise, he was kept under follow-up with hormonal replacement alone. After 6 months of the treatment his ptosis improved partially (Fig. 4).

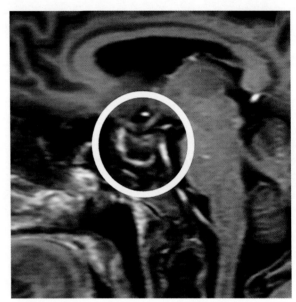

Fig. 2: MRI of pituitary done 2 months prior to the event.

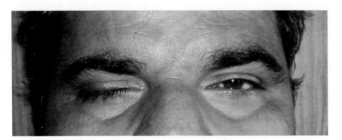

Fig. 1: Clinical picture of the patient with ptosis.

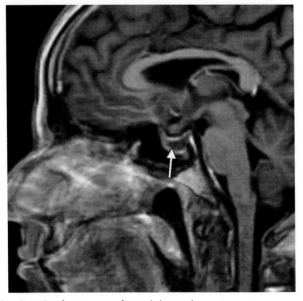

Fig. 3: MRI of pituitary performed during the acute event.

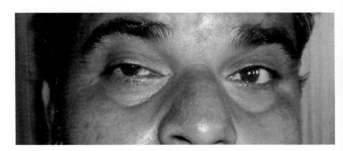

Fig. 4: Clinical picture of the patient after 6 months of the initial episode.

DISCUSSION

Percival Bailey was the first to describe a patient with pituitary apoplexy, resulting from a catastrophic hemorrhage of a pituitary adenoma in 1896. Pituitary apoplexy (PA) is heralded by an abrupt onset of severe headache, deterioration of visual acuity, restriction of the visual fields, disorders of ocular motility, and altered sensorium caused usually by hemorrhagic infarction of the tumor leading on to rapid enlargement of a pituitary adenoma. These symptoms are attributed to the rapid expansion of an infarcted and/or hemorrhagic pituitary adenoma which extends laterally into the cavernous sinus to compress the cranial nerves: III, IV, V, VI and may extend superiorly compressing the optic chiasm. The initial management of patients presenting with PA includes stabilization of the patient with hormonal replacement followed by surgical decompression, if necessary. Early surgical decompression must be considered in cases with severe visual impairment or cranial neuropathy.[1,2]

REFERENCES

1. Cho WJ, Joo SP, Kim TS, et al. Pituitary apoplexy presenting as isolated third cranial nerve palsy with ptosis : two case reports. J Korean Neurosurg Soc. 2009;45(2):118-21.
2. Kim SH, Lee KC, Kim SH. Cranial nerve palsies accompanying pituitary tumor. J Clin Neurosci. 2007;14(12): 1158-62.

CASE 7

A 24-year-old gentleman presented with holocranial headache for eight years, coarsening of the face and enlargement of the hands and feet for the past six years (Figs. 1A to C). He had undergone a microscopic transsphenoidal excision of a pituitary adenoma elsewhere, a year before presenting to us. His preoperative growth hormone level was more than 40 ng/mL and was 31.7 ng/mL postoperatively. He also had history of Diabetes mellitus since the past 2 years and on regular medications.

On examination, his vital signs were normal. He had enlarged hands, acral enlargement (Figs. 1A to C). Visual acuity and the visual fields were normal in both the eyes. Fundoscopy was normal.

Now, on investigating, the basal serum growth hormone (GH) was 21.8 ng/mL, 8 am Serum cortisol was 9.19 µg%. An Magnetic Resonance Imaging (MRI) pituitary with gadolinium was done (Shown in Figs. 2A to D).

WHAT IS THE DIAGNOSIS?

The MRI pituitary showed a small residual tumor in the right half of the sella measuring 17 × 10 × 7 mm with compression of the normal pituitary gland to the left side. The mass was encasing the right internal carotid artery. The mass was iso-intense on T1-weighted images and hyperintense on T2-weighted images.

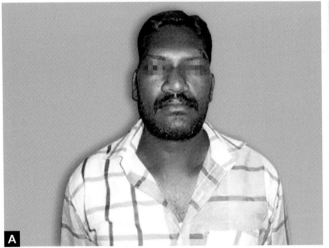

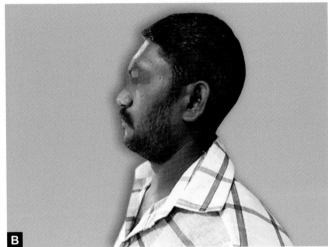

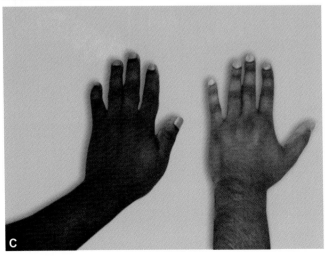

Figs. 1A to C: Clinical picture showing coarsening of the face, frontal bossing and acral enlargement on comparing a normal hand on the right side.

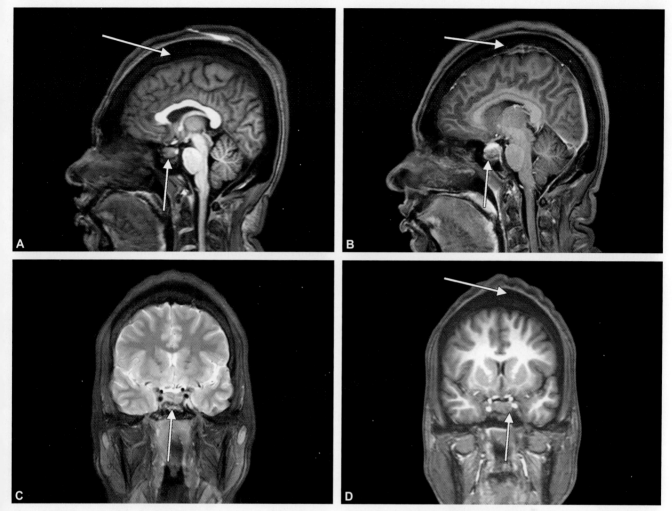

Figs. 2A to D: MRI of the brain showing pneumosinus dilatans and a pituitary macroadenoma (shown with the arrows).

He was diagnosed to have acromegaly due to a recurrent Hardy's Grade B residual growth hormone secreting pituitary macroadenoma.

The patient underwent a binostril endoscopic near total excision of residual pituitary adenoma. Postoperatively on the first day his random GH level was 5.56 ng/mL. On the 7th postoperative day, his 2-hour post glucose suppression GH level was 1.43 ng/mL. He was advised to come after 3 months for reassessment and was started on Cabergoline 0.5 mg twice weekly, since he could not afford for octreotide therapy.

DISCUSSION

Acromegaly is a clinical syndrome that results from excessive secretion of GH. The most common cause of acromegaly is a somatotroph (growth hormone-secreting) adenoma of the anterior pituitary.[1] These patients may present in the following ways: direct effects of tumor and effects of GH/IGF1 excess. The treatment of choice is almost always surgery. In patient who is in-operable or who are waiting for surgery shall be started on medical management or offer radiotherapy.[2]

REFERENCES

1. Katznelson L, Laws ER, Melmed S, et al. Acromegaly: An Endocrine Society Clinical Practice Guideline. J Clin Endocrinol Metab. 2014:30.
2. Neggers SJCMM, van der Lely AJ. Medical approach to pituitary tumors. Handb Clin Neurol. 2014;124:303–16.

CASE 8

A 54-year-old gentleman presented with chief complaints of progressive visual deterioration in the left eye, excessive height, and enlargement of the head, hands, feet, tongue and holocranial headache since the past 4 years. He had prognathism, frontal bossing and enlarged tongue (Figs. 1A to E). His visual acuity was 6/18 in the right eye and only perception of light in the left eye. He had bitemporal hemianopia. Fundus examination demonstrated optic atrophy in the left eye. He was operated for the same problem, 2 years before and was referred for further management.

His investigations revealed a Growth Hormone (GH): 326 ng/mL, Insulin like growth factor-1 (IgF-1): 1212 ng/mL,

Thyroid-Stimulating Hormone (TSH): 0.747 mU/L, Luteinzing Hormone (LH): 0.399 mIU/mL, Follicle-Stimulating Hormone (FSH): 1.01 mIU/mL, Testosterone: 31.0 ng/dL, Prolactin (HPRL) 184.91 ng/mL. An Magnetic Resonance Imaging (MRI) pituitary was done and the images are shown in Figures 2A to F.

WHAT IS THE DIAGNOSIS?

The preoperative images prior to the first surgery were not available for comparison. The clinical and the biochemical features were suggestive of Acromegaly due to a GH secreting pituitary macroadenoma residual/recurrent

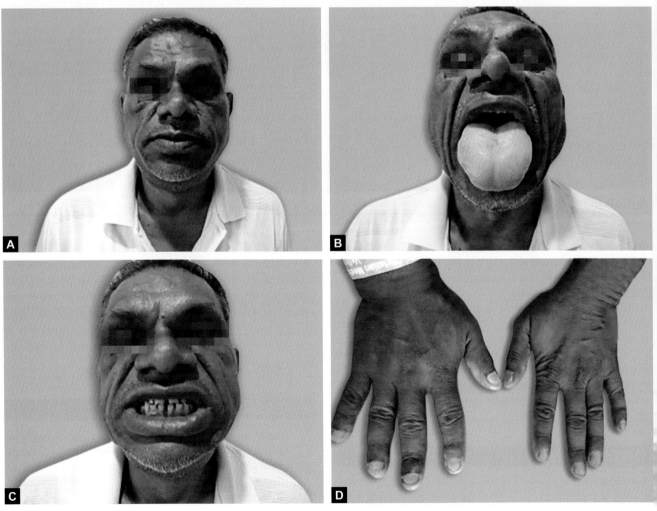

Figs. 1A to D

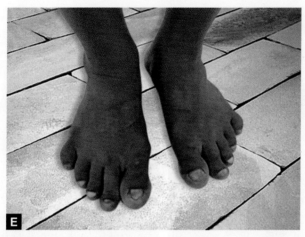

Figs. 1A to E: Clinical images showing coarsened facial features, an enlarged tongue, mal-occluded teeth, acral enlargement and large feet, respectively.

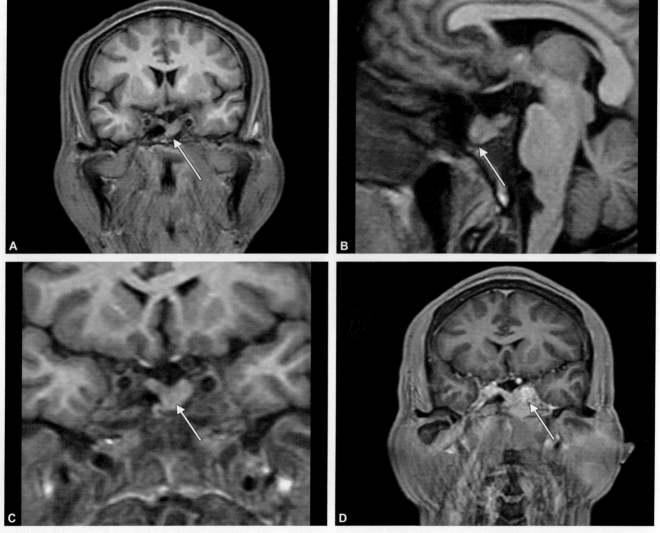

Figs. 2A to D

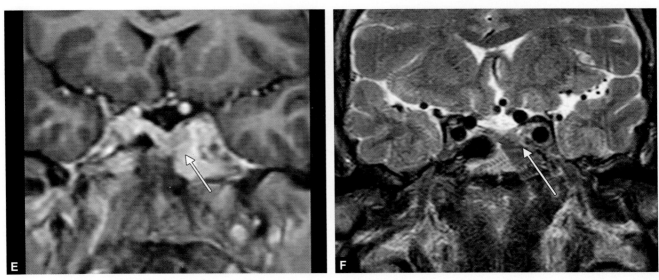

Figs. 2A to F: Preoperative MRI images showing a residual pituitary lesion, shown with arrow.

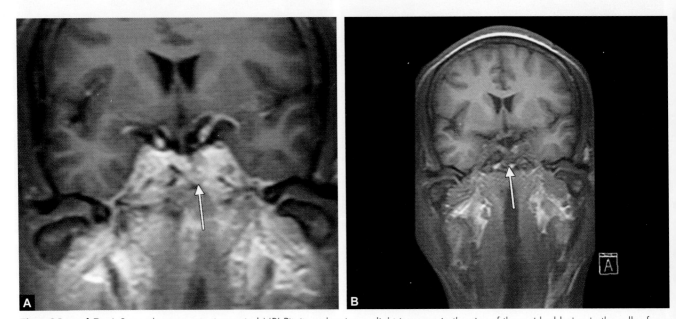

Figs. 3A and B: A 3 months postoperative period MRI Pituitary showing a slight increase in the size of the residual lesion in the sellar fossa (shown with arrow).

disease. He underwent a Transnasal transsphenoidal excision for the residual lesion. After one week postoperative period, his basal GH levels were still high (6.80 ng/mL). In view of the same he was started on cabergoline 1 mg twice weekly and advised to follow up after 3 months duration.

He was re-evaluated after 3 months and found to have high basal and post 1- and 2-hour glucose GH levels (5.66, 4.66 and 4.62 ng/mL respectively). He was also found to have high serum Insulin like growth factor(IGF-1) levels

(643 ng/mL). His repeat MRI pituitary showed a residual lesion (Figs. 3A and B). He was referred to the Department of Radiotherapy for stereotactic radiotherapy.

DISCUSSION

The symptoms of acromegaly are due to the increase in the growth hormone levels as well as an action of the insulin like growth factor-1 (IGF-1) levels.[1] In addition to the over growth of soft tissue and skin which can be clinically seen as an increase in the foot pad thickness, visceral enlargement, reversible prostatic enlargement is also common, even in men with hypogonadism. Thyroid enlargement may be diffuse or multinodular. Cardiovascular abnormalities include hypertension, left ventricular hypertrophy, and cardiomyopathy. Obstructive sleep apnoea may represent an additional risk factor for cardiovascular complications and excess mortality in patients with acromegaly. Overt diabetes mellitus is seen in up to 10–15 percent of cases and impaired glucose tolerance in a further 50 percent of patients with acromegaly. Colonic neoplasia and diverticulae are also commonly seen in acromegaly.[2]

Growth hormone (GH)-producing adenomas may respond to dopamine agonists, either alone or in combination with somatostatin analogs, although at lower response rates than in patients with prolactinomas. Response to cabergoline is better in acromegaly patients with mildly elevated insulin like growth factor 1 (IGF-1) levels and in those with prior radiation treatment. Pasireotide is a new somatostatin agonist with a high affinity for somatostatin receptors that may hold a promise in the treatment of acromegaly. Stereotactic radiosurgery and fractionated stereotactic radiation have both been shown to be effective in preventing the tumor growth after surgery and are typically well tolerated. Stereotactic radiosurgery is the most commonly used technique to deliver radiation to the pituitary tumors. Rates of biochemical response to radiation for growth hormone (GH)-producing adenomas and prolactinomas are probably near 90% and higher in 10 years time with radiation and medical therapy combined.[1,2]

REFERENCES

1. Neggers SJCMM, van der Lely AJ. Medical approach to pituitary tumors. Handb Clin Neurol. 2014;124:303–16.
2. Katznelson L, Laws ER, Melmed S, et al. Acromegaly: An Endocrine Society Clinical Practice Guideline. J Clin Endocrinol Metab.2014;30; jc20142700.

CASE 9

A 24-year-old gentleman presented with a history of progressive acral and foot enlargement since the age of 15-years with associated increase in the height over the same duration. He also had history of headache and difficulty in going through narrow pathways with associated vomiting and giddiness off and on. His height was 200 cm with an expected target height of 174+/10 cm. Magnetic resonance imaging (MRI) of the pituitary gland are shown below (Figs. 1A to D). His postoperative image is shown in Figure 2.

WHAT IS THE DIAGNOSIS?

This patient had clinical features suggestive of Gigantism. His MRI Pituitary showed a giant pituitary adenoma measuring 83 × 70 × 60 mm in the sellar region extending superiorly into the suprasellar region (shown with arrow) and into the middle cranial fossa. It was isointense on T1 and hyper intense on the T2-weighted image. The mass also encased the left Internal Carotid Artery (ICA) and proximal left Middle Cerebral Artery (MCA) and Anterior Cerebral Artery (ACA). The mass also had displaced the left temporal and frontal lobes (Figs. 1A to D). Furthermore it had also caused a midline shift of 17 mm. He had Human Growth Hormone (HGH) basal 150 ng/mL with IGF-1 levels of 1300 ng/mL. He did not have features of the syndromic cause for gigantism. He was found to have central hypothyroidism with hypocortisolemia for which he was started on prednisolone and thyroxine preoperatively.

He underwent a left fronto-temporal craniotomy and partial excision of the pituitary adenoma. The surgical specimen was reported as an atypical, mixed, sparsely granulated growth hormone and prolactin producing pituitary adenoma. Postoperatively his vision in the left eye improved to finger counting at 2 feet distance and the vision in the right eye improved to 6/12. After 2 weeks the GH levels dropped to 100 ng/mL.

He was also started on cabergoline 1 mg twice a week and long acting injectable octreotide. He was then called for follow-up after 3 months for the radiation therapy.

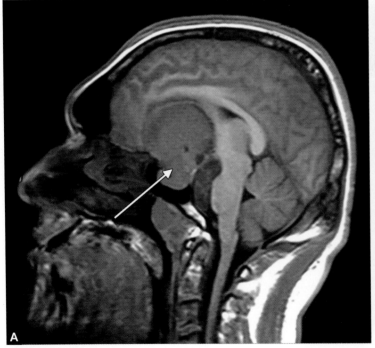

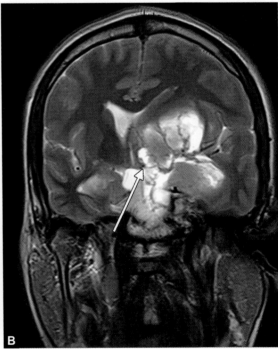

Figs. 1A and B

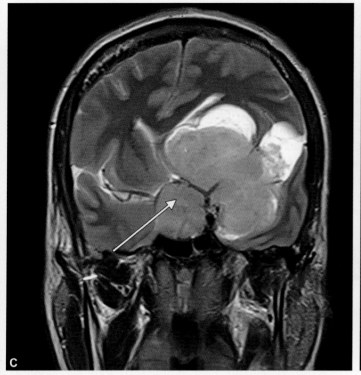
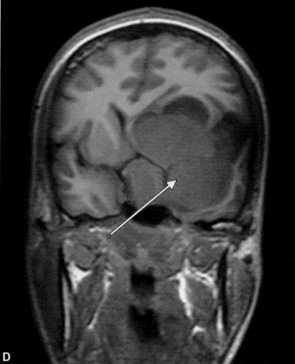

Figs. 1A to D: Magnetic resonance imaging (MRI) of the brain.

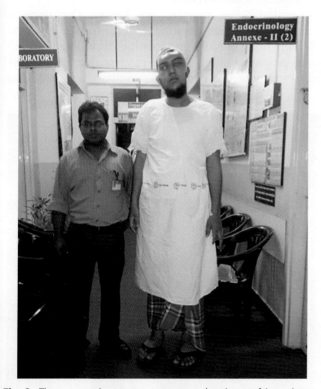

Fig. 2: The patient with gigantism postoperatively with one of the authors.

DISCUSSION

Pituitary gigantism refers to GH excess that occurs before fusion of the epiphyseal growth plates. Therefore, by definition the condition is only seen in growing children. In this setting, elevated levels of serum GH and IGF-I cause rapid, excessive linear growth and, if unchecked, extremely tall adult stature. In contrast, GH excess that begins in adulthood, after complete epiphyseal fusion, has no effect on stature and is called acromegaly. Pituitary gigantism typically is a sporadic and isolated condition. However, it may occur within the context of a coexisting disorder or arise according to a pattern of familial inheritance. Syndromes in which gigantism is a well-recognized feature include McCune Albright Syndrome (MAS), multiple endocrine neoplasia type I (MEN-1), and Carney complex.[1,2]

REFERENCES

1. Bhattacharjee R, Roy A, Goswami S, et al. Pituitary Gigantism: A Case Report. Indian J Endocr Metab 2012;16, (Suppl S2):285-7
2. Mammis A, Eloy JA, Liu JK. Early descriptions of acromegaly and gigantism and their historical evolution as clinical entities. Neurosurg Focus. 2010;29(4):E1

CASE 10

A 38-year-old gentleman presented to the emergency services with history of sudden onset headache, visual disturbance, followed by loss of consciousness. Magnetic Resonance Imaging (MRI) Brain showed a sellar—suprasellar mass with a cystic area within (Figs. 1A to C). His wife explained, she noticed that his footwear size had increased to "size 12" from "9" and he was also not able to wear their wedding ring. His growth hormone (GH) levels just preoperatively and a year later were well suppressed after an oral glucose load.

WHICH OF THE FOLLOWING ARE FALSE?

1. He may have acquired GH deficiency after apoplexy
2. Octreotide may not have a role in this patient at present
3. Hypogonadism is likely
4. Diabetes mellitus is unlikely to improve
5. The enlarged shoe size is unlikely to decrease.

This patient has presented with acromegalic features, with subsequent history suggestive of a pituitary apoplexy (hemorrhagic infarction). The serial photographs show the evolution of acromegaly over a period of 10 years, with subsequent regression of some of his features following apoplexy in the final photograph (Figs. 1A to C).

The MRI showed a T1-weighted image with a large mass about 3 cm in vertical diameter and an anteroposterior diameter of 1.8 cm. It appeared to be brightly enhancing and had a hypointense cystic zone in the inferior part. The coronal T2-weighted image revealed a hyperintense cystic zone with the same density as cerebrospinal fluid (CSF). These findings are consistent with that of an acute pituitary apoplexy in a large macroadenoma (Figs. 2 and 3).

The histological section showed an absence of normal pituitary tissue or any pituitary adenoma for that matter, what is seen is necrotic material and a few red blood cells, a finding that is reminiscent of a previous pituitary apoplexy. There are no distinctive pituitary adenocytes on the photomicrogram (Fig. 4).

DISCUSSION

Growth hormone deficiency after apoplexy is fairly common. Octreotide has no role unless there is active production of GH with elevated IGF-1 levels. Bony changes in acromegaly are unlikely to improve in patients with normalization of GH levels, it is only the soft tissue changes which regress as conceived in the photographs viewed above, hence the shoe size remained the same. Most patients with pituitary apoplexy recover spontaneously though occasional cases do require surgery. In a large series of patients with acromegaly, pituitary apoplexy occurred in 3.5% of all cases and spontaneous recovery occurred in 75–88% of cases.

Occasional late relapses are known. Occasionally, acromegaly has been reported to occur for the first time following infarction of a pre-existing clinically non-functional pituitary tumor. It is of interest that the empty-sella syndrome can occur after pituitary apoplexy and

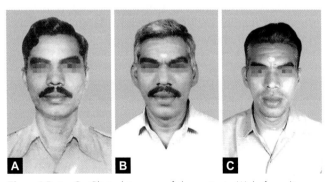

Figs. 1A to C: Clinical images of the patient. (A) before disease. (B) at the time of symptoms (C) after treatment.

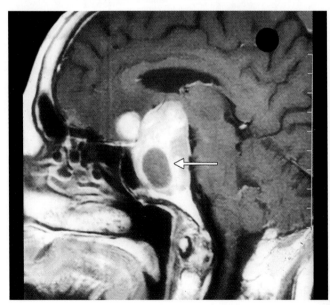

Fig. 2: MRI T1-weighted image with a cystic zone (shown with arrow).

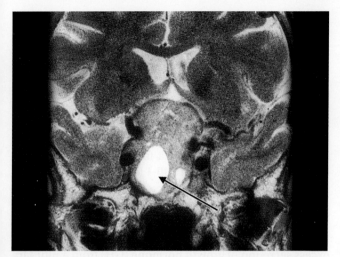

Fig. 3: MRI T2-weighted image with a cystic zone (shown with arrow) within the tumor.

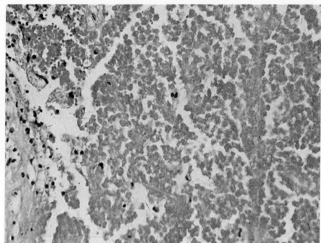

Fig. 4: Histopathology of the surgical specimen showing gross necrosis.

that the commonest functioning tumor encountered in patients with an empty-sella syndrome is GH producing tumor. With the advent of MRI it may be possible to pick up pituitary apoplexy more often in asymptomatic or only mildly symptomatic patients. Occasionally the infarction is so selective, so as to leave behind normal residual pituitary function.[1,2]

REFERENCES

1. Nabarro JD. Acromegaly. Clin Endocrinol (Oxf). 1987;26 (4):481-512.
2. Thomas N, Simon R, Chacko G, et al. Regression of acromegaly following pituitary apoplexy. Neurol India. 1999; 47(2):161-2.

CASE 11

Mrs R presented with increase in the size of the nose and hoarseness of voice for three years. She also complained of headache and also had past history of loss of consciousness once. The clinical image of the lady before and after the symptoms were shown in Figures 1A and B.

WHAT IS THE DIAGNOSIS?

She had clinically acromegalic features. Her visual acuity was normal and her visual fields were satisfactory. The rest of the neurological examination was normal. Her Human Growth Hormone (HGH) was elevated, 45.2 ng/mL as well as the Insulin like growth factor-1 (IgF-1) which was 759 ng/mL.

Her magnetic resonance imaging (MRI) brain showed a 1.3 cm Hardy's grade A pituitary macroadenoma with extension into the sphenoid sinus (Figs. 2A to C).

She underwent an endoscopic transsphenoidal radical excision of the adenoma. On the postoperative day 1, her HGH level was 1.23 ng/mL and on the 7th day post-suppression Growth Hormone (GH) was 1.49. On the 7th postoperative she also had symptoms of nausea, vomiting and was also feeling tired. She was started on oral glucocorticoids with which her symptoms subsided. A 2-week postoperative GH level was 1.7 ng/mg supporting

a partial remission. Subsequently, she was stared on oral cabergoline 0.5 mg once a week. The histopathological biopsy was reported as a sparsely granulated growth hormone secreting pituitary adenoma with the cells staining for GH. She was advised a follow-up after 3 months to check the serum GH and IGF-1 levels.

DISCUSSION

In most of the patients, acromegaly is due to the chronic, excess secretion of growth hormone (GH) from a pituitary adenoma. However, ectopic source of GH and GHRH also been described in causing acromegaly. GH induces the synthesis of hepatic insulin-like growth factor 1(IGF-1); thereby the elevated GH and IGF-1 levels cause metabolic complications of acromegaly. There is a linear correlation between the mortality rates in acromegaly with the GH and IGF-1 levels. So, the current definition for a cure includes GH levels < 0.4 µg/L after an oral glucose load, and IGF-1 levels within the normal age and gender-adjusted range. The mortality is less if the random GH levels is <2.5 µg/L or, more recently a level of less than <1 µg/L. The therapeutic goals in acromegaly can be achieved by modalities, such as pituitary surgery (removing the adenoma), medical therapy, and radiotherapy or in combination.[1,2]

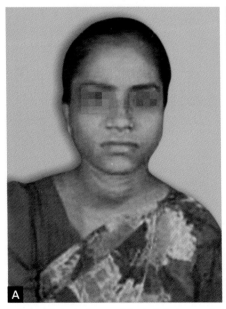 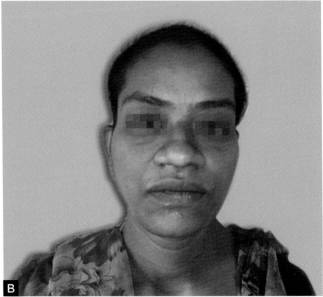

Figs. 1A and B: Clinical picture of the lady before and after development of facial symptoms.

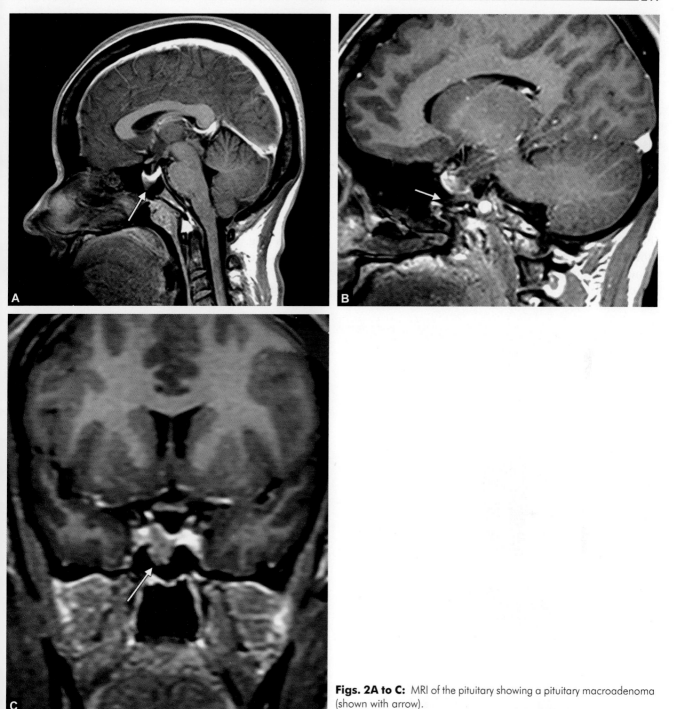

Figs. 2A to C: MRI of the pituitary showing a pituitary macroadenoma (shown with arrow).

REFERENCES

1. Melmed S, Casanueva FF, Klibanski A, et al. A consensus on the diagnosis and treatment of acromegaly complications. Pituitary. 2013;16(3):294-302.

2. Thanabalasingham G, Grossman AB. Acromegaly: Beyond surgery. Indian J Endocrinol Metab. 2013;17(4):563.

CASE 12

Mr. U, 40-year-old gentleman presented our Endocrine clinic at the age of 28 years with complaints of enlarging hands and feet with prognathism and bifrontal headache. His preoperative lateral X-ray of the skull is shown in Figure 2. He was evaluated and found to have clinical and biochemical features of acromegaly with a sellar and suprasellar mass measuring 5 × 4.5 × 3 cm with partial encasement of internal carotids bilaterally. Subsequently, he underwent a transsphenoidal excision of the mass. The MRI pituitary done after 3 months of the operation is shown in Figure 3. He was given stereotactic radiotherapy following that year. He came for follow-up after 10 years. His clinical images are shown in Figures 1A to F. His present MRI Brain is displayed in Figure 4. His bone scan is shown in Figure 5.

WHAT IS YOUR DIAGNOSIS?

He was on oral prednisolone and thyroxine during the present visit. His hormonal evaluation did not show any abnormalities. However his clinical examination revealed that he has asymmetrical facial features and café au lait spots (Fig. 1). His bone scan showed an increased uptake in the both parietal bones and left mandibule (Fig. 5). With the clinical and the radiological features, in the back ground of acromegaly he was diagnosed to have

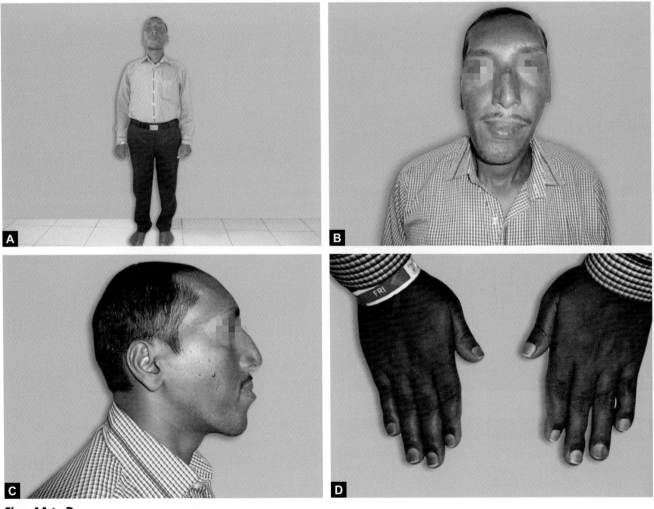

Figs. 1A to D

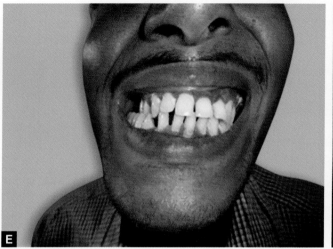

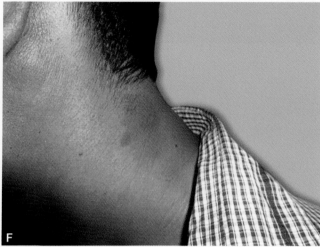

Figs. 1A to F: Acromegalic features: Prognathism, enlarged hands and widespread teeth with asymmetry of the face and a cafe au lait spot in the neck are suggestive of the McCune Albright Syndrome (MAS) clinically.

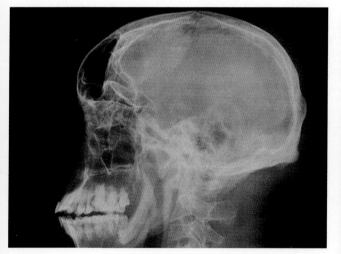

Fig. 2: X-ray skull lateral showing an enlarged frontal sinus, widened sella fossa, thickened skull table and prognathism.

McCune Albright syndrome. He, however did not have fibrous dysplasia of any of the bones at present.

DISCUSSION

McCune-Albright syndrome was first described in 1936 as the triad of café au lait spots of the skin, polyostotic fibrous dysplasia, and multiple endocrine abnormalities including precocious puberty. The diagnosis is generally accepted if 2 of the 3 symptoms are present because of the wide spectrum of disease phenotypes. The syndrome is due to a mutation in the GNAS gene that causes a persistent

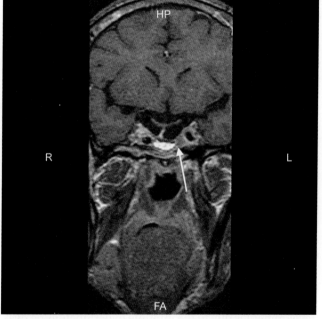

Fig. 3: MRI of the pituitary showing a residual lesion in the left side of the pituitary gland (Shown with arrow), done after 3 months of the surgery.

activation of the G stimulatory-alpha subunit of the G protein cellular signaling complex. The asymmetrical" bony and organ distribution as well as a hyperpigmentation distribution follows the "lines of Blaschko" or nevus lines. One of the first characteristics of McCune Albright syndrome is osteitis fibrosa disseminata, a form of fibrous dysplasia. The histopathological nature of the disease are

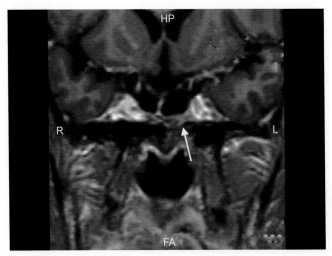

Fig. 4: MRI of the pituitary showing a slight reduction of the left side residual lesion, on comparing the MRI pituitary done in 2004 (shown with arrow).

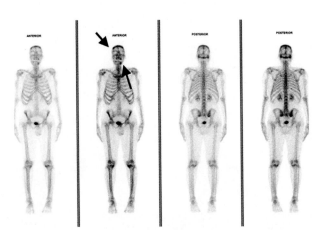

Fig. 5: Bone scan showing a diffusely increased tracer uptake in the both parietal bones and a focal area of the left mandible (shown with the arrows) with no fibrous dysplasia changes.

described in 3 common patterns - a Chinese writing" form, a Pagetoid" form, and a hypercellular form.

The café au lait spots can be faint at birth and often are missed, the lesions gradually darken as the patient gets older. The "Coast of Maine" appearance of the café au lait spot which emphasizes the "irregularity"of the borders of these lesions is an another hallmark for this syndrome. Kim et al. in 1999 isolated the melanocytes, fibroblasts, and keratinocytes from these pigmented lesions and determined that the G stimulatory alpha mutation was present solely in the melanocytes and not in the other two cell lines. This mutation was eventually found to increase the tyrosinase activity. Tyrosinase catalyzes the hydroxylation of tyrosine, the first step towards melanin biosynthesis. Over time, the faint café au lait spots evolve to darker and more visible lesions due to the persistent accumulation of melanin via this mechanism.

The third hallmark of McCune Albright's disease is the involvement of the endocrine system, of which precocious puberty is common affecting the girls. This early sexual development is due to the multiple hyperfunctioning ovarian cysts which form and regress spontaneously, there-by producing large amounts of estradiol in the process. Thus, it is a peripheral precocious puberty.

Non-endocrine organs can also be affected by McCune Albright"s syndrome. In the liver, it can produce nodular hyperplasia, biliary dysfunction, and in neonates can cause severe jaundice. Gastrointestinal polyps and hyperplasia of the spleen and pancreatic islet cells are other intestinal expressions of the disease.

In the heart, hypertrophic cardiac myocytes can be seen. Kidney involvement often presents with nephrocalcinosis. Hypophosphatemic phenotype in these patients also been described. Microcephaly, developmental delay, and failure to thrive are the other manifestations of neonatal disease.[1,2]

REFERENCES

1. Boyce AM, Collins MT. Fibrous dysplasia/McCune-Albright syndrome. In: Pagon RA, Adam MP, Ardinger HH, et al, Editors. GeneReviews® [Internet]. Seattle (WA): University of Washington, Seattle; 1993. Available from: http://www.ncbi.nlm.nih.gov/books/NBK274564/

2. Shetty S, Varghese RT, Shanthly N, et al. Toxic thyroid adenoma in McCune-Albright Syndrome. J Clin Diagn Res. 2014; 8(2):281-2.

CASE **13**

A 24-year-old gentleman came with a history of acral and pedal enlargement over 4 years. His height was 202 cm (Figs. 1A and B) with a height centile more than 97 centiles. His mid-parenteral height was around 170 cm. His clinical examination revealed spotty pigmentation in the sclera and lentiginous spots over the face (Fig. 1C). He had axillary freckling in addition. Spotty pigmentation of the eyes and the lentiginous spots over the face (Figs. 1C to E).

WHAT IS THE DIAGNOSIS?

In view of the features suggestive of gigantism, he was investigated further and was found to have Human Growth Hormone (GH), basal and 1 hour post 100 grams oral glucose levels 12.1 and 11.7 ng/mL respectively with Insulin like growth factor-1(IGF-1) of 1000 ng/mL {116 to 358}. The Magnetic Resonance Imaging (MRI) of the pituitary revealed a 23 × 20 × 30 mm (AP × TR × CC) well defined sella - suprasellar mass, which was heterogeneously hyperintense on T2 weighted image and predominantly hypointense on T1 weighted image with focal area of T2W hypointensity and T1W hyperintensity on the inferior aspect, representing an area of hemorrhage suggestive of an apoplexy (Figs. 2A to F). Since the clinical examination also revealed a mass in the left testes, an ultrasound of the testes was ordered. It showed a heterogeneous hypoechoic small ill defined hypoechoic lesion measuring 9 × 7 mm in the

inferior pole of the left testes suggesting a testicular germ cell tumor (Fig. 3). However, echocardiography did not reveal atrial myxomas.

He underwent a transnasal transsphenoidal excision of the sellar and suprasellar mass and postoperatively he had transient diabetes insipidus which was managed conservatively with oral desmopressin. The histopathological report showed a sparsely granulated growth hormone secreting pituitary adenoma. Postoperatively the HGH basal and post 1 hour glucose levels were 2.56 and 1.42 ng/mL. In view of the non suppression of the HGH levels, he was started on Cabergoline and advised to review after 3 months. His immediate postoperative MRI pituitary showed a T1 hyperintense foci suggestive of blood products (Figs. 4A and B). He was referred to Department of Urology for the treatment for the probable germ cell tumor of the left testes. In view of the clinical features of gigantism with spotty pigmentation of the sclera, lentinginous spots with a testicular mass a, clinical diagnosis of Carney's complex was made.

DISCUSSION

Carney's complex as described by J Aiden Carney in 1985 is an autosomal dominant disorder characterized by neoplasia involving heart, central nervous system and endocrine organs. Presence of pigmented skin and mucosal

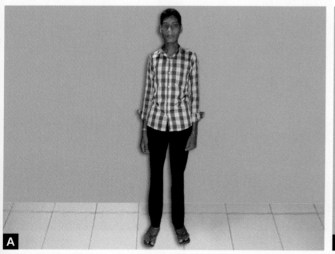

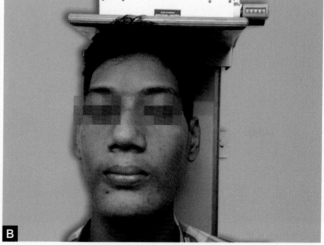

Figs. 1A and B

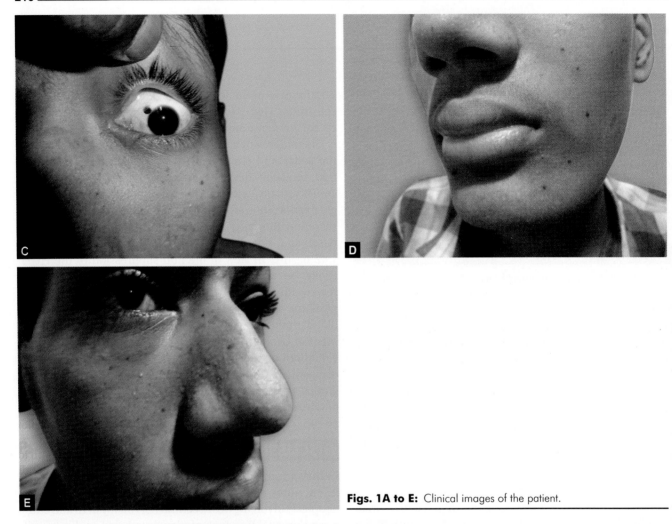

Figs. 1A to E: Clinical images of the patient.

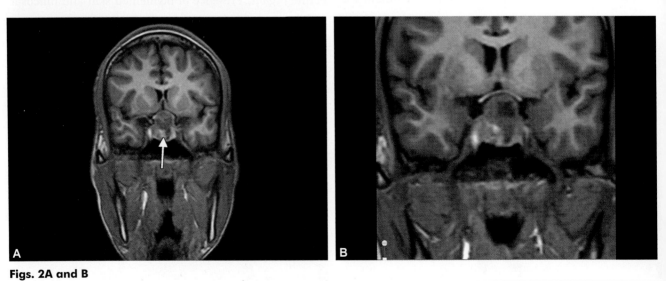

Figs. 2A and B

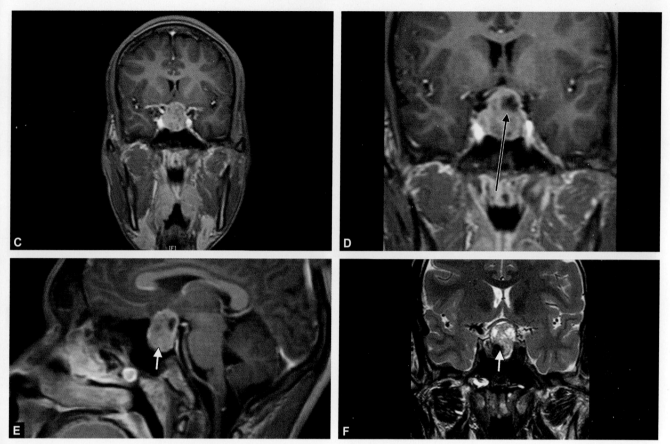

Figs. 2A to F: MRI Pituitary showing a pituitary macroadenoma with an apoplexy (shown with arrow).

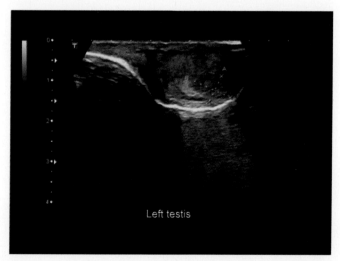

Fig. 3: Ultrasound of the left testes.

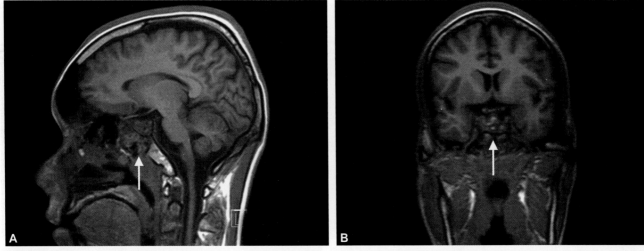

Figs. 4A and B: Postoperative MRI of the pituitary showing blood products in the sellar region (shown with arrow).

lesions along with these tumors is an important hallmark of this syndrome.[1] Carney's complex can manifest itself as a spotty cutaneous pigmentation, cutaneous myxomas, cardiac myxomas, psammomatous melanotic schwannoma (PMS), acromegaly, large cell calcifying sertoli cell tumor (LCCSCT), thyroid carcinoma or nodule and breast adenoma. PRKAR 1 alpha is a tumor suppressor gene that is found to be mutated in almost 50% of cases with Carney's complex.[2]

REFERENCES

1. Carney Complex: case report and review - 1749-8090-6-25.pdf [Internet]. Available from: http://www.cardiothoracic-surgery.org/content/pdf/1749-8090-6-25.pdf
2. Microsoft Word - 0032007033.doc - kcj-37-183.pdf [Internet]. Available from: http://synapse.koreamed.org/Synapse/Data/PDFData/0054KCJ/kcj-37-183.pdf

CASE 14

An important differential diagnosis for acromegaly is Pachydermatoperiostosis. Pachydermoperiostosis (PDP) or primary hypertrophic osteoarthropathy is a rare syndrome with diverse radiological and clinical features. This patient had periodontal disease; anaemia; clubbing, and deformities of the hands and feet; swelling without acute inflammatory signs at the wrist, ankle, and knee joints; and thickening and folding of the facial skin (Figs. 1 and 2). Lingual enlargement was not noted (Figs. 2A and B). The patient had hyperhidrosis and complained of a feeling

of heat in the palms and soles. He denied any history of trauma. A family history of similar disease was negative. Three forms of PDP are described, *classic or complete form*, with skin and skeletal changes; *incomplete form*, with skeletal changes but no dermal findings; and *forme fruste* with dermal changes but no skeletal findings.

Facial involvement occurs in the form of thickening of the facial skin and scalp, with prominent folds on the forehead and cheek. A leonine facies is usually a late feature (Fig. 2A). Sometimes, the scalp takes on an undulating

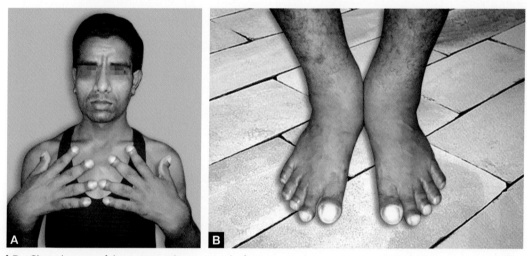

Figs. 1A and B: Clinical image of the patient with acromegalic features.

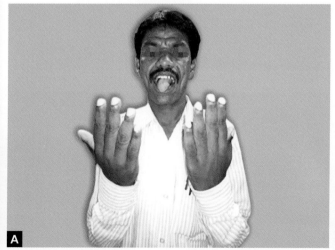 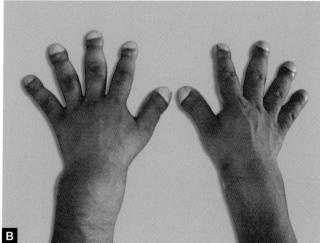

Figs. 2A and B: Clinical image showing acromegaloid features and no tongue enlargement.

appearance and shows prominent grooves, the appearance being referred to as *cutis vertices'gyrata* because of its resemblance to the sulci and gyri of the brain. These can also be a so-called *bull-dog appearance.*

Differential diagnoses include variants of PDP, secondary hypertrophic osteoarthropathy, thyroid acropachy, acromegaly, van Buchem's disease (in which there is absence of clubbing and skin changes), diaphyseal dysplasia (endosteal and periosteal proliferation), and syphilitic periostosis.

Variants of PDP include *Rosenfeld-Kloepfer syndrome* (characterized by enlargement of the jaws, especially mandible, and of the hands and feet, nose, lips, tongue, and forehead, along with cutis vertices gyrata and corneal leucoma); *Currarino idiopathic osteoarthropathy* (an incomplete form of PDP seen in children and adolescents and characterized by the presence of eczema and sutural diastases); and a *localized form* with only the radiographic features of PDP. Treatment is limited to nonsteroidal anti-inflammatory drugs (NSAID), steroid, or colchicine therapy to alleviate arthralgias and retinoids for the dermal changes. Surgical treatment is limited to plastic surgery for cosmetic indications or correction of associated deformities of the lower extremities.[2]

REFERENCES

1. Bhaskaranand K, Shetty RR, Bhat AK. Pachydermoperiostosis:Three case reports. J OrthopSurg (Hong Kong) 2001; 9:61–6
2. Auger M, Stavrianeas N. Pachydermoperiostosis. Orphanet Encylcopedia. Available from: http://www.orpha.net

CASE 15

A 45-year-old, Ms. S presented with complaints of recent onset weight gain and increased hair over the upper lip. She had a moon face, centripetal obesity, dorsal pad of fat and excessive deposition of fat over the shoulder and upper limbs (Figs. 1A and B). Facial hirsutism was also noticed. There was diffuse hyperpigmentation over the body mainly over the face, knuckles and neck. Her visual acuity and visual field were clinically normal.

WHAT IS THE DIAGNOSIS?

Investigations revealed a basal 8 am serum cortisol of 23.66 mcg% and 24-hour basal urinary cortisol of 544 mcg/day. The sleeping Midnight cortisol was 20 mcg/dL with a simultaneous Adrenocorticotropic Hormone (ACTH) level of 24 pmol/mL. This elevation of midnight serum cortisol is highly sensitive for endogenous Cushing's syndrome. Her 8 am serum ACTH was 54 pmol/mL. The overnight post 1 mg and 8 mg dose Dexamethasone suppression serum Cortisol levels were 3.7 mcg% and 1.7 mcg% respectively. The non-suppression of serum cortisol with post 1 mg overnight dexamethasone and more than 50% suppression of the basal cortisol with 8 mg overnight dexamethasone were highly suggestive of ACTH dependent Cushing's disease. Her rest of the hormonal evaluation revealed features suggestive a central hypothyroidism.

A magnetic resonance imaging (MRI) of the pituitary was done for the localization of the ACTH source.

The MRI pituitary showed a mild asymmetry of the left side of the pituitary gland (Figs. 2A to C) and the dynamic imaging showed a lesion measuring 6 × 5 mm towards the left with a mild delayed enhancement (Fig. 2C).

She underwent a endoscopic transnasal transsphenoidal excision of the left microadenoma. Postoperatively her serum cortisol levels were monitored daily which was 40, and 16.69 ug% respectively at 6 hours, and 24 hours postoperatively. On the 3rd postoperative day she had vomiting and excessive tiredness and her simultaneous serum cortisol was 1.20 mcg/dL suggestive of a remission. She was started on parenteral hydrocortisone and was over lapped with oral prednisolone. It was planned to evaluate her Hypothalamo-pituitary-adrenal axis after tapering and stopping oral the glucocorticoids over a period of three months. Histopathology was reported as an atypical ACTH producing sparsely granulated pituitary microadenoma, sellar region with an MIB-1 labelling index of 4% and occasional tumor nuclei are positive for p53. Crooke's hyaline change was also highlighted in the adjoining adenohypophysis.

DISCUSSION

Cushing's disease is caused by a discrete ACTH-secreting tumor in the majority of cases: diffuse corticotroph hyperplasia is rarely encountered. As a result, optimal treatment is surgical resection by selective adenomectomy, performed by an experienced surgeon, as long as the

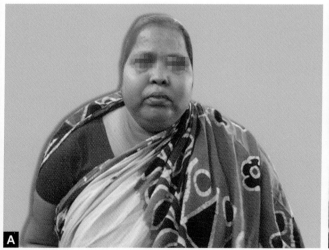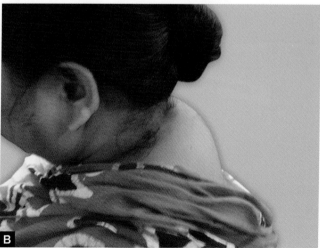

Figs. 1A and B: Clinical image of the patient with a moon face and a dorsal pad of fat.

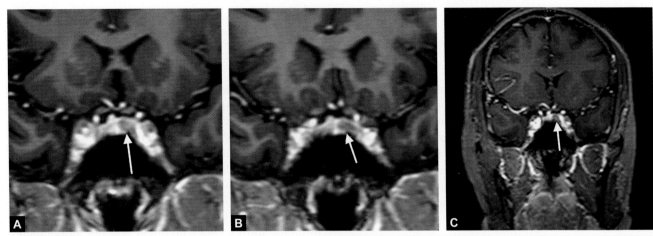

Figs. 2A to C: MRI of the pituitary showing a microadenoma in the left side of the pituitary gland (shown with arrow).

tumor can be identified. Careful sectioning through the pituitary gland may be required to locate the tumor, because some tumors have an identifiable pseudo-capsule, whereas others do not exhibit a discrete border between the tumor and normal pituitary tissue. If the tumor was pathologically identified at initial surgery, the probability of a subsequent successful resection is higher than if no tumor was found initially. Trans-sphenoidal micro-surgery is still the most widely used technique.[1]

Favorable prognostic factors associated with successful adenomectomy include detection of the microadenoma by MRI, a well-defined tumor that is not invading either the basal dura or cavernous sinus, histological confirmation of an ACTH-secreting tumor, low postoperative serum cortisol levels, and long-lasting adrenal insufficiency.

For patients in whom a discrete microadenoma cannot be located by sellar exploration, total or partial (central core or hemi-) hypophysectomy may be indicated. However, total or partial hypophysectomy induces remission less often (approximately 70% of patients) than selective tumor resection and is associated with a higher rate of complications and hypopituitarism than selective adeno-mectomy.[2]

REFERENCES

1. Woo YS, Isidori AM, Wat WZ, et al. Clinical and biochemical characteristics of adrenocorticotropin-secreting macroadenomas. J Clin Endocrinol Metab 90:4963–69
2. De Tommasi C, Vance ML, Okonkwo DO, et al. Surgical management of adrenocorticotropic hormone-secreting macroadenomas: outcome and challenges in patients with Cushing's disease or Nelson's syndrome. J Neurosurg 103:825–30

CASE 16

A 55-year-old, postmenopausal lady with a background history of hypertension and uncontrolled diabetes mellitus with micro vascular complications diagnosed in the recent past presented with progressive weight gain of 30 kg over 12 months. She also noticed reddish lesions over the arms and legs over last 6 months with history of difficulty in climbing stairs. Examination showed the findings which are shown in the pictures below (Figs. 1A to C).

WHAT IS THE DIAGNOSIS?

With the recent worsening of glycaemic status, hypertension and gaining of weight over the past few months, the problem most probably is due to the steroid excess which either could be a external steroid intake or an endogenous origin. This patient denies any history of steroid intake in any of the forms since or before the symptoms started. Her baseline 8 am serum cortisol was markedly raised (24 mcg/dL) with an associated 24-hour urine free cortisol also markedly high. Midnight serum cortisol (26 mcg/dL) and serum Adrenocorticotropic hormone (ACTH) (40 pg/mL) levels were also elevated suggestive of ACTH dependent Cushing's syndrome. Her 8 am serum cortisol did not get suppressed with an overnight 1 mg dexamethasone. After an overnight 8mg dexamethasone, the serum 8 am cortisol and the 24 hour urine free cortisol were suppressed more

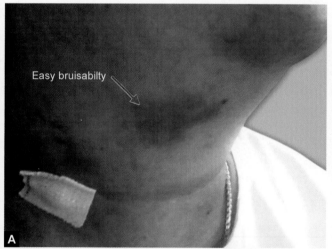

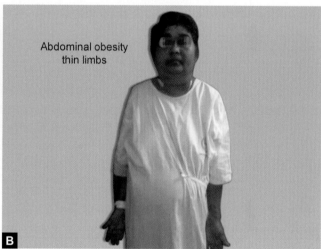

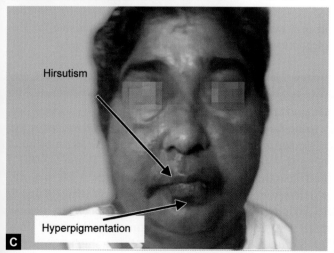

Figs. 1A to C: Clinical features showing Cushingoid features.

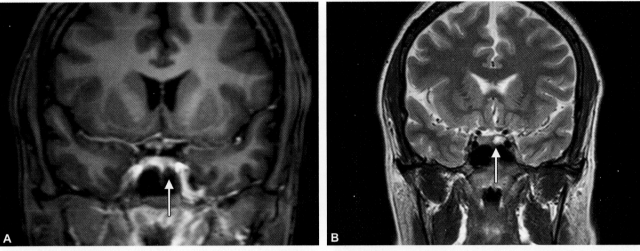

Figs. 2A and B: MRI Pituitary showing a 10 x 9 x 7 mm sized (AP x Tr X CC) well defined T1 hypointense and T2 hyperintense lesion in the left side of the pituitary gland (shown with arrow).

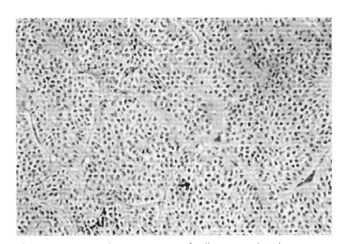

Fig. 3: Histopathology of the tumor showing monomorphic appearance of cells arranged in sheets.

than 50% that of the baseline parameters, suggestive of ACTH dependent Cushing's syndrome of pituitary origin or Cushing's disease

With the clinical and biochemical findings listed above, the patient was diagnosed to have an ACTH dependent Cushing's disease. Her magnetic resonance imaging (MRI) pituitary showed a microadenoma in the left side of pituitary in the anterior lobe (Figs. 2A and B, shown with an arrow). She underwent a trans-sphenoidal microadenoma removal and her glycemic control improved markedly in the postoperative period. Histopathology of the microadenoma showed cells positive for ACTH immuno histochemistry, confirming an ACTH dependent pituitary adenoma (Fig. 3) She had lost 25kgs weight after the 3 months postoperative period. She required a small dose of oral antidiabetic agents and antihypertensive for the glycemic and blood pressure control respectively.

DISCUSSION

Diagnostic criteria that suggest Cushing's syndrome are a urine free cortisol greater than the normal range for the assay, serum cortisol greater than 1.8 µg/dL (50 nmol/liter) after an 1 mg overnight dexamethasone (1-mg ONDST), and sleeping late-night cortisol greater than 1.8 mcg/dL. The awake midnight serum cortisol greater than 7.5 µg/dL (> 207 nmol/liter) has a sensitivity and specificity greater than 96%. A single sleeping serum cortisol greater than 1.8 µg/dL (>50 nmol/liter) also has a high sensitivity (100%) for the diagnosis of Cushing's syndrome.[1]

Selective trans-sphenoidal pituitary adenomectomy remains the treatment of choice for cushings disease. However the rate of cure at long-term follow-up is suboptimal with a high recurrence rates, even in the hands of an expert neurosurgeon. A measurement of 8 am serum cortisol during the first postoperative week below 2 µg/dL is considered as the best index of remission. When the serum cortisol is between 2 and 5 µg/dL the patient can be considered in remission. A postoperative serum cortisol above 5 µg/dL for up to 6 weeks is indicative of a persistent disease and requires further evaluation. Medical treatment, a second-line treatment option, have either a primary or adjunctive role in patients who cannot safely undergo a surgery, if the initial surgery fails, or if the tumor recurs. Drugs directed at reducing ACTH levels in Cushing's disease include the dopamine agonist, Cabergoline (off-label use), and the parenteral somatostatin analogue-pasireotide. Ketoconazole and Mitotane are the best of the choices at present. Bilateral adrenalectomy provides an immediate cure in patients where other treatments fail or in patients with moribund Cushing's syndrome. Radiation therapy (conventional or stereotactic radiosurgery) should be reserved as the third-line treatment.[2]

REFERENCES

1. Nieman LK, Biller BMK, Findling JW, et al. The Diagnosis of Cushing's Syndrome: An Endocrine Society Clinical Practice Guideline. J Clin Endocrinol Metab. 2008;93(5): 1526–40.
2. Guignat L, Bertherat J. The diagnosis of Cushing's syndrome: an Endocrine Society Clinical Practice Guideline: commentary from a European perspective. Eur J Endocrinol. 2010;163(1):9–13.

CASE 17

A 12-year-old, girl presented with history of inability to gain height since the past 4 years duration. She also gave history of non-development of the secondary sexual characters, but was noticing excessive facial hair growth for the past few months. Her height was 134 cms with a target height of 147.5 ± 8 cm (Fig. 1). She was short statured with a height less than the 5th centile for her age in Agarwals growth chart. Clinical examination showed hyperpigmentation of the knuckles.

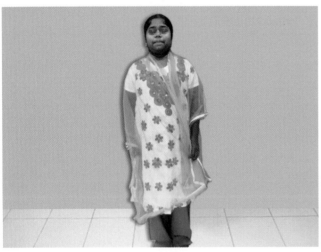

Fig. 1: Clinical image showing obesity, stunted growth and hirsutism.

WHAT IS THE DIAGNOSIS?

The post 1 mg and 8 mg overnight dexamethasone serum cortisol were not suppressed in this patient. The MRI of the pituitary showed a doubtful centrally located pituitary microadenoma (Figs. 2A and B). The patient underwent a transnasal transsphenoidal excision of the microadenoma; however the histopathology showed only a adenohypophyseal tissue with Crooke's hyaline change. As she did not undergo a remission postoperatively, she was started on oral Ketoconazole. She is on regular follow-up since then.

DISCUSSION

In comparison to adult Cushing's syndrome (CS), growth failure with associated weight gain is one of the most reliable indicator of hypercortisolemia in pediatric CS.[1] Clinical features may occur gradually over a period of time and may go unrecognized by parents and care givers. For example, the change in facial appearance, which is almost always present, can often be missed. Two consecutive 24-hour urine collections for urinary free cortisol levels (UFC) are usually the first line investigation. The UFC measurements have high sensitivity but relatively low specificity. If repeated UFC excretion is normal then CS is

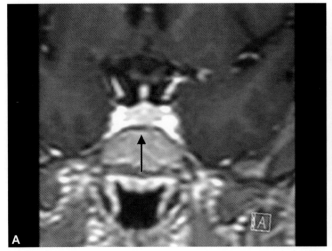

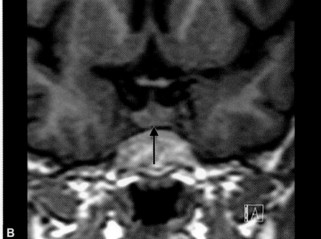

Figs. 2A and B: MRI pituitary showing a doubtful sellar mass in the center of the pituitary gland (shown with arrow).

unlikely. As a result, tests for Cushing's syndrome are not indicated in obese children unless their stature related growth rate has slowed down. The dose for overnight dexamethasone suppression is 10 mcg/kg or 0.5–1 mg/m^2.

A dexamethasone dosage of 0.5 mg 6-hourly is generally used to perform the low dose dexamethasone suppression test in children weighing ≥ 40 kg, while, in patients < 40 kg, a dosage of 30 mcg/kg/ day is recommended. The cut off for the diagnosis of cushings syndrome is otherwise same as that of the adults.

Transsphenoidal adenomectomy is the treatment of choice for children with Cushing's disease, as it is in adults.[2]

Under 7 years, of age, tumors related to adrenal gland causing CS (adenoma, carcinoma, bilateral hyperplasia, and McCune Albright syndrome) are the most frequent ones.

REFERENCES

1. Chan LF, Storr HL, Grossman AB, et al. Pediatric Cushing's syndrome: clinical features, diagnosis, and treatment. Arq Bras Endocrinol Amp Metabol. 2007;51(8):1261–71.
2. Magiakou MA, Mastorakos G, Oldfield EH, et al. Cushing's syndrome in children and adolescents. Presentation, diagnosis, and therapy. N Engl J Med. 1994;8;331(10):629–36.

CASE 18

A 55-year-old gentleman has had headache for 5 years. He complained of pain mainly over the vertex and back of the head. There were no history of associated vomiting or loss of consciousness or a visual disturbance. He gave no history of enlargement of hands and feet or striae, ecchymoses, proximal myopathy and weight gain. However, he noticed erectile dysfunction for the past 2 years and also a reduction in the shaving frequency during the same duration.

His clinical examination revealed a testicular volume: 20 ml bilateral with pubic hair of Tanner's stage 5. His rest of the clinical examination being grossly normal.

WHAT IS THE DIAGNOSIS?

Clinical examination revealed that he had a sparse body hair with dry skin. His investigations were: Prolactin in dilution (HPRL): 1000 ng/mL, Serum Cortisol-8 am: 16.6 µg%, FSH: 5.71 mIU/mL, Testosterone: 162 ng/dL with a normal thyroid function tests. Magnetic Resonance Imaging (MRI) of the pituitary gland showed a mass lesion in the left cavernous sinus and left side of the sella, isointense with grey matter, with a dural tail. So an ectopic Prolactinoma in the left cavernous sinus was considered (Figs. 1A and B).

He was started on cabergoline-orally 0.5 mg twice weekly and was called for a review after 3 months. The Erectile dysfunction improved subsequently after the treatment with cabergoline.

DISCUSSION

Prolactin secretion by the pituitary Lactotroph cells is suppressed by hypothalamic dopamine that traverse through the portal venous system. Factors that induce prolactin synthesis as well as the secretion are estrogen, thyrotrophin-releasing hormone (TRH), epidermal growth factor (EGF) and dopamine receptor antagonists especially antipsychotic medications. Symptoms of hyperprolactinemia ranges from asymptomatic to features of hypogonadism, infertility, and galactorrhoea.[1] A single non stress vene-puncture sample of serum prolactin more than the

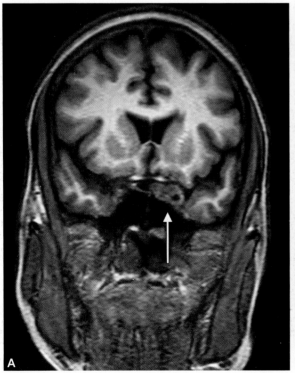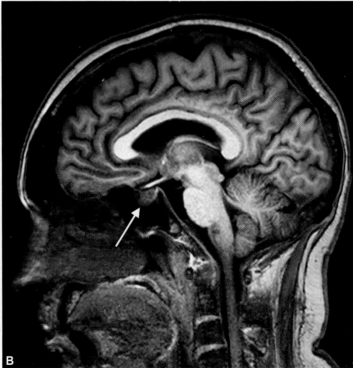

Figs. 1A and B: MRI of the brain showing a mass lesion in the left side of the sella encasing the left carotid artery (shown with arrow).

upper limit of normal is recommended as a diagnosis of hyperprolactinemia. A serum prolactin level greater than 500 ng/ml is diagnostic of a prolactinoma. However, a serum prolactin level greater than 250 ng/ml may indicate the presence of a Prolactinoma. Selected drugs such as risperidone and metoclopramide can cause prolactin elevations above 200 ng/ml in patients without an evidence of pituitary adenoma. At times these drugs can elevate the prolactin levels to more than 500 ng/ml also.[1,2]

REFERENCES

1. Halperin Rabinovich I, Cámara Gómez R, García Mouriz M, et al. Clinical guidelines for diagnosis and treatment of Prolactinoma and hyperprolactinemia. Endocrinol Nutr Engl Ed. 2013;60(6):308–19.
2. Melmed S, Casanueva FF, Hoffman AR, et al. Diagnosis and Treatment of Hyperprolactinemia: An Endocrine Society Clinical Practice Guideline. J Clin Endocrinol Metab. 2011; 1;96(2):273–8.

CASE 19

A 26-year-old unmarried girl presented with history of chronic headache with a progressive decline in vision over the past 1-year and secondary amenorrhea during the same duration. She also had galactorrhea which she noticed over the past 8 months. On fundus examination, the optic disc was pale with both the eyes showing bitemporal hemianopia.

WHAT IS THE PROBABLE DIAGNOSIS?

In this patient, the serum prolactin level was 7310 ng/mL with the other hormonal levels within normal range. The Magnetic Resonance Imaging (MRI) of the pituitary gland showed a mass in the sellar, suprasellar region (42 × 34 × 23 mm) with right parasellar extension and infiltration of the right cavernous sinus, superiorly the lesion compresses and stretches the optic chiasm (Figs. 1A and B, shown with arrow). So she was diagnosed a prolactin secreting pituitary macroadenoma or a macroprolactinoma. Figure 2 shows the MRI of the pituitary gland done after 5 months of cabergoline treatment with definite tumor regression to 25 mm size on comparing the prior MRI.

DISCUSSION

The most common pituitary adenoma which causes infertility, menstrual irregularity and galactorrhoea in women and hypogonadism, decreased libido, infertility, erectile dysfunction and gynecomastia in men is Prolactinoma. Therapy in patients with prolactinomas is dependent on the tumor size and the effects of hyperprolactinemia. 95% of patients with microprolactinomas do not enlarge over a 4–6 year period.[1]

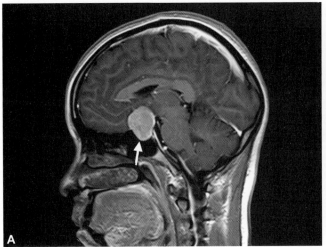
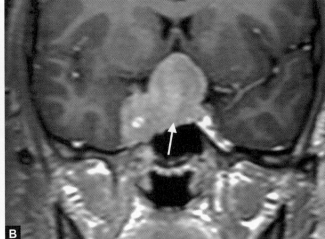

Figs. 1A and B: MRI scans of the patient.

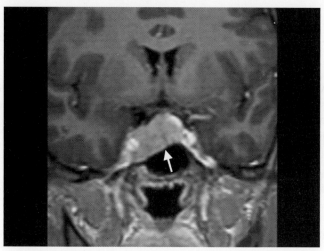

Fig. 2: Post-treatment MRI pituitary done after 5 months of Cabergoline.

Pituitary tumors larger than 4 cm in size are termed as "giant adenomas". "Invasive giant Prolactinoma" is defined as: 1) tumor diameter of >4 cm; 2) serum prolactin >1000 ng/mL; and 3) clinical symptoms induced by the hyperprolactinemia or mass effect.

Patients with microadenomas and those with macroadenomas and negative MRI scans after treatment are good candidates for drug withdrawal. In patients with macroadenomas and negative MRI scans, for at least after 2 years of medical treatment the drug should be slowly tapered before withdrawal. During the first year after drug withdrawal, serum prolactin levels and clinical symptoms should be assessed at 3-month intervals because recurrence rates are highest in 12 months after withdrawal.[2]

REFERENCES

1. March CM, Kletzky OA, Davajan V, et al. Longitudinal evaluation of patients with untreated prolactin-secreting pituitary adenomas. Am J Obstet Gynecol. 1981;1;139(7):835-44.
2. Siddiqui A, Chew N, Miszkiel K. Unusual orbital invasion by a giant Prolactinoma. Br J Radiol. 2008;81:259-62.

CASE 20

A 33-year-old lady presented with amenorrhea, galactorrhea and occasional vomiting and headache for 10 years. She had elevated prolactin levels in the blood. She was started on a weekly tablet. Displayed images are that of Magnetic Resonance Imaging (MRI) brain (Figs. 1A to C).

WHAT IS THE DIAGNOSIS?

Discussion

Prolactinomas can cause symptoms in 2 ways. Symptoms can happen when:
1. Due to excess production of prolactin hormone levels.
2. Due to pressure levels over the adjacent brain tissues.

Symptoms in premenopausal women:
1. Hypogonadism—Infertility, oligomenorrhea, or amenorrhea.
2. Galactorrhoea.

Symptoms in Men:
1. Hypogonadotropic hypogonadism
2. Erectile dysfunction
3. Infertility
4. Galactorrhoea

Diagnosis
1. Serum prolactin concentration

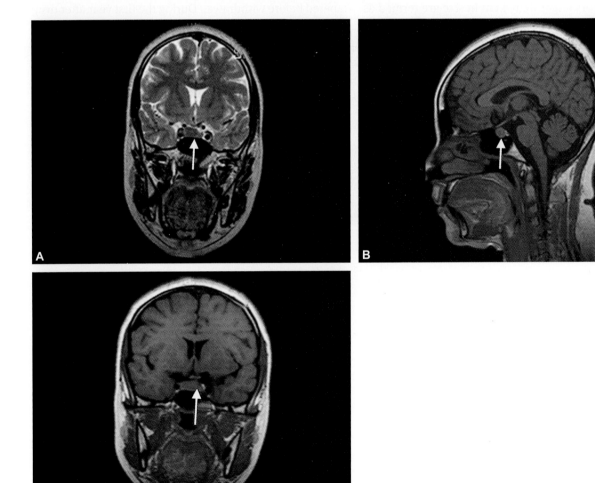

Figs. 1A to C: MRI of the brain showing a pituitary lesion (shown with arrow).

Levels	Condition
5–20 ng/mL	Normal
20–200 ng/mL	Hyperprolactinemia due to any cause.
> 200 ng/mL	Lactotroph adenoma

2. Imaging—MRI pituitary is the choice of investigation to detect adenoma arising from hypothalamo-pituitary region.

TREATMENT

Indications for treatment in patients with hyperprolactinemia

1. Existing or impending neurologic symptoms due to the large size of a Lactotroph adenoma, and
2. Hypogonadism or other symptoms due to hyperprolactinemia, such as galactorrhoea

Agents used to treat hyperprolactinemia

1. Dopamine agonists—Bromocriptine, Cabergoline, Pergolide, Quinagolide

2. Oestrogen therapy in patient with microadenomas and who do not tolerate dopamine agonists.

Trans-sphenoidal surgery is indicated in

1. Unsuccessful treatment with dopamine agonists.
2. Post cabergoline treatment induced CSF leak
3. Persistent visual compromise even after adequate medical therapy

Postoperative radiation therapy is indicated in

1. Radiation is primarily used to prevent regrowth of residual tumor in a patient with a very large macroadenoma after transsphenoidal debulking of Lactotroph adenomas that are resistant to cabergoline.[1,2]

REFERENCES

1. Casanueva FF, Molitch ME, Schlechte JA, et al. Guidelines of the Pituitary Society for the diagnosis and management of prolactinomas. Clin Endocrinol (Oxf). 2006;65(2): 265–73.
2. Schlechte JA. Long-term management of prolactinomas. J Clin Endocrinol Metab. 2007;92(8):2861–5.

CASE 21

A 25-year-old Ms. Z was seen in the endocrinology OPD for the complaints of chronic headache associated with visual difficulty. She also was amenorrheic over a year. She did not give history to suggest hypothyroidism or hypercortisolemia. Clinically other than for the bitemporal hemianopia, rest was otherwise unremarkable.

WHAT IS THE DIAGNOSIS?

Her investigation revealed a Serum 8 am Cortisol of 12.67 ug%, Total Thyroxine level of 4.8 ug% and Free thyroxine levels of 0.86 ng/dL and Prolactin in dilution of 7310 ng/mL. The Magnetic Resonance Imaging (MRI) Pituitary showed a Lobulated T2 hyperintense and T1 iso-hypointense lesion in the sellar suprasellar region measuring 32 × 34 × 23 mm with a right parasellar extension and evidence of infiltration of the right cavernous sinus (Figs. 1A to E). So a diagnosis of invasive Prolactinoma was made and was started on 0.5 mg twice weekly Cabergoline which was hiked up to 1 mg twice weekly after 1 week.

The repeat serum prolactin in dilution after 4 months of cabergoline was 349 ng/ml and the MRI pituitary showed a homogeneously enhancing lesion measuring ~25 × 20 × 16 with the evidence of right parasellar extension into the cavernous sinus and partial encasement of the right internal carotid artery (Figs. 2A to E). However comparing to the previous image the lesion had regressed considerably. She was found to be having central hypothyroidism during this visit and she was started on oral thyroxine.

After 7 months of cabergoline, she was found to have a serum prolactin in dilution of 244.5 ng/mL. However the MRI was not repeated at this time and was advised to review after 6 months.

Her serum prolactin decreased to 164 ng/mL after 18 months of therapy with Cabergoline and the repeat MRI Pituitary showed a significant resolution of the right cavernous sinus component of the tumor with region of probable necrosis (Figs. 3A to E). She was advised to continue Cabergoline and to follow-up after 1 year.

DISCUSSION

Dopamine is the chemical that inhibits prolactin secretion normally. So prolactinoma can be treated medically with Bromocriptine, Cabergoline (both ergot derivatives) or Quinagolide which are dopamine agonist. Dopamine agonists are the primary therapy for both microadenomas that require treatment and macroprolactinomas. They rapidly normalize prolactin levels, restore reproductive function, reverse galactorrhoea, and decrease tumor size in most patients. Bromocriptine is associated with side-effects such as nausea and dizziness and hypotension in view of the side effects to start slowly.

Prolactin levels often rise again in most patients when the drug is discontinued. Recent studies have shown increased success in remission of prolactin levels after discontinuation, in patients having been treated for at least 2 years prior to cessation of dopamine agonist treatment.

Cabergoline is also a dopamine agonist which also has side-effects such as nausea and dizziness, but these are less common than with Bromocriptine. This drug has a long half-life of 4–7 days. Its long duration of action is due to the fact that it is slowly eliminated from pituitary tissue, has greater binding to pituitary receptors and more extensive enterohepatic recycling.

Higher doses and a longer duration of cabergoline therapy were associated with a higher risk of valvulopathy. The mechanism of its development has been postulated to be $5HT_{2b}$-receptor stimulation leading to fibromyoblast proliferation of the heart valves. The appropriate duration of dopamine agonist therapy in a given patient is uncertain.[1,2]

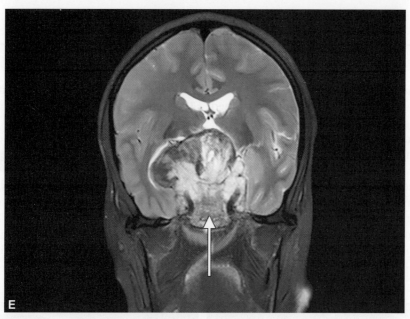

Figs. 1A to E: MRI of the pituitary done during the initial assessment.

Cabergoline 1 mg twice weekly. He advised to come for a follow up after 3 months.

DISCUSSION

Given the efficacy of medical therapy for prolactinomas, only a small minority of patients with prolactinomas require a trans-sphenoidal surgery or a radiation therapy. Indications for surgery are, increasing in size with refractory or resistant to the medical therapy, pituitary apoplexy, persistent visual compromise even after adequate medical therapy, cerebrospinal fluid (CSF) leak while on a dopamine agonist, psychiatric patient's whom the dopamine agonist are contraindicated.

Dopamine agonists should be discontinued once the pregnancy is confirmed. However, re-initiation of treatment with Bromocriptine is recommended if the patient has optic compressive symptoms. Visual assessment has to be done every 2 months in patients with prolactinoma who are pregnant.[1,2]

REFERENCES

1. Klibanski A. Prolactinomas. N Engl J Med. 2010;362 (13): 1219–26.
2. Witek P, Zieliński G. Management of prolactinomas during pregnancy. Minerva Endocrinol. 2013;38(4):351–63.

CASE 23

A 42-year-old gentleman presented to endocrine clinic with history of generalized tiredness. He also complained of some intermittent headache. There were no history suggestive of a pituitary apoplexy (vomiting, diplopia or ptosis). He is a known hypertensive and on regular medication for the same.

On examination, he was alert and oriented. His visual acuity was 6/6 in both the eyes. Examination of the visual fields did not reveal any findings with normal fundoscopy. There were no other focal neurological deficits.

His biochemistry investigation showed: Total T4–5.2 ug%, Free thyroxine - 0.57 ng%, 8AM cortisol-1.44mcg%

LH - 0.773 mIU/mL, FSH - 1.26 mIU/mL, Testosterone-101.60 ng/dL, Prolactin in dilution (HPRL) - 31.89 ng/mL, HGH - 0.092 ng/mL.

WHAT IS THE DIAGNOSIS?

In view of the deranged hormones, the diagnosis of panhypopituitarism was made and an Magnetic Resonance Imaging (MRI) brain was done. The MRI of the brain showed a 2.4 × 2.8 cm sellar mass with suprasellar extension upto the floor of the 3rd ventricle with extension into the left cavernous sinus (Figs. 1A to C). There were no

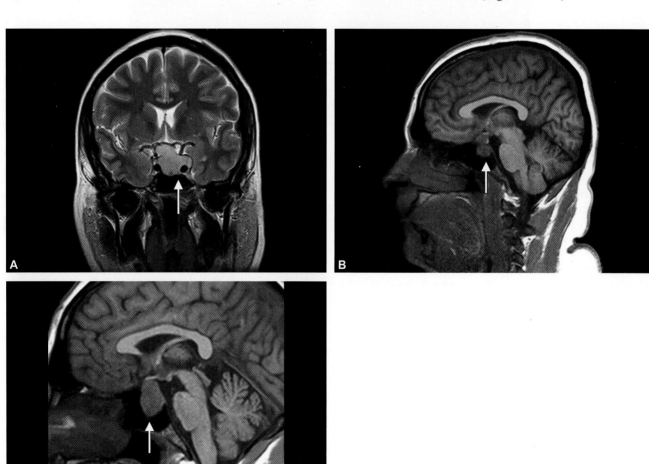

Figs. 1A to C: MRI of the pituitary showing a sellar mass with a suprasellar extension (shown with arrow).

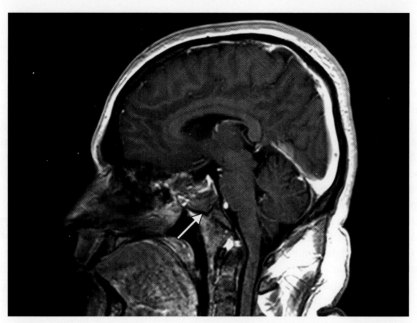

Fig. 2: Three months postoperative MRI of the brain with contrast showing a residual lesion (shown with arrow).

cysts or haemorrhage. The diagnosis of Hardy's Grade B/E and Knosps Grade 3 invasive non-functioning pituitary macrodenoma with panhypopituitarism was made. He was started on oral thyroxine and prednisolone. He was referred to the Department of Neurosurgery for further management.

He was started on oral tri-iodothyronine, 25 mcg thrice daily for 2 days prior to the surgery and advised to continue for 2 days postoperatively. Subsequently, he underwent a endoscopic transnasal trans-sphenoidal subtotal excision of the pituitary macroadenoma leaving behind tumor that is extending into the left cavernous sinus. His vision improved postoperatively and he was continued on thyroxine and prednisolone replacement.

The histopathology of the tumor showed features suggestive of an atypical null cell adenoma with focal LH positivity. He was planned for stereotactic radiosurgery, in case he has a residual tumor at 3 months follow up.

In his review after 3 months, he was asymptomatic and the MRI pituitary showed a minimal enhancing tissue in the superior aspect of the left cavernous sinus which was suggestive of residual lesion (Fig. 2). He was planned to be kept in follow-up by repeating a MRI Pituitary after a year as the tumor was non-functioning in nature.

DISCUSSION

Non-functioning pituitary adenomas are relatively common pituitary tumors. A large number of these tumors are incidentally found pituitary microadenomas (< 1 cm) which are of not much clinical importance. In general macroadenomas present with a history suggestive of mass effect in the form of visual compromise and/or hypopituitarism. At the time of diagnosis visual field defects roughly seen in 70% of patients with non-functioning macroadenoma. A large majority of these tumors are positive for glycoprotein (Alpha subunit) production going by immunocytochemistry. However, only a minority of these tumors actively secrete intact gonadotropins or glycoprotein subunits. The therapy aims at improving the vision or acuity and/or correcting the hypopituitarism.[1,2]

REFERENCES

1. Jaffe CA. Clinically non-functioning pituitary adenoma. Pituitary. 2006;9 (4):317–21.
2. Rogers A, Karavitaki N, Wass JAH. Diagnosis and management of prolactinomas and non-functioning pituitary adenomas. BMJ. 2014;10; 349 (sep10 7):g5390–g5390.

CASE 24

A 65-year-old, Mrs. S presented with progressively increasing holo-cranial headache and diminution of vision for the past one year duration. There were no history of coarsening of facial features, or hirsuitism, abnormal gain or loss of weight, heat or cold intolerance. Also, there were no history of altered behaviour or seizures, sudden episodes of headache, vomiting or loss of consciousness. She is a known patient with type 2 diabetes mellitus and hypertension since the past four-year and on regular medications. She was a postmenopausal lady for the past 10 years time. Her visual acuity was 6/12 in the right eye and 6/9 in the left eye with bi-temporal hemianopia

Her investigations revealed: Serum 8 am Cortisol- 14.09 ug/dL, Total T4- 6.1 ug%, Free thyroxine - 0.79 ng%, Thyroid-Stimulating Hormone (TSH) - 1.64 uIU/mL, Lute- inizing Hormone (LH) - 1.84 mIU/mL, Follicle-Stimulating Hormone (FSH) - 4.14 mIU/mL, Prolactin in dilution (HPRL) < 0.30ng/mL. In view of her symptoms and abnormal blood parameters, a magnetic resonance imaging (MRI) of the brain was ordered. Shown below are the images Figures 1A to E.

WHAT IS THE DIAGNOSIS?

The MRI of the pituitary with gadolinium contrast revealed a contrast enhancing sellar and suprasellar mass measuring 2.3 × 2.4 × 3.6 cm and distorting the floor of the third ventricle with involvement of the bilateral cavernous

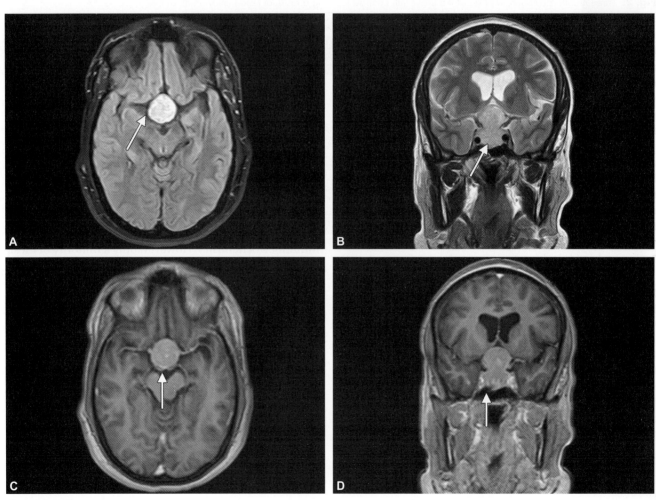

Figs. 1A to D

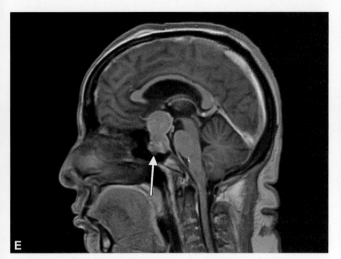

Figs. 1A to E: MRI of the brain showing a sellar mass with suprasellar extension (shown with arrow).

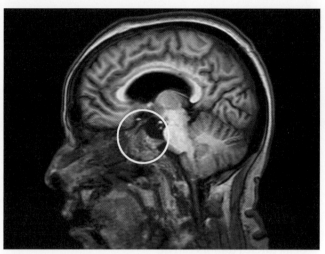

Fig. 2: Immediate postoperative MRI showing post operative changes with no obvious residual lesion (shown with a circle).

sinus. The lesion also had eroded the sphenoid sinus floor inferiorly too (Figs. 1A to E).

The patient clinically presented with features of a suprasellar mass with chiasmatic compression without any features of raised intracranial pressure. Her hormonal evaluation revealed a low FTC with normal TSH suggestive of a central hypothyroidism and was started on oral thyroxine. Her FSH and LH levels were inappropriately low for her postmenopausal status, however her serum cortisol was normal. Her MRI brain showed a Hardy grade C/E with Knosps grade 3 invasive pituitary macroadenoma. So, the diagnosis of non-functional pituitary macroadenoma with partial hypopituitarism was made. She underwent a radical excision (transnasal transsphenoidal endoscopic excision) of the pituitary macroadenoma.

The surgical specimen, histopathologically showed features suggestive of a gonadotroph adenoma (FSH and alpha subunit positive). Her immediate post operative MRI of the brain showed no residue in the sellar or suprasellar region (Fig. 2)

Postoperatively, there was a significant improvement in her visual acuity and the visual fields. She was given perioperative steroids for three days. However after the steroid withdrawal her 8 AM serum Cortisol on the 7th postoperative day was 6.96 ug% with a post 1 hour synacthen (Co-synthropin) serum Cortisol levels of 33.11 ug%. She was advised her to come back for a repeat check-up with a MRI pituitary after 3 months.

DISCUSSION

Patients presenting with a suspected or known pituitary adenoma need to undergo a complete radiographic and endocrine assessment prior to the initiation of either medical or surgical therapy. MRI of the pituitary is the modality of choice and should be requested with a localized pituitary protocol involving thin cuts in the coronal and sagittal planes. In addition to the radiographic imaging, the patient's baseline endocrine panel should include serum Growth Hormone (GH), Insulin-like growth factor (IGF-I), TSH, Free-T4, T3, Prolactin(PRL), Adrenocorticotropic Hormone (ACTH), 8 am cortisol, LH, FSH, and testosterone levels.

Hardy's classification system.

Sella turcica tumors can be

1. Noninvasive
   a. Grade 0, intact with normal contour;
   b. Grade I, intact with bulging floor
   c. Grade II, intact, enlarged fossa

2. Invasive
   d. Grade III, localized sellar destruction
   e. Grade IV, diffuse destruction

The other classification is

1. Grade A, suprasellar cistern only
2. Grade B, upto the recess of the third ventricle not compressing
3. Grade C, compressing the whole anterior third ventricle
4. Grade D, intracranial extradural
5. Grade E, extracranial extradural [cavernous sinus][1,2]

REFERENCES

1. Chacko A G, Chandy M J. Transsphenoidal line of vision on MRI for pituitary tumor surgery. Neurol India 2002;50:136
2. Di Ieva A, Rotondo F, Syro LV, et al. Aggressive pituitary adenomas—diagnosis and emerging treatments. Nat Rev Endocrinol. 2014;10(7):423–35.

CASE 25

Mr. M, a 35-year-old gentleman, presented to us with progressive diminution of vision in the both eyes for the past 6 months with lethargy and tiredness for the past 2 months. There were no history to suggest a hormonal excess or a deficiency. He had no co-morbidities.

His examination was within normal limits except for a vision of 6/18 in both the eyes with bitemporal hemianopia. However there were no focal neurological deficits.

The blood tests revealed: Serum 8 am Cortisol 16.88 ug/dL with all the other hormonal investigations been normal. Further a magnetic resonance imaging (MRI) pituitary was ordered, the images of which are shown in Figures 1A and B.

WHAT IS THE PRELIMINARY DIAGNOSIS?

His MRI of the pituitary with gadolinium revealed a contrast enhancing mass measured 3.46 × 3.5 × 2.5 cm in the sella with suprasellar extension with right cavernous sinus involvement. Superiorly the mass was compressing the floor the third ventricle. Laterally it was abutting the medial wall of the internal carotid artery bilaterally (Figs. 1 and 2).

So, the diagnosis of a Hardy's grade C/E pituitary macroadenoma was made. He underwent a binostril endoscopic transsphenoidal excision of the non-functional pituitary adenoma. The biopsy was reported as an atypical pituitary adenoma with MIB-1 labelling index of 3–4%.

Postoperatively the vision in both eyes showed an improvement The postoperative images are shown in Figures 3A and B. On the 3rd postoperative day, he had symptoms of hypocortisolemia in the form of vomiting, excessive tiredness and low blood pressure with a significant postural drop in blood pressure. He was found to have hyponatremia with low serum cortisol level, 3.87 ug%. He was started on parenteral steroids followed by oral prednisolone. He was kept on Tab. Prednisolone 5-0–2.5 mg at discharge and advised to review after 3 months.

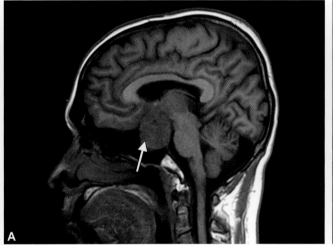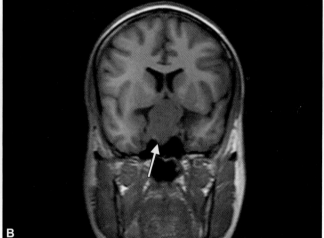

Figs. 1A and B: MRI of the pituitary showing a sellar mass with suprasellar extension (shown with arrow).

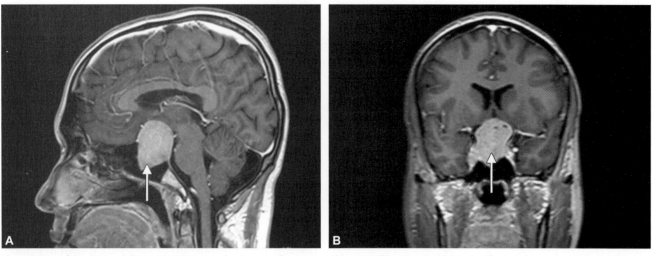

Figs. 2A and B: Postgadolinium MRI Pituitary showing a sellar mass with suprasellar extension (shown with arrow).

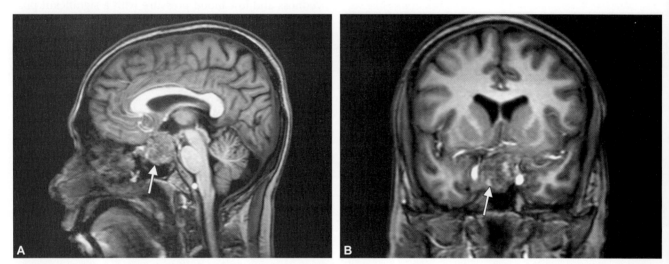

Figs. 3A and B: Immediate postoperative MRI Brain showing postoperative changes (Hematoma and fat packing) in the sellar suprasellar region (shown with arrow).

DISCUSSION

The Knosp classification system has been used to quantify invasion of the cavernous sinus, in which only grades 3 and 4 define true invasion of the tumor into the cavernous sinus. Grade 0, no cavernous sinus involvement; grades 1 and 2, the tumor pushes into the medial wall of the cavernous sinus, but does not go beyond a hypothetical line extending between the centres of the two segments of the internal carotid artery (grade 1) or it goes beyond such a line, but without passing a line tangent to the lateral margins of the artery itself (grade 2); grade 3, the tumor extends laterally to the internal carotid artery within the cavernous sinus; grade 4, total encasement of the intra-cavernous carotid artery.[1,2]

REFERENCES

1. Chacko A G, Chandy M J. Transsphenoidal line of vision on MRI for pituitary tumor surgery. Neurol India 2002;50:136
2. Di Ieva A, Rotondo F, Syro LV, et al. Aggressive pituitary adenomas—diagnosis and emerging treatments.Nat Rev Endocrinol. 2014;13;10(7):423–35.

CASE 26

A 55-year-old, Mrs. K presented with progressive decrease in vision bilaterally, left more than the right eye since the past 4 years, which had worsened more rapidly over the last two years. There was a history of intermittent holocranial headache for the last one year, but had no associated vomiting or loss of consciousness. There was no history suggestive of any hormonal dysfunctions or any urinary complaints. She was seen by the Endocrinologist earlier and was told to have abnormal thyroid function tests, for which she was started on once daily 100mcg of oral thyroxine. She also had history of loss of memory since the past few months. Her visual acuity was 6/9 in the right eye and 2/60 in the left eye (counting fingers at 3 feet). There was temporal pallor seen in the left optic disc with bitemporal hemianopia.

She was investigated further for a pituitary lesion and for imbalanced pituitary hormonal axes which revealed T4 - 6.8 ug%, FTC - 0.64 ng% with Thyroid-Stimulating Hormone (TSH) - 1.049 uIU/mL. 8 am Cortisol -5.80 ug%. Post 1 hour synacthen serum cortisol -32.63, Luteinizing Hormone (LH) 0.394 mIU/mL, Follicle-Stimulating Hormone (FSH) -1.54 mIU/mL.

An magnetic resonance imaging (MRI) brain was done and showed the following changes (Figs. 1A to E).

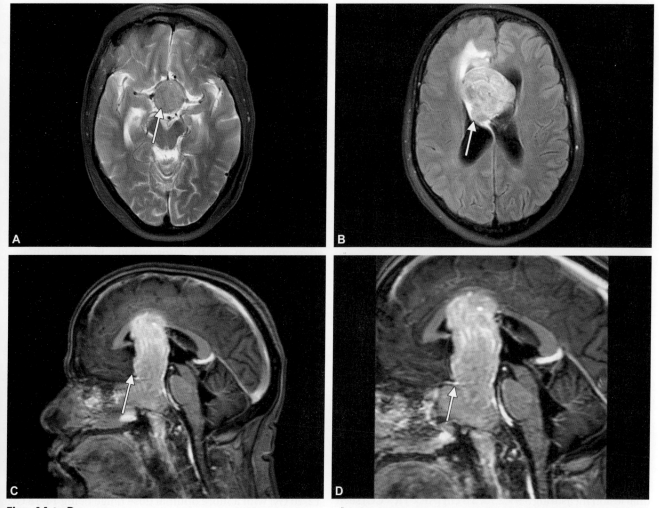

Figs. 1A to D

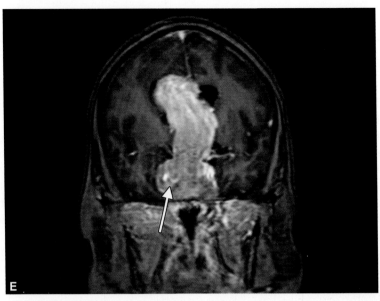

Figs. 1A to E: Massive lesion in the sellar and suprasellar region (shown with arrow).

WHAT IS THE DIAGNOSIS?

The MRI of the brain showed a well defined sella-suprasellar mass measuring 7.8 × 4.8 × 4 cm, eroding the sella and extending into the sphenoid sinus and posterior ethmoid sinus, and also infiltrating the clivus inferiorly. Superiorly the tumor extended into third ventricle in the midline and also along the right side of the third ventricle, reaching upto the undersurface of the body of the corpus callosum, pushing it upwards suggestive of a giant pituitary macroadenoma (Figs. 1A to E). The nature of the disease was discussed with the relatives and she was planned for a transcranial resection of the tumor, in view of its large size and the extent of suprasellar extension. A right frontal craniotomy and transcortical approach to subtotal excision of the giant non-functional pituitary adenoma was done. She developed diabetes insipidus postoperatively which was managed with the Desmopressin. The histopathology report showed a silent corticotroph adenoma with weak FSH staining. Thus the patient was diagnosed to have Hardy's Grade D/E giant invasive silent corticotroph pituitary macroadenoma. She was discharged with phenytoin (300 mg Once daily), Prednisolone (5 mg Once daily) thyroxine (100 mcg once daily) and oral Desmopressin (50 mcg Once daily at bedtime). Stereotactic radiotherapy for the residual tumor was planned for the residual after 3 months.

The MRI Pituitary after 3 months demonstrated a residual lesion measuring 3.9 × 2.7 × 3.5 cm (AP × TR × CC) seen in the sellar and cavernous sinus region with extension into the ethmoid air cells anteriorly encasing the right internal carotid artery and cavernous sinus bilaterally (Figs. 2A to F). She was referred to the Department of Radiotherapy as previously planned in view of the massive residual tumor.

DISCUSSION

Radiation is given an adjuvant to the subtotal resection of the nonfunctioning pituitary macroadenoma or as a primary therapy in the setting of surgical inaccessibility, medical inoperability, or eventually that of the patient's choice. The goal of radiation therapy in nonfunctioning adenomas is to arrest tumor growth. Even though the radiation therapy clearly reduce the risk of recurrence of nonfunctioning adenomas, this decision must be made depending on the histological and molecular analyses of tumors, such as tumor proliferative index. The tumor proliferation index has the ability to predict whether these tumors can recur also can be used as a guide for the choice of adjuvant radiation therapy in the future. Radiation can be delivered either by single fraction stereotactic radio surgery (SRS) (with Gamma knife, linear accelerator SRS, or proton SRS) or by any of a number of fractionated radiation therapy modalities (linear accelerator-based therapies of stereotactic radiotherapy, three-dimensional conformal radiation therapy, intensity-modulated radiation therapy, or proton therapy). Common SRS doses are 12-20 Gy, with a more optimal dose range being 14-18 Gy. The common fractionated doses are 45-54 Gy at 1.8 Gy per fraction, with adequate doses being 45-50.4 Gy.[1,2]

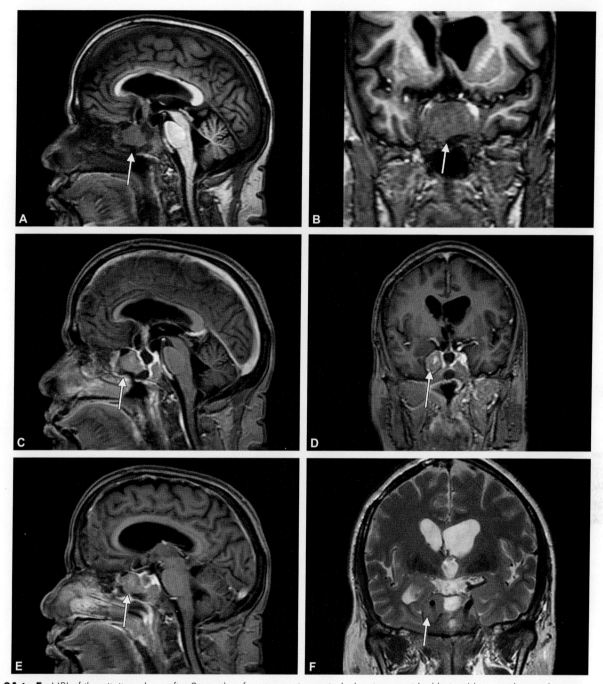

Figs. 2A to F: MRI of the pituitary done after 3 months of postoperative period, showing a residual lesion (shown with arrow).

REFERENCES

1. Sheehan JP, Starke RM, Mathieu D, et al. Gamma knife radiosurgery for the management of nonfunctioning pituitary adenomas: a multicenter study. J Neurosurg. 2013; 119(2):446-56.

2. Loeffler JS, Shih HA. Radiation therapy in the management of pituitary adenomas. J Clin Endocrinol Metab. 2011;96 (7):1992-2003.

CASE 27

A 45-year-old gentleman was diagnosed to have Hardy's grade C pituitary adenoma of size 2.2 cm × 2.6 cm × 1.4 cm with apoplexy and was subsequently discharged on Prednisolone and Thyroxine 15 years back. The surgery was deferred as he did not have any field defects. A repeat computed tomography (CT) scan done after 15 years had shown a suprasellar mass, demonstrated in Figure 1.

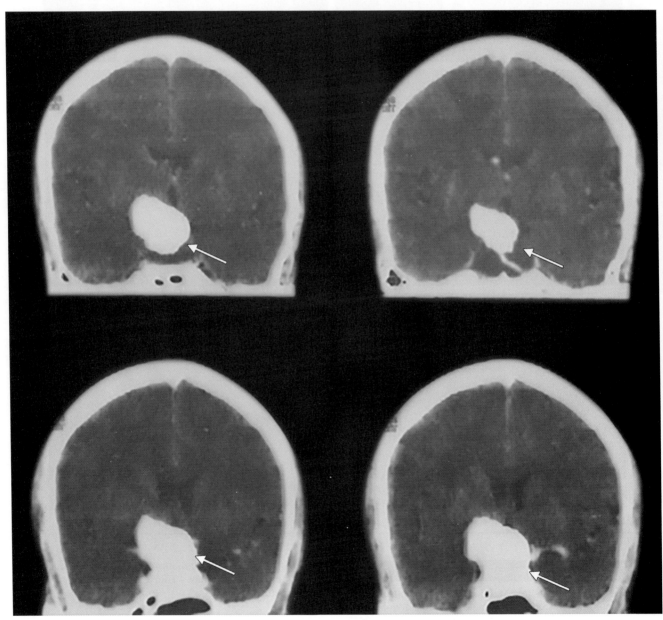

Fig. 1: CT brain -Coronal image showing a calcified mass in the sellar-suprasellar region (shown with arrow).

WHAT IS THE DIAGNOSIS?

He was diagnosed to have calcified craniopharyngioma or pituitary stone due to a calcified pituitary macroadenoma.

DISCUSSION

Calcification is a well recognized but relatively uncommon feature of functional and non-functional pituitary tumors. The differential diagnosis of calcified lesions in the sellar region includes craniopharyngioma, meningioma, aneurysm, optic/hypothalamic glioma, germ cell tumors and rarely a Rathke's cleft cyst. Prolactinomas tend to undergo dystrophic calcification, which can appear microscopically as Psammoma bodies or encompass the entire mass ("pituitary stone"). The radiological appearance of calcification in pituitary adenomas has been found to be either an intratumoural "pituitary stone" or capsular "egg-shell like calcification."[1,2]

REFERENCES

1. Kumar V, Abbas AK, Fausto N. Robbins and Cotran Pathologic Basis of Disease, 7th Ed. Elsevier; 2005:1156-64
2. Webster J, Peters JR, John R, et al. Pituitary stone: two cases of densely calcified thyrotrophin-secreting pituitary adenomas. Clin Endocrinol (Oxf). 1994;40(1):137–43.

CASE 28

A 25-year-old gentleman from Bangladesh presented to our pituitary clinic with history of headache and history of bumping to the sides of the door while walking even during the daytime. He did not give history of any endocrine dysfunction. Magnetic resonance imaging (MRI) done is displayed in Figures 1 and 2.

WHAT IS THE DIAGNOSIS?

Magnetic resonance imaging (MRI) pituitary showed a large sellar and suprasellar mass that was T1 hypointense and T2 heterogeneously hyperintense lesion measuring ~64 × 64 × 56 mm—giant pituitary macroadenoma/clival chordoma (shown with a circle) (Figs. 1 and 2). He underwent transnasal transsphenoidal excision of the mass. The histopathological biopsy was reported as an atypical pituitary adenoma (Silent Adrenocorticotropic Hormone [ACTH] and focal follicle stimulating hormone [FSH]) with a MIB-1 labelling index of 7%. The postoperative MRI—Pituitary images are shown in Figures in 3 and 4, which showed a residual tumor along the periphery, in the region of the cavernous sinuses bilaterally and a component in the central basal frontal region and in the right clival region is noted (shown with circles and arrow). He was referred to the Department of Radiotherapy for further management.

Thus, the patient was diagnosed to have Non functioning pituitary macroadenoma—Hardy's grade -D/E and Knosps Grade 4.

DISCUSSION

The main aim for the treatment of patients with clinically non-functioning pituitary macroadenomas are the preservation or restoration of the visual function and also adequate long-term tumor control. In case of a conservative approach, i.e in patients who are kept in follow up, the hormonal assessments should be done every 6 months because of the chance of remaining pituitary functions been compromised by growth of the macroadenoma. A MRI of the pituitary should be repeated within 1 year. Thereafter, radiological assessment by MRI is recommended with yearly intervals, which may be extended to two yearly intervals in the absence of progression of the pituitary macroadenoma.

Follow-up of the patients post surgery should include an intial ophthalmological assessment within 3-4 months after surgery, and subsequent assessments after 1 and 2 year, to estimate the final effect of surgical treatment on visual function. However, it is recommended to assess with a MRI pituitary the effectiveness of surgery about 3-4 months, because it takes such an amount of time for the resolution of blood clots and the packed items done during the surgery. A second postoperative MRI should be performed about 1 year after the surgery. Thereafter, the frequency of MRI's depends on the volume of the residual tumor and the distance between the residual adenoma and the optic chiasm. Often radiotherapy can cause delayed decrements in the pituitary functions

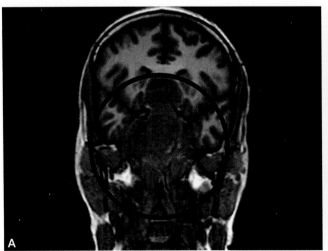
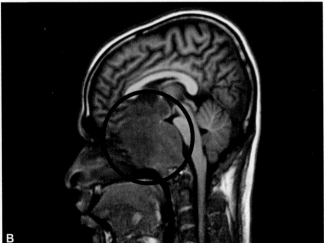

Figs. 1A and B: MRI of brain showing-T1 weighted images.

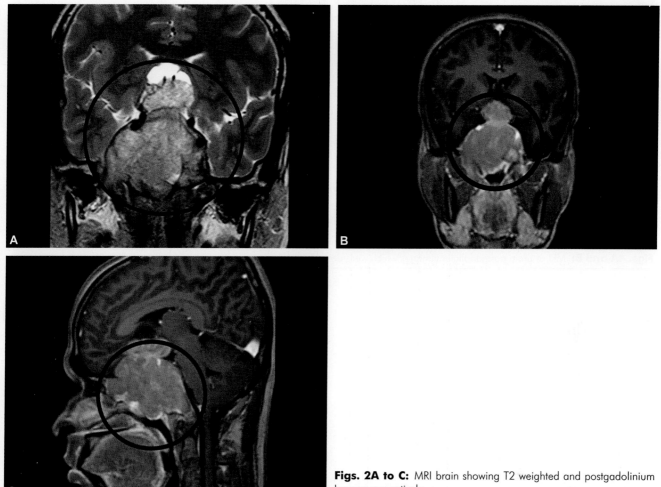

Figs. 2A to C: MRI brain showing T2 weighted and postgadolinium Images respectively.

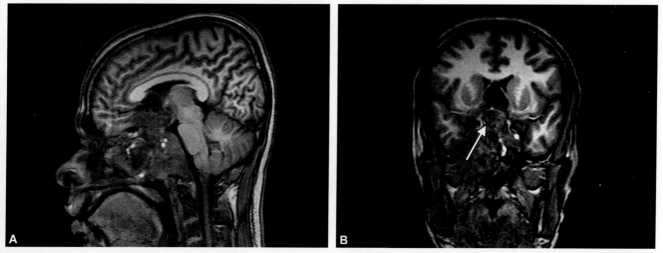

Figs. 3A and B: Immediate postoperative, MRI brain with T1 weighted images.

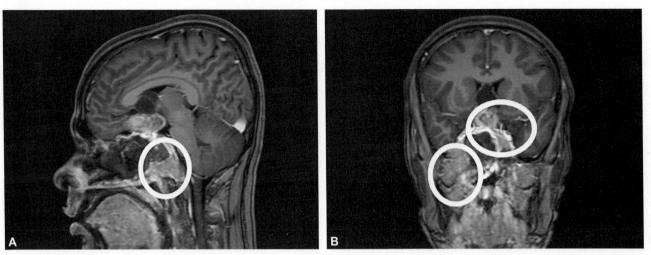

Figs. 4A and B: MRI of brain postgadolinium Images which were done during the immediate postoperative period.

upto 5–10 years after the radiotherapy. Therefore, in the absence of panhypopituitarism, patients treated with the concomitant RT/Radiosurgery should be evaluated every 6 months.[1,2]

REFERENCES

1. Dekkers OM, Pereira AM, Romijn JA. Treatment and Follow-Up of Clinically Non-functioning Pituitary Macroadenomas. J Clin Endocrinol Metab. 2008;93(10):3717–26.
2. Rieken S, Habermehl D, Welzel T, et al. Long-term toxicity and prognostic factors of radiation therapy for secreting and non-secreting pituitary adenomas. Radiat Oncol. 2013; 8(1):18.

CASE 29

A 40-year-old, Mrs. S presented with history of polydipsia and polyuria and bi-frontal headache for 9 months duration. There were no symptoms suggestive of an anterior pituitary hormonal dysfunction or a pituitary apoplexy. She was diagnosed to have Diabetes Insipidus and on oral Desmopressin. A Magnetic Resonance Imaging (MRI) brain demonstrated the features which are shown in Figures 1 and 2.

WHAT IS THE DIFFERENTIAL DIAGNOSIS?

The MRI pituitary showed a hypointensity on T1W images with peripheral enhancement on post contrast images, however in T2 weighted image the lesion was hyperintense in nature, measuring 15 × 10 × 11 mm (TR × AP × CC) (Figs. 1 and 2 shown with arrow). The differentials considered were Rathke's cleft cyst, Pituitary abscess, cystic craniopharyngioma, cystic pituitary adenoma or pituitary apoplexy. The patient underwent transnasal transsphenoidal excision of the pituitary lesion. The histopathological specimen revealed adenohypophyseal tissue with parts of a cyst wall composed of hyalinised fibro collagenous tissue lined focally by single layer of flattened to cuboidal epithelium which is immuno positive for pancytokeratin, features suggestive of a Rathke's cleft cyst. She was advised to continue the desmopressin postoperatively and she was advised to be on regular follow up.

DISCUSSION

Rathke's cleft cysts are congenital, non-neoplastic sellar and suprasellar cysts derived from remnants of Rathke's pouch. The lumen of Rathke's pouch develops as a rostral out pouching of the primitive oral cavity during the third or fourth week of gestation.

A Rathke's pouch has an anterior and a posterior wall and a central embryonic cleft. The anterior wall of the pouch proliferates to form the anterior lobe of the pituitary gland and the pars tuberalis; the posterior wall becomes the pars intermedia. The residual lumen of the pouch is reduced to a narrow Rathke's cleft, which generally regresses. It is the persistence and enlargement of this cleft that is said to be the cause of a symptomatic Rathke's cleft cyst. These lesions are more commonly diagnosed preoperatively or discovered incidentally with the availability of modern imaging techniques. Often, it is difficult to differentiate

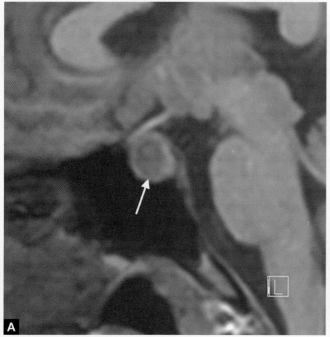
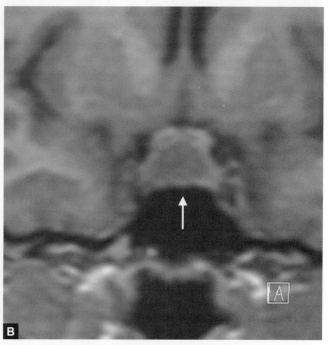

Figs. 1A and B: MRI of the pituitary showing T1 weighted images.

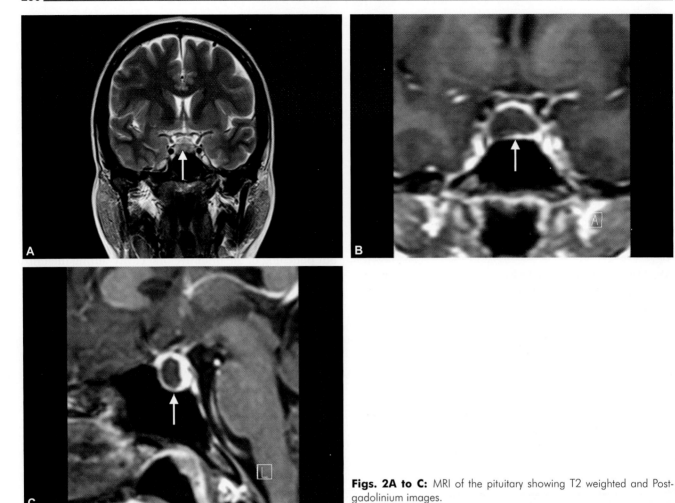

Figs. 2A to C: MRI of the pituitary showing T2 weighted and Post-gadolinium images.

Rathke's cleft cysts from a craniopharyngioma or cystic pituitary adenomas by radiologic studies. Because of the cystic fluid of Rathke's cleft cyst, cystic craniopharyngioma, and cystic pituitary adenoma which show variable signal intensities in MR images, the diagnosis of Rathke's cleft cyst is not possible based on signal intensity of cyst fluid on MR images alone.[1,2]

REFERENCES

1. Nemoto Y, Inoue Y, Fukuda T, et al. MR appearance of Rathke's cleft cysts. Neuroradiology. 1988;30(2):155–9.
2. Byun WM, Kim OL, Kim D sug. MR Imaging Findings of Rathke's Cleft Cysts: Significance of Intracystic Nodules. Am J Neuroradiol. 2000;21(3):485–8.

CASE **30**

A 74-year-old gentleman was apparently normal till 1 year ago, when his relatives noticed irrelevant speech and was evaluated, found to have hyponatremia. He was evaluated in his hometown initially and was referred here. In view of the recent onset altered sensorium he was advised a Magnetic Resonance Imaging (MRI) brain which is shown in Figures 1 and 2.

WHAT IS THE DIAGNOSIS?

His investigations revealed an undetectable level of serum 8 am cortisol with a low thyroxine and Thyroid-Stimulating Hormone (TSH) levels, suggesting hypocortisolemia and central hypothyroidism respectively. He also was found to have undetectable levels of serum testosterone with suppressed LH and FSH levels. The MRI brain revealed a T1 weighted hyperintense and T2 weighted hypointense sellar-suprasellar lesion with a small posteroinferior hypointense component, suggestive of a Rathke's cleft cyst or a cystic craniopharyngioma with panhypopituitarism.

In view of his age and also no compromise of the vision, he was kept under follow-up regarding the probable Rathke's cleft cyst.

DISCUSSION

The signal characteristics of Rathke's cleft cyst vary according to the cyst composition which may be mucoid or serous. In T1 weighted image 50% are hyperintense (high protein content), 50% are hypointense. However in T2 weighted image 70% are hyperintense and 30% are iso or hypointense. In postcontrast Gadolinium T1 weighted image no contrast enhancement of the cyst is seen, however a thin enhancing rim of surrounding compressed pituitary tissue may be apparent. In 70–80% of cases a small non-enhancing intracystic nodule can be identified which is

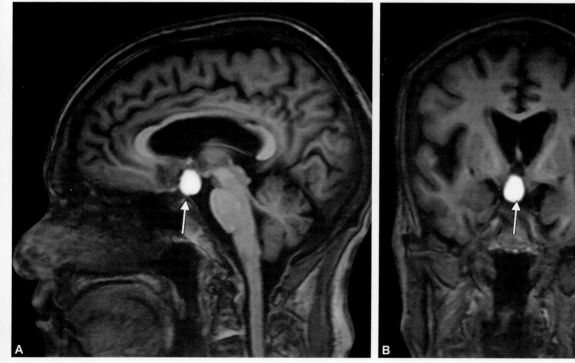

Figs. 1A and B: MRI of the brain-T1 weighted images.

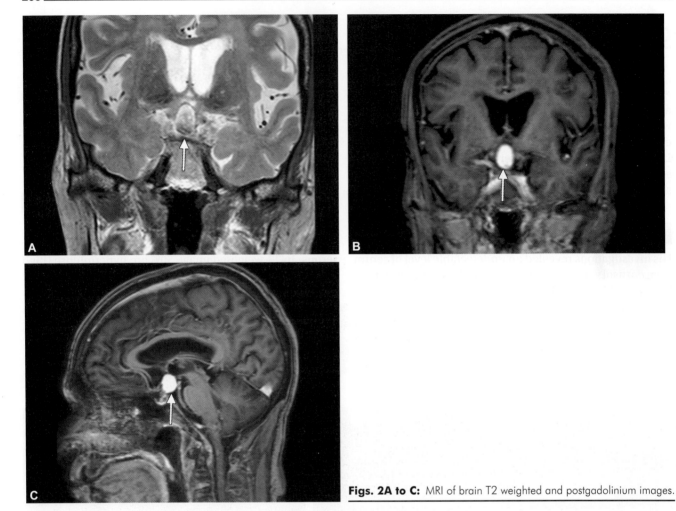

Figs. 2A to C: MRI of brain T2 weighted and postgadolinium images.

virtually pathognomic of a Rathke's cleft cyst. When seen it is hyperintense to surrounding fluid on T1 and hypointense on T2. Depending on the signal of the surrounding fluid it may be inapparent on one or other sequence. Occasionally, a fluid-fluid level may be seen (particularly if there has been a hemorrhage).[1,2]

REFERENCES

1. Rajaratnam S. Pituitary gland imaging. Indian J Endocrinol Metab. 2013;17(7):100.
2. Chacko G, Chacko AG, Lombardero M, et al. Clinicopathologic correlates of giant pituitary adenomas. J Clin Neurosci Off J Neurosurg Soc Australas. 2009;16(5):660–5.

CASE 31

A 33-year-old lady presented with history of holocranial headache since the past one year. She also revealed that she takes 7 litres of fluids per day and also having amenorrhoea for the same duration. However, 3 months prior to admission she had sudden onset vomiting with associated severe headache and she was diagnosed to have hypocortisolemia. She was started on oral prednisolone by her family physician.

WHAT ARE THE DIFFERENTIAL DIAGNOSES?

Investigations done are shown below: Serum sodium 143 meq/dL. Luteinizing hormons (LH)-5.4 Miu/mL, Follicle-Stimulating Hormone (FSH) 5 Miu/ml, Total T4-13.4 mcg/mL, Free T4-1.1 ng/mL and Prolactin in dilution-44 ng/mL. She underwent a water deprivation test which showed a failure of concentration of the urine (Urine osmolality <200 mOsm) with high serum sodium

(>145 mq/dL) levels, which were responding to the subcutaneous vasopressin, suggestive of central diabetes Insipidus.

The magnetic resonance imaging (MRI) Brain demonstrated a well-defined T1 hypointense and T2 hyperintense sellar-suprasellar lesion measuring ~16 × 14 × 14 mm (TR × AP × CC) which had a peripheral rim of enhancement on post-contrast images (Figs. 1 and 2, shown with arrow). The differentials considered were Rathke's cleft cyst, Pituitary abscess, cystic craniopharyngioma, cystic pituitary adenoma or pituitary apoplexy.

She underwent a transnasal transsphenoidal excision of the sellar-suprasellar mass. The histopathology specimen had fragments of adeno-hypophyseal tissue with parts of a lesion composed of dense infiltrates of lymphocytes, plasma cells, histiocytes and foamy macrophages set in a sclerotic stroma suggesting a pituitary abscess. MRI of the brain which was done after 3 months of the postoperative

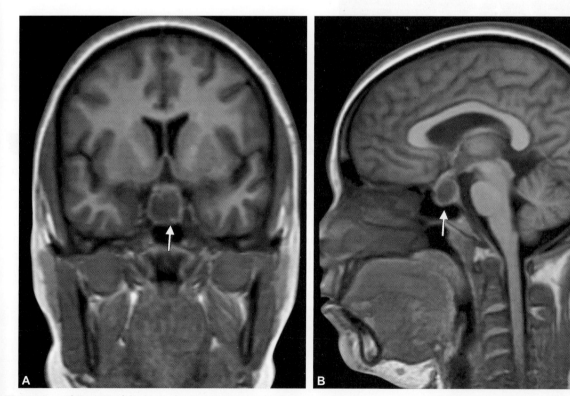

Figs. 1A and B: MRI of the brain showing T1 weighted images.

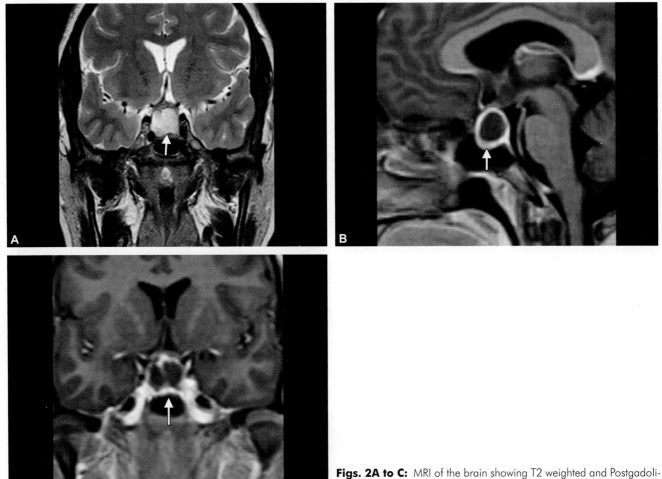

Figs. 2A to C: MRI of the brain showing T2 weighted and Postgadolinium images.

period showed a thickened optic nerve and chiasm, with an evidence of small enhancing residual lesion (Figs. 3 and 4).

She was advised for a close follow as she was asymptomatic. At 6 months postoperative period her Hypothalamic Pituitary Adrenal axis recovered, however she was continued on oral hormone replacement therapy and oral desmopressin.

DISCUSSION

Pituitary abscess represents less than 1% of all cases of pituitary disease. Pituitary abscess is caused either by a hematogenous seeding to the pituitary gland or by direct extension of an adjacent infection such as sphenoid sinusitis, Cavernous sinus thrombophlebitis or a contaminated CSF fistula. The most common infectious agents are

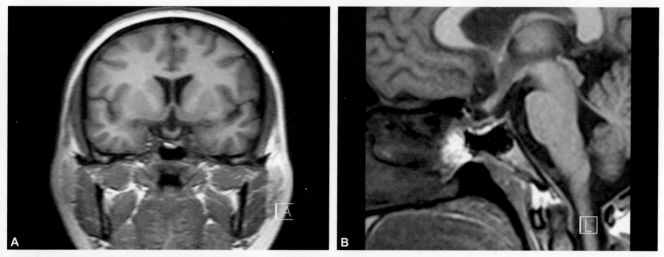

Figs. 3A and B: MRI of the brain done after 3 months postoperative period.

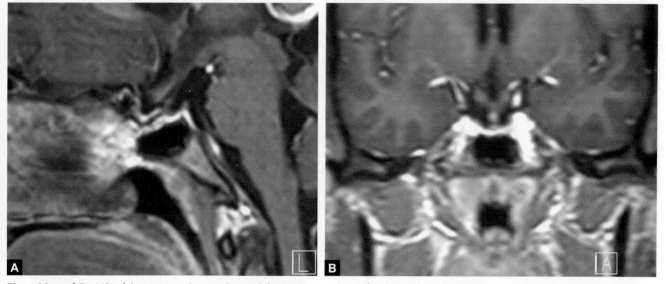

Figs. 4A and B: MRI of the pituitary showing Postgadolinium Images done after 3 months postoperative period.

Gram-positive cocci. Sterile cultures are frequent due to the antibiotic therapy initiated before or during surgery. The most common presenting clinical features of pituitary abscess are headache, visual complaints, and pituitary dysfunction ranging from hyperprolactinemia to panhypopituitarism.[1,2]

REFERENCES

1. Vates GE, Berger MS, Wilson CB. Diagnosis and management of pituitary abscess: a review of twenty-four cases. J Neurosurg. 2001;95(2):233–41.
2. Thomas N, Wittert GA, Scott G, et al. Infection of a Rathke's cleft cyst: a rare cause of pituitary abscess. Case illustration. J Neurosurg. 1998;89(4):682.

CASE 32

A 34-year-old gentleman presented with a 6-month history of polydipsia and polyuria with a daily consumption of 7–8 liters of fluids. Historically, he had holocranial headache but with no symptoms of raised intracranial hypertension.He also did not give any history to suggest anterior pituitary hormonal dysfunction. The water deprivation test confirmed the patient having a partial central diabetes insipidus. The Initial Magnetic Resonance Imaging (MRI) brain is shown in Figure 1. After 1 year of therapy, the MRI brain was repeated (Fig. 2).

WHAT IS THE DIAGNOSIS?

Figure 1 showed a homogenous contrast-enhancing mass with the pituitary stalk thickening (shown with arrow). Based on the clinical (diabetes insipidus), laboratory, and radiologic features (symmetric mass with homogenous enhancement and stalk thickening), the diagnosis of lymphocytic hypophysitis was made. The repeat MRI Brain shown in Figure 2 showed a complete resolution of the stalk thickening after treatment. After 1 year of steroid treatment, the patient had a marked resolution of stalk thickening with a normal-sized pituitary gland. Even though he did not develop any deficiency of anterior pituitary hormones

during follow-up there was no resolution of diabetes insipidus for which he was treated with desmopressin.

DISCUSSION

The differential diagnoses such as sarcoidosis, histiocytosis, lymphoproliferative disorders and other granulomatous lesions need to be ruled out before diagnosing autoimmune hypophysitis. Hypophysitis is of five types depending on the histology. They are Lymphocytic, inflammatory, granulomatous, xanthogranulomatous and necrotizing hypophysitis. Lymphocytic hypophysitis is a rare inflammatory disorder of the pituitary with a definite female predilection usually during the post-partum period. Lymphocytic hypophysitis is extremely rare in men, presenting with headache and visual disturbances with a wide range of symptoms such as anterior pituitary hormonal deficiency or an isolated diabetes insipidus to panhypopituitarism. The etiology of the disease is unknown, but it is associated with autoimmune diseases like thyroiditis and adrenalitis, which suggests an auto immune cause with IgG4 antibody been implicated in patients. Glucocorticoid therapy has been successful for the remission of symptoms and for reducing the lesion size. Transsphenoidal surgery is reserved for patients who do not respond to medical therapy.[1,2]

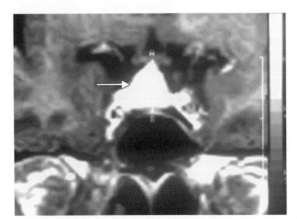

Fig. 1: MRI of the brain done during the first visit.

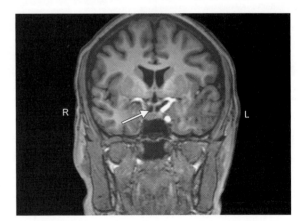

Fig. 2: MRI of the brain done after 1 year of the treatment.

REFERENCES

1. Paul T, Koshy G, Asha HS, et al. Visual vignette. Autoimmune hypophysitis (lymphocytic hypophysitis). Endocr Pract. 2008;14(8):1064.

2. Caturegli P, Newschaffer C, Olivi A, et al. Autoimmune hypophysitis. Endocr Rev. 2005;26:599-614.

CASE 33

A 38-year-old gentleman was apparently well 6 months ago, when he started developing decrease in vision of the left eye which progressively worsened followed by involvement of the right eye. He had a history of numbness on the left half of the face. He also complained of reduced beard growth and sexual dysfunction with occasional projectile vomiting and associated headache. He had cranial nerve deficits in the form of bilateral 6th nerve involvement with left 5th Cranial nerve ophthalmic and mandibular division involvement (Fig. 1). Magnetic Resonance Imaging (MRI) brain is displayed in Figures 2A and B.

WHAT IS THE DIAGNOSIS? WHAT DO YOU THINK SHOULD BE DONE?

The biochemistry investigations were suggestive of central hypothyroidism with other hormonal axes been normal. Pituitary imaging was suggestive of an inflammatory pituitary lesion with extensive dural thickening and involvement of the left cavernous sinus and optic nerve (shown with the arrows) (Figs. 2A and B).

The differential diagnoses considered were inflammatory conditions like sarcoidosis, histiocytosis, granulomatous

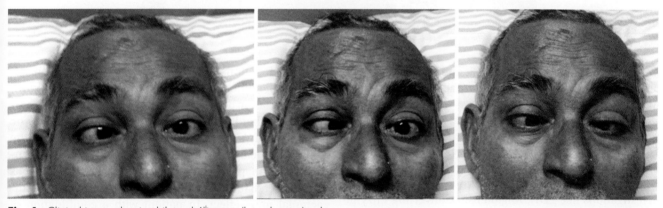

Fig. 1. Clinical image showing bilateral 6th nerve (lateral rectus) palsy.

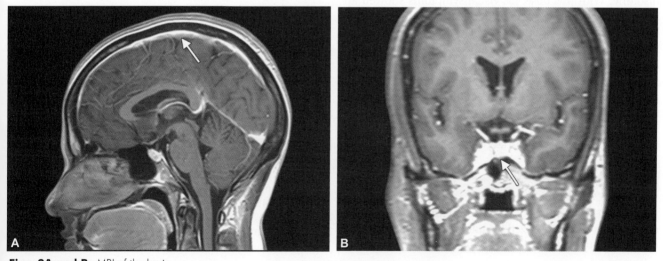

Figs. 2A and B: MRI of the brain.

Fig. 3: Histopathological image showing a lymphocytic infiltration of the pituitary gland.

infectious diseases like tuberculosis and chronic meningitis, hematological conditions like lymphoma or a metastasis to the pituitary gland.

Further investigations revealed an elevated levels of proteins, lymphocytic pleocytosis in the CSF. GeneXpert PCR for TB, of the CSF was negative. A Bone marrow biopsy, done to look for infiltrative or hematological conditions did not show any definite pathology. Other investigations like LDH, Angiotensin Converting Enzyme levels , Pulmonary Function Tests and chest X-ray were normal.

He was started on thyroxine and 1mg/kg of oral prednisolone. With this dose, his visual symptoms showed an improvement. However, in order to establish the etiological diagnosis, a pituitary biopsy was planned and a neurosurgery consult was obtained. The biopsy of the lesion showed a lymphocytic infiltration of the pituitary gland (Fig. 3). He was discharged and asked to follow-up after 3 months on a tapering schedule of oral steroids. A repeat MRI pituitary done after three months showed a significant reduction in size of the pituitary gland as well as meningeal lesions due to steroids.

DISCUSSION

Lymphocytic hypophysis (LYH) is a neuroendocrine disorder which is characterized by autoimmune inflammation of the pituitary gland with varying degrees of pituitary gland dysfunctions. The histopathology usually consists of an initial monoclonal lymphocytic infiltrates. The clinical presentation varies depending on the pituitary hormonal axis that is more severely affected. In lymphocytic adenohypophysis (LAH) an early destruction of the ACTH-producing cells is characteristic. Lymphocytic infundibuloneurohypophysis (LINH) typically presents as acute onset diabetes insipidus (DI) with symptoms of intracranial mass-effect. In patient with a combination of extensive anterior pituitary involvement with DI, lymphocytic Infundibulopanhypophysis (LIPH) should be suspected. Coexistence of other autoimmune conditions was reported in up to 25–50% of cases and in biopsy-proven cases, the pituitary autoantibodies had been detected in up to 70%. The therapeutic approach in lymphocytic hyphophysis is controversial, although transsphenoidal surgery is often performed. Given the self-limiting nature of the inflammatory process, a conservative medical management is justified in most of the patients.[1,2]

REFERENCES

1. Rivera J-A. Lymphocytic hypophysis: disease spectrum and approach to diagnosis and therapy. Pituitary. 2006;9 (1):35-45.
2. Nakata Y, Sato N, Masumoto T, et al. Parasellar T2 dark sign on MR imaging in patients with lymphocytic hypophysis. Am J Neuroradiol. 2010;31(10):1944-50.

CASE **34**

A 25-year-old lady presented to the endocrinology OPD with complaints of increased thirst and increased frequency of micturition since the past 2 years. She also complained of intermittent nonspecific backache, irregular menstrual cycles, constipation, and non-quantifiable weight loss over the past 2 years. She also had diminution of vision and severe headache during the same duration. She had previously been treated for Multidrug resistant pulmonary Kochs for 18 months.

Her investigation revealed 8 am Serum Cortisol: 5.24 µg%, thyroid-Stimulating Hormone (TSH): 0.480 µIU/mL T4-5 mcg%, Free T4-0.2 ng., Prolactin: 24.40 ng/mL, Luteinizing Hormone (LH): <0.10 mIU/mL, Follicle-Stimulating Hormone (FSH): 0.631 mIU/mL.

To further investigate an MRI of the brain was done (Figs. 1A and B).

WHAT DO YOU THINK IS THE DIAGNOSIS?

Her Water deprivation test revealed a central diabetes insipidus. The MRI of the brain demonstrated multiple ring-enhancing hypointense lesions in the suprasellar region encasing the pituitary stalk (Shown with arrow in Figs. 1A and B). With the combination of symptoms, investigations and MRI findings, the possibility of a calcified tuberculoma was considered. However for the confirmatory diagnosis the biopsy of the suprasellar mass was done which showed the histological features shown in Figure 2. She was started on Anti-tubercular medications. She was also started on oral prednisolone and thyroxine. She is on regular follow up with us since then.

DISCUSSION

The causes of granulomatous hypophysitis include tuberculosis, syphilis, sarcoidosis, mycotic granuloma, foreign body granuloma due to the rupturing of a Rathke's cleft cyst and idiopathic giant cell granulomatous hypophysitis (GGH) all of which appear with the similar histological findings. Wegener's granulomatosis is another cause for granulomatous inflammation of the pituitary. In developing countries, tuberculoma may be still the common cause for intracranial space occupying lesions. On CT intrasellar tuberculoma appears as a hyperdense mass brightly enhancing with contrast with suprasellar extension. On MRI Brain a thickened infundibulum and hypophyseal

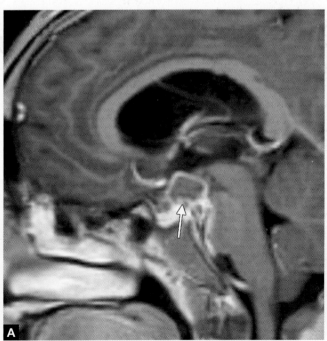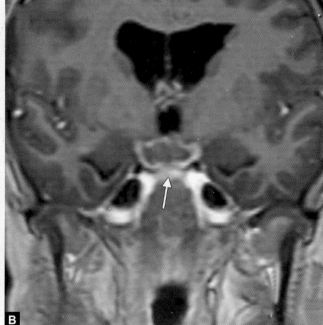

Figs. 1A and B: MRI of the brain.

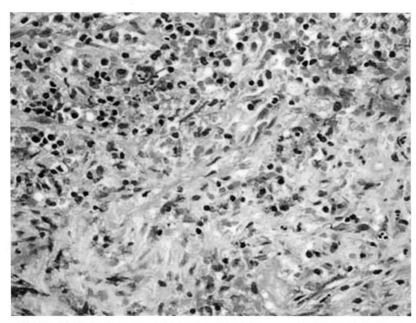

Fig. 2: Histopathological image showing granulomatous inflammation.

stalk is seen. However, this finding can also be seen in neoplastic or infiltrative diseases such as sarcoidosis and syphilis, apart from the sellar tuberculomas. Transsphenoidal biopsy is a safe and effective technique for obtaining the diagnosis. The anti-tuberculous drugs usually result in a good outcome, thereby surgery may be avoided.[1,2]

REFERENCES

1. Arunkumar MJ, Rajshekhar V. Intrasellar tuberculoma presenting as pituitary apoplexy. Neurol India 2001;49:407.
2. Singh S. Pituitary tuberculoma: Magnetic resonance imaging. Neurol India 2003;51:548-50.

CASE 35

A 42-year-old gentleman presented with headache, diplopia over 5 months duration and an episode of altered sensorium. Tuberculous meningitis was diagnosed previously, based on cerebrospinal fluid (CSF) studies and was started on anti-tuberculous therapy. He had two recent episodes of epistaxis too. He had history of constipation with decreased frequency of shaving and erectile dysfunction. On examination, a left lateral rectus palsy was noted. Computerized tomography of the brain revealed a mass in the sphenoid sinus with erosion of the surrounding bone and left parasellar extension. Magnetic resonance imaging (MRI) Brain showed an internal carotid pathology with flow void lesions, corresponding to the left parasellar and petrous region, indicated by the arrow (Fig. 1).

WHAT IS THE DIAGNOSIS?

Biochemistry confirmed the presence of panhypopituitarism: an 8:00 am serum cortisol <1 mcg/dL, total thyroxine: 3.45 mcg/dL and free thyroxine 0.63 ng/dL, serum testosterone <20 ng/dL, follicle-stimulating hormone (FSH) 0.74 mIU/mL, LH 0.55 mIU/ml and Prolactin 0.65 ng/mL.

Cerebral angiography of the brain showed two aneurysms from the left internal carotid artery, (a) a fusiform aneurysm in the petrous segment, measuring 16×13 mm^2 [shown with small arrow] and (b) a giant saccular aneurysm of the cavernous segment, projecting into the enlarged sella, measuring 31×14 mm^2 [shown with large arrow] (Fig. 2).

Coil embolization of the left internal carotid artery was done which reduced the flow into the aneurysm, resulting in thrombosis. The patient was discharged in a stable state and subsequently the anti-tuberculous drugs were stopped. He was started on Prednisolone 5 mg and 2.5 mg, thyroxine (100 mcg/day) and testosterone (250 mg intramuscularly once monthly). He is on regular follow-up.

DISCUSSION

The aneurysm in the neighboring sella turcica which can cause hypopituitarism is a known etiology. The presentation is wide-spread due to the pressure effects of the thrombosis, apoplexy of the pituitary adenoma, or following a subarachnoid hemorrhage. Pituitary dysfunction may involve a single hormonal axis or panhypopituitarism. Most intra-sellar aneurysms arise from the internal carotid artery. Hypopituitarism following surgery of aneurysms has also been described. In patients with headache, cranial nerve palsy and altered sensorium, tuberculous meningitis is one of the important differential diagnoses. Even the rupture of a sellar aneurysm and pituitary apoplexy can

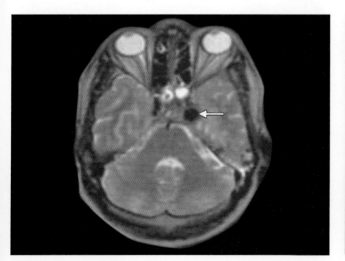

Fig. 1: MRI of the brain.

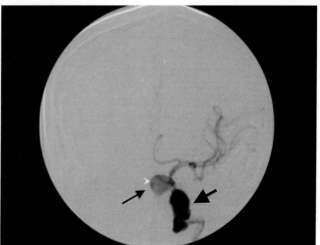

Fig. 2: MR angiogram of the brain.

have a similar presentation. An elevated protein in the CSF is seen in all the conditions that have been mentioned. In case of a sellar aneurysm (following a subclinical rupture) and pituitary apoplexy, xanthochromia with a high protein is seen in the CSF. Computed Tomography (CT) angiography of brain necessitates the diagnosis of the aneurysm of carotid artery, thereby preventing an inaccurate diagnosis and treatment.[1,2]

REFERENCES

1. Gondim J, Schops M, Ferreira E. Hypopituitarism and amenorrhea galactorrhea syndrome caused by thrombosis of both internal carotid artery and giant intrasellar aneurysm. Arq Neuropsiquiatr 2004;62:158-61.
2. Kreitschmann-Andermahr I, Hoff C, Niggemeier S, et al. Pituitary deficiency following aneurysmal subarachnoid haemorrhage. J Neurol Neurosurg Psychiatr 2003;74:1133-5.

CASE 36

A 64-year-old gentleman presented to an another tertiary care center, with visual impairment and altered sensorium. A visual field assessment was done which revealed bitemporal hemianopia. Investigations showed a serum sodium of 125 mEq/dL. A magnetic resonance imaging (MRI) brain was done which revealed the findings seen below (Fig. 1).

A transsphenoidal surgery was done and the mass was incompletely excised. Biopsy of the surgical specimen was suggestive of a pituitary adenoma, which was reported by a pathologist in that center. Following the procedure, the patient was subjected to radiotherapy of the sella turcica.

He was well until 6 months later, when he presented again with generalized tonic-clonic seizures and loss of consciousness. The pathological diagnosis was reviewed, which showed sheets of cancer cells (Fig. 2). He was sent for a repeat MRI Brain and the images are displayed in Figures 3A and B.

WHAT IS THE DIAGNOSIS?

The patient presented with a primary pituitary gland lesion that was initially misdiagnosed to be a pituitary macroadenoma. Subsequently he developed metastases to other parts of the cerebral cortex as seen in the MRI brain

done 6 months later (Fig. 3). The primary malignancy had an unknown source. He was referred to the Department of Radiotherapy for further management.

DISCUSSION

Pituitary metastases have been reported in up to 2% of autopsied cases of patients with a known underlying carcinoma. The primary origin of these malignancies was carcinoma breast in women and lung in men. However other malignancies such as prostate, pancreas, leukemia, lymphoma, ovary, melanoma are also noted to cause metastases to the pituitary gland. There are cases where adenocarcinoma involving the pituitary gland has been identified but the primary origin remains undetermined. The posterior pituitary gland is involved in 70% of the cases, alone or in combination with the anterior pituitary gland. Hence the common clinical presentation is diabetes insipidus, which in its partial form can be easily missed. Other features of hypopituitarism are less likely, since the posterior pituitary is affected more that than the anterior compartment. The reason for this is that the posterior pituitary receives a direct systemic blood supply.

Non-hematogenous mechanisms of spread of the tumor include an extension from juxtasellar metastases and

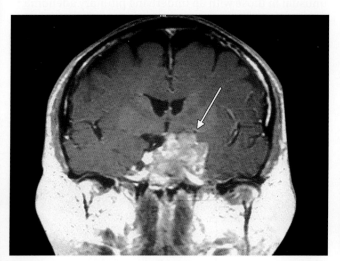

Fig. 1: MRI of the brain with a mass arising from the pituitary region (shown with arrow).

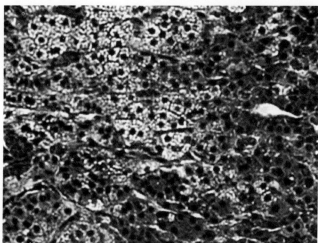

Fig. 2: Histopathology specimen.

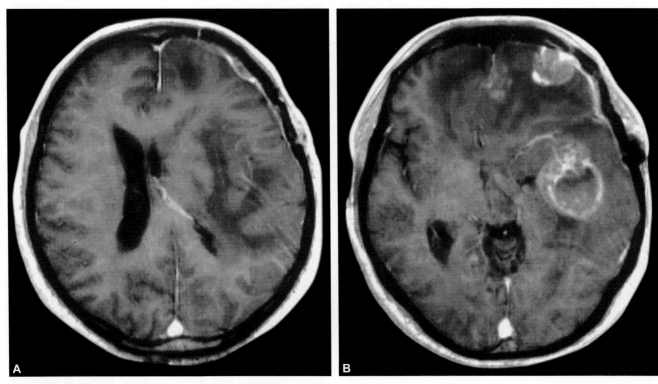

Figs. 3A and B: MRI of the brain repeated 6 months later.

an invasion of the suprasellar cistern by leptomeningeal metastases. On imaging, coincident metastatic deposits at other sites of the brain are seen in 30-70% of these patients at the time of identification of the primary pituitary lesion. Imaging can localize the degree of sellar or suprasellar extension, but may not help in differentiating metastases from a pituitary adenoma. Sclerotic change of the sellar margins on a skull X-ray, aggressive bony destruction of the sellar, clivus and clinoids and extensive vascularity of the mass could be a pointer towards metastases, but a sellar meningioma must be considered as a differential diagnosis.

The rapid growth of the lesion postoperatively or after radiation, should be a reason to review the initial pathological diagnosis and suspect metastases, so also the progression to develop cranial nerve palsies which is more unusual in those with an underlying pituitary adenoma.[1,2]

REFERENCES

1. Abrams HL, Spiro R, Goldstein N. Metastases in carcinoma; analysis of 1000 autopsied cases. Cancer. 1950;3(1):74-85.
2. Houck WA, Olson KB, Horton J. Clinical features of tumor metastasis to the pituitary. Cancer. 1970;26(3):656-9.

CASE 37

A 16-year-old, boy came to the endocrinology OPD with history of failure of linear growth. Physical examination showed his height of 134 cm and failure to attain the expected height of about 164 cm ± 8 cm. He was also noticed to have central obesity with puffy face and a dry skin (Fig. 1). He was also noticed to have a hoarseness of voice.

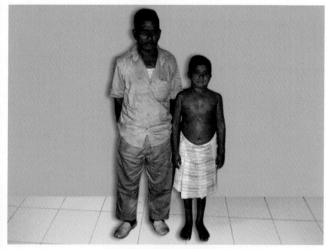

Fig. 1: Clinical picture of the patient with his father.

WHAT IS THE DIAGNOSIS?

Investigations revealed features of central hypothyroidism, low cortisol, suppressed Luteinizing Hormone (LH), Follicle-Stimulating Hormone (FSH), and Testosterone. Bone age was markedly delayed (Fig. 2).

So a diagnosis of short stature due to panhypopituitarism was made. The Magnetic Resonance Imaging (MRI) brain showed a mass in the suprasellar region with extension into the parasellar and infra-sellar area (Fig. 3) with cystic and calcified content (shown encircled).

The T1 weighted MRI images showing an extensive calcification in the suprasellar region is often called as a pituitary stone. The patient underwent a transnasal transsphenoidal excision of the mass and intraoperatively found to have machine oil like fluid from the mass. So the final diagnosis in this patient was short stature with panhypopituitarism due to craniopharyngioma.

DISCUSSION

Craniopharyngiomas are rare solid or mixed solid-cystic tumors that arise from remnants of Rathke's pouch along the line from the nasopharynx to the diencephalon. There

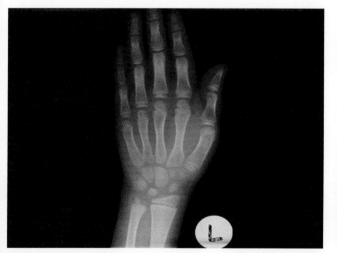

Fig. 2: X-ray of the left hand showing a bone age of around 8–9 years.

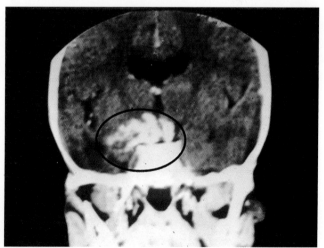

Fig. 3: MRI of the brain.

is a bimodal age distribution, with one peak in children between the age of 5 and 14 years and a second peak in adults between 50 and 75 years of age. Craniopharyngiomas are epithelial tumors that usually arise in the pituitary stalk in the suprasellar region, adjacent to the optic chiasm. A small percentage of these tumors arise within the sella, and a few tumors have been described within the optic system or the third ventricle.

Although benign histologically, these tumors frequently shorten the life span and should be considered as low-grade malignancies. Most Craniopharyngiomas contain both solid and cystic components. The cysts are filled with turbid fluid that contains cholesterol crystals.

In the World Health Organization classification of central nervous system tumors, craniopharyngiomas are divided into two categories, adamantinomatous Craniopharyngiomas and papillary Craniopharyngiomas. The prognostic factors for both types are visual symptoms, endocrine abnormalities and headache. Surgery and radiotherapy are indicated in almost all the cases.[1,2]

REFERENCES

1. Pratheesh R, Swallow DMA, Rajaratnam S, et al. Incidence, predictors and early post-operative course of diabetes insipidus in paediatric craniopharygioma: a comparison with adults. Pediatr Neurosurg. 2013;29(6):941–9.
2. Selvan AS, Jebasingh KF, Rajaratnam S, et al. Craniopharyngioma: a single institutional experience from South India. 2008 Apr 1; Available from: http://www.endocrine-abstracts.org/ea/0015/ea0015p208.htm

CASE 38

A 40-year-old, gentleman presented with history of decreased shaving frequency and erectile dysfunction since the past 2 years. However, he did not seek any medical attention for the same. Prior to admitting in the hospital he experienced severe headache with several episodes of vomiting. Retinal evaluation showed bilateral papilledema. The investigations revealed a suppressed follicle-stimulating hormone (FSH) and Luteinising hormone (LH) with an undetectable serum testosterone level. His serum cortisol was not checked because he was on oral prednisolone after the episodes of vomiting. The thyroid-stimulating hormone (TSH) was low with suppressed total and Free thyroxine levels. Magnetic resonance imaging (MRI) brain revealed a mass which is shown circle in Figures 1 and 2A to C.

WHAT IS THE DIAGNOSIS?

Magnetic resonance imaging (MRI) of the brain revealed a 3.5 × 3 × 3.6 cm sized lobulated fairly well-defined lesion in the suprasellar cistern, interpeduncular fossa, compressing the third ventricle which was mildly hyperintense on both T1- and T2-weighted images suggestive of third ventricular craniopharyngioma (Fig. 1 and 2, shown with a circle).

From the clinical and biochemical findings he was diagnosed of having panhypopituitarism. He was started on oral thyroxine (100 mcg) and triiodothyronine for 3 days (25 mcg thrice daily) and was cleared for surgery with perioperative hydrocortisone stress cover. He underwent a decompression of the cyst and partial excision of the cyst wall via a medial frontal craniotomy and an anterior inter-hemispheric approach. Intraoperatively the cyst consisted of machine oil like fluid within. The histopathological biopsy was found to have features suggestive of an adamantinomatous craniopharyngioma. He was referred to the Department of radiotherapy for radiation of the residual tumor. He was given 54 Gy in 30 fractions by a 3D conventional radiotherapy.

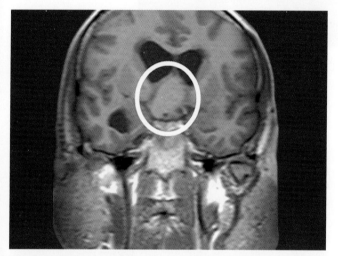

Fig. 1: MRI of the brain showing T1 weighted image.

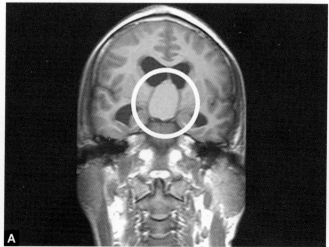

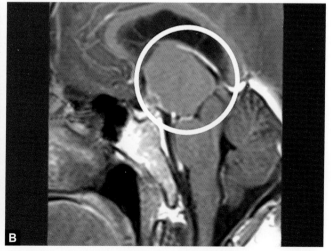

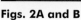

Figs. 2A and B

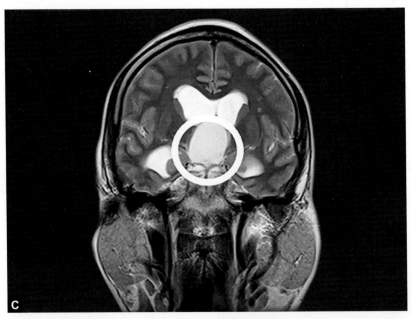

Figs. 2A to C: MRI of the brain showing T1 weighted postgadolinium and T2 weighted images.

DISCUSSION

Craniopharyngioma is a common suprasellar tumor of the children, wherein they most commonly present with short stature or delayed puberty. The other most common presentation is central diabetes insipidus. Owing to the location of these tumors they may present with varying visual field symptoms. Depending on the histology, Craniopharyngiomas can be of three types. (1) Adamantinomatous: epithelial mass forming a reticulum - most common in children, (2) Mucoid epithelial cyst, (3) Squamous papillary. Classic findings on a Computed Tomography (CT) are calcified suprasellar mass with cysts. Post surgery the radiation therapy is targeted to the tumor volume, encompassing all its components. Current radiation techniques that are used in the treatment of craniopharyngioma include stereotactic radiotherapy and radiosurgery, intensity modulated radiation therapy (IMRT), and proton beam therapy. The prescribed radiation dose is 50-60 Gy. If beyond 60 Gy is administered; optic neuropathy and brain necrosis can be expected. Even patient with absent pituitary hormonal deficiencies should be followed up regularly as they have the high chance of hormonal deficiency which evolves over the time period post radiation. So the follow-up includes yearly hormonal evaluation, visual field assessment and imaging.[1,2]

REFERENCES

1. Joseph V, Chacko AG. Suprabrow minicraniotomy for suprasellar tumours. Br J Neurosurg. 2005;19(1):33-7.
2. Asirvatham JR, Deepti AN, Chyne R, et al. Paediatric tumours of the central nervous system: a retrospective study of 1,043 cases from a tertiary care centre in South India. Childs Nerv Syst ChNS Off J Int Soc Pediatr Neurosurg. 2011; 27(8):1257-63.

CASE 39

A 23-year-old, Mrs. S presented with oligomenorrhea for two years, followed by amenorrhea for one year, progressive diminution of vision in the both eyes for seven months. Her right eye vision was worse than the left eye with bilateral primary optic atrophy. There was no history of galactorrhea, apoplexic symptoms or any symptoms to suggest any other endocrine dysfunction. There were no associated co-morbid illnesses. Her biochemical Investigations revealed hCG levels which were elevated, 456.7 mIU/mL (Normal upto 5) and also alpha fetoprotein of 75.4 IU/mL (Normal upto 5.5). Magnetic resonance imaging (MRI) brain was done, which is shown in Figures 1A to E. She was on cabergoline 0.5 mg twice weekly when she was admitted.

WHAT IS THE DIAGNOSIS?

Investigations also revealed T4 (Total T4 and Free T4)-7.5 ug% and 0.75 ng% respectively, Cortisol (8 AM) – 2.39 ug%., LH – 0.691 mIU/mL, follicle-stimulating hormone (FSH)-0.375 mIU/mL, Prolactin (HPRL) [In dilution] – 99 ng/mL.

Magnetic resonance imaging (MRI) brain showed a sellar with suprasellar mass, which was enhancing with contrast and also with areas of blooming on susceptibility weighted imaging (Fig. 1E) within the mass. The differential

diagnoses considered after seeing the MRI images were a meningioma, a prolactinoma or a germinoma. Pre-operatively, she was started on oral Triiodothyronine (T3) 25 mcg thrice daily for 2 days with a plan to continue post-operatively for 2 days along with oral prednisolone.

Subsequently, she underwent a right frontotemporal craniotomy and a partial excision of the mass. Intraoperatively, a frozen section was sent which was reported as a germinoma; hence the surgery was limited to a partial excision of the suprasellar germinoma. The histopathology specimen was immunopositive for OCT3/4 suggestive of a germinoma. Post surgery she had polyuria and polydipsia with serum sodium rising up to 162 mEq and the corresponding urine osmolarity less than 100 mOsm/L. She was given oral desmopressin and also continued prednisolone and thyroxine supplementation. As the biopsy report was confirmatory of germinoma, she was given four cycles of Etoposide and Cisplatin based chemotherapy and she is on regular follow up.

DISCUSSION

Intracranial germinomas (also known as dysgerminomas or extragonadal seminomas) are a germ cell type of tumor, and are predominantly seen in pediatric populations.

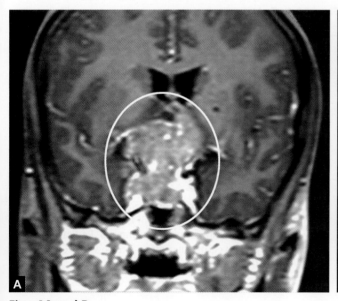
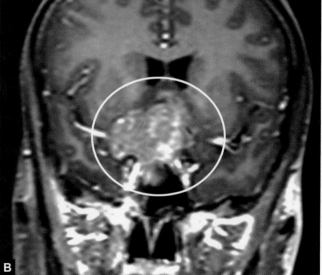

Figs. 1A and B

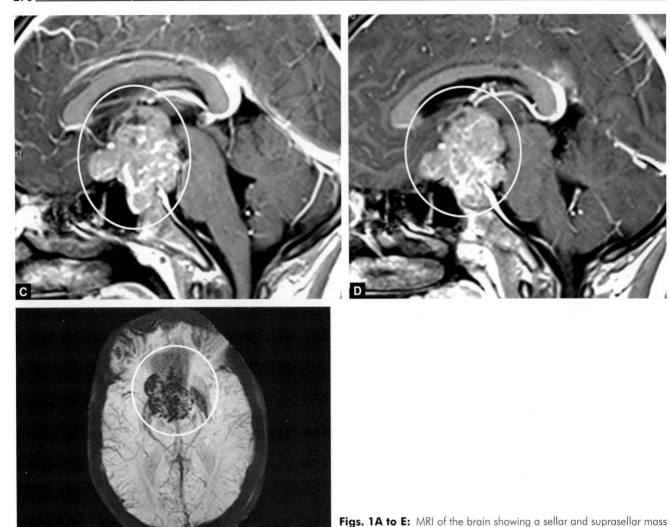

Figs. 1A to E: MRI of the brain showing a sellar and suprasellar mass (shown with a circle).

They tend to occur in the midline, either at the pineal region (majority) or along the floor of the third ventricle/suprasellar region. They are the most common tumor of the pineal gland. Presentation depends on location of the tumor, with compression of the tectal plate leading to obstructive hydrocephalus and Parinaud syndrome, whereas involvement on the pituitary infundibulum, leads to diabetes insipidus (most common), hypopituitarism (common) or optic chiasm compression or signs of raised intracranial hypertension. On Computed Tomography (CT) the high cellularity results in a degree of hyperdensity compared to adjacent brain which usually enhances brightly with contrast. The prognosis for patients with germinomas is quite good, with many series reporting survival rates of greater than 90% in five years following diagnosis and treatment. Radiotherapy or Cisplatin based chemotherapy are tried with greater success in patients with germinoma.[1,2]

REFERENCES

1. Packer RJ, Cohen BH, Cooney K. Intracranial germ cell tumors. The Oncologist. 2000;1;5(4):312–20.
2. Echevarría ME, Fangusaro J, Goldman S. Pediatric central nervous system germ cell tumors: A review. The Oncologist. 2008;1;13(6):690–9.

CASE **40**

A 5-year-old boy, born of a non-consanguineous marriage was brought by his parents with history of increase in size of external genitalia (Figs. 1A and B) with a rapid increase in height for the past one year and episodes of spontaneous spells of laughing of the same duration. There were no history of crying episodes, headache or visual disturbance. The mother also noticed acnes over the face for the past 3 months.

On examination, his height was 136 cm (> 97th centile: 120 cm with a height age for 10.5 years) and weight of 30.3 kg (> 97th centile: 23 kg with a weight age for 11 years). His systemic examination was normal. Sexual Maturity rating was done and the findings were: pubic hair: Tanner stage 3. Axillary hair: nil. Genital stage: G4. Testicular volume: right 20 ml and left 15–20 ml. Stretched Penile Length (SPL): 8 cm. Voice: cracked (low pitch).

WHAT IS THE DIAGNOSIS?

On investigating, Thyroid-Stimulating Hormone (TSH): 0.6 μIU/ with Normal TFT, Luteinizing Hormone (LH): 1.71 mIU/mL, Follicle-Stimulating Hormone (FSH): 1.10 mIU/mL, Testosterone: 200 ng/dL, Prolactin (HPRL): 11.71 ng/mL and Cortisol [8 am]: 8.29 μg%. A Magnetic Resonance Imaging (MRI) was done and showed the following features (Figs. 2A and B).

His bone age was 9–11 years (Fig. 3). The post 100 mcg Triptorelin showed an LH increment of 22 mIU/mL. Hence the patient was diagnosed to have isosexual central precocious puberty due to a hypothalamic hamartoma (Fig. 2). He was started on Leuprolide Depot 11.25 mg intramuscularly. It was planned to administer Leuprolide Depot 11.25 mg once every 3 months till around 12–14 years of age. He was started on Sodium Valproate for control of the gelastic seizures.

DISCUSSION

Hypothalamic or a tuber cinereum hamartomas are non-neoplastic nodules, which consists of mature glial and neurons cells. The site of hamartomas may either embedded in the hypothalamus (intrahypothalamic) or in the ventral hypothalamus situated anywhere from the tuber cinereum to the mammillary bodies (parahypothalamic). The degree of clinical presentation may vary from central precocious puberty to compressive symptoms due to the parahypothalamic hamartoma or rarely features of acromegaly. Hypothalamic displacement correlates with the findings on clinical presentation.

These hamartomas are generally non-disabling. The intrahypothalamic variety is associated with intractable seizures, which may be focal or gelastic ("laughing") seizures

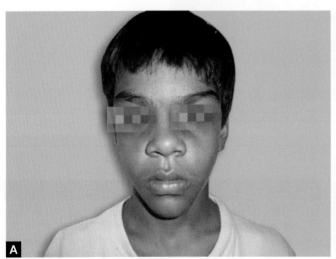
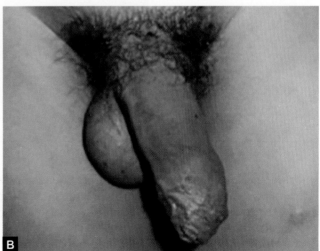

Figs. 1A and B: Clinical picture of the patient.

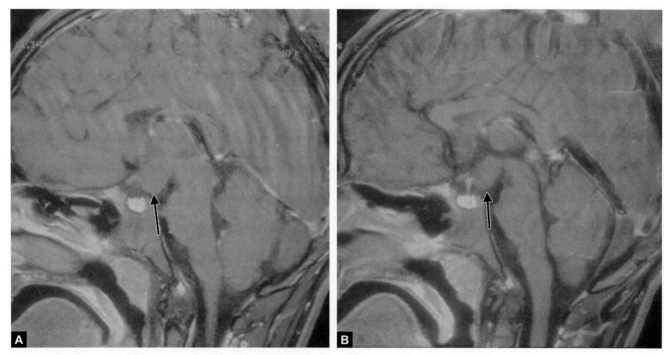

Figs. 2A and B: MRI of the brain showing a lesion in the region of hypothalamus (shown with arrow).

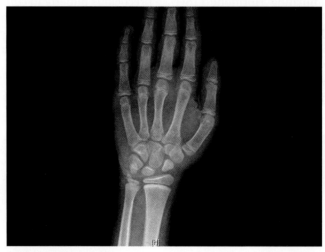

Fig. 3: X-ray of the wrist showing a bone age of 9–11 years.

with secondary generalization. Central precocious puberty can easily be treated medically with gonadotropin-releasing hormone agonist therapy (GnRH agonist). Surgical therapy is indicated rarely. Antiepileptic drugs are used as a first-line treatment for the control of seizures. In patients with retractable seizure, the surgical management of hypothalamic hamartomas is important.[1,2]

REFERENCES

1. Jacob JJ, Koshy TG, Paul TV. Visual vignette. Tuber cinereum hamartoma. Endocr Pract. 2007;13(2):204.
2. Kotwal N, Yanamandra U, Menon AS, et al. Central precocious puberty due to hypothalamic hamartoma in a six-month-old infant girl. Indian J Endocrinol Metab. 2012; 16(4): 627–30.

CASE 41

A 55-year-old gentleman was known to have carcinoma of the colon for which he underwent a right hemicolectomy a year prior and was on salvage chemotherapy with 5-fluorouracil and Irinotecan. Histopathology of the operated colon specimen showed a moderately differentiated adenocarcinoma (Fig. 1). He was referred to Department of Endocrinology for the evaluation of polydipsia and polyuria. He was also known to have diabetes mellitus with good glycemic control, achieved with oral antidiabetic therapy and insulin. On biochemical evaluation: serum sodium, potassium, urinary osmolality were 160 mEq/L, 3.2 mEq/L and 140 mOsm/L respectively. All the anterior pituitary hormonal axes assessed were normal. Computed Tomography (CT) Chest (Fig. 2) showed a nonhomogenous opacity consistent with lymphangitis carcinomatosa. Subsequently the Magnetic Resonance Imaging (MRI) brain was done which is displayed in Figure 3. Computed Tomography (CT) of the abdomen also showed a mass in the right ascending colon (Fig. 4).

WHAT IS THE DIAGNOSIS?

This patient had polyuria and hypernatremia with a normoglycemic status making central diabetes insipidus the likely diagnosis. Biochemical features such as high serum sodium with a low urinary osmolarity further supported the diagnosis. With MRI pituitary showing a thickened stalk and a lesion in the posterior pituitary, features suggestive of pituitary metastasis, which could explain the central diabetes Insipidus (DI). He was started on oral desmopressin tablets, 50 mcg twice daily after which he improved symptomatically. On discharge, the patient was

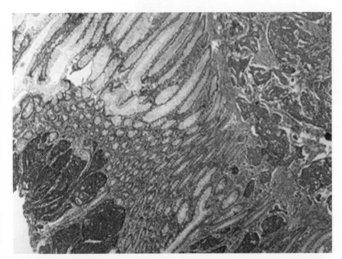

Fig. 1: Histopathological examination (HPE) showing the wall of large bowel infiltrated by moderately differentiated adenocarcinoma.

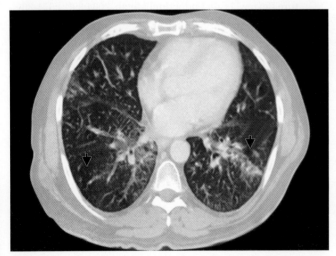

Fig. 2: CT of lung showing multiple tiny nodules and reticulonodular appearance (black arrowheads) suggestive of lymphangitis carcinomatosa.

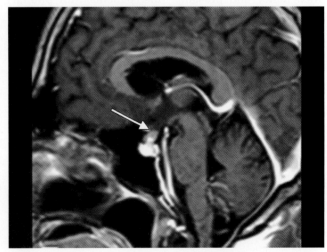

Fig. 3: Magnetic resonance imaging (MRI) (sagittal section) showing a hypo intense nodular focus in the posterior gland and along the infundibulum with enhancement postgadolinium (shown with arrow), consistent with metastasis.

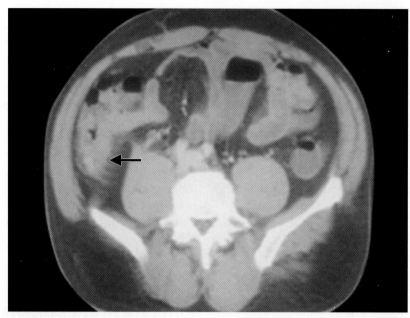

Fig. 4: Computed tomography (CT) abdomen showing a diffuse wall thickening of the caecum suggestive of carcinoma colon (shown with arrow).

asked to continue medications, maintain an output chart and to monitor the serum sodium periodically.

DISCUSSION

Pituitary metastasis is quite an uncommon disorder, responsible for less than 1% of the pituitary tumors. Malignancies metastasizing to the pituitary gland in descending order are carcinoma lung, breast, gastrointestinal tract malignancy and prostate. Most patients with pituitary metastasis are symptomatic. Posterior pituitary metastasis is more common due to the direct arterial blood supply and also it is outside the blood brain barrier. The patients with pituitary metastasis usually have a poor prognosis. The primary modalities of treatment are radiation and chemotherapy. Hence a metastatic central DI should be considered in any patients with polyuria or hypernatremia with present or past history of carcinoma elsewhere.[1,2]

REFERENCES

1. Komninos J, Vlassopoulou V, Protopapa D, et al. Tumors metastatic to the pituitary gland: Case Report and Literature Review. J Clin Endocrinol Metab. 2004;89(2):574-80.
2. Turcu AF, Erickson BJ, Lin E, et al. Pituitary stalk lesions: the mayo clinic experience. J Clin Endocrinol Metab. 2013; 8(5):1812–18.

CASE 42

A 65-year-old man presented with polyuria and polydipsia of sudden onset along with weight loss of 4 kg over a period of a month with associated headaches. His past history was uneventful. His height was 168 cm and weight was 61 kg. Physical examination did not provide any clues except for tenderness over the occiput.

Basic investigation revealed a 2 hour postprandial plasma glucose of 145 mg/dL, serum creatinine of 0.9 mg/dL, sodium 147 mEq/L, potassium: 4.0 MEq/L, Total calcium: 9 mg/dL, Phosphorus: 3 mg with normal complete blood count, erythrocyte sedimentation rate and liver function tests.

On admission to hospital he was found to have a urine output of 7 liters over 24 hours. A water deprivation test was performed. Within 8 hours of starting the test his weight dropped to 57 kg. The urine osmolality at this point was 120 mOsmol/L and the serum sodium is I56 mmol/L. After subcutaneous desmopressin (5 units), the urine osmolality in 2 hours was 430 mOsmol/L.

The patient's skull X-ray and technetium bone scans are displayed in Figures 1 and 2 respectively.

WHAT IS THE DIAGNOSIS?

This patient had clinical features of central diabetes insipidus along with a positive water deprivation test. The differential diagnoses for central diabetes insipidus would include: sarcoidosis, metastases to the pituitary gland and histiocytosis (Langerhans cell granulomatosis). Considering his age and the presence of honey lesions (as evidenced by a lytic lesion on the X-ray skull and the increased uptake over the skull on the technetium bone scan), the most likely possibilities would be either histiocytosis X or a metastatic lesion in the pituitary gland. The biopsy from the lytic lesion was suggestive of histiocytosis X. He was treated with melphalan and prednisolone and radiotherapy.

DISCUSSION

Classification of causes for diabetic insipidus:
- Familial:
  - Hereditary (autosomal dominant)
  - DIDMOAD syndrome (Diabetes insipidus, diabetes mellitus, optic atrophy, nerve deafness, Atonia of bladder and ureters)
- Acquired:
  - Head trauma
  - Neurosurgery
  - Tumors (craniopharyngioma, germinoma, metastatic deposits)
  - Granulomatous disease (TB, sarcoidosis, histiocytocis, Wegener's granulomatosis)
  - Infections (meningitis, encephalitic)
  - Vascular disorders (Sheehan's syndrome, aneurysms, thrombotic thrombocytopenic purpura)

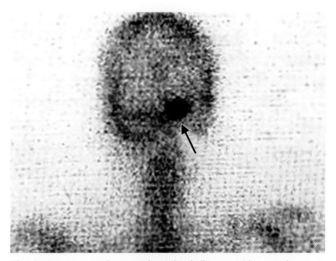

Fig. 1: X-ray skull showing a lytic lesion (shown with arrow).

Fig. 2: Bone scan with an uptake in the skull occiput (shown with arrow).

- Circulating antibodies to vasopressin (secondary to pitressin injection)
- Autoimmunity
- Idiopathic

Nephrogenic:
- Familial:
  - Hereditary (X-linked recessive)
- Acquired:
  - Chronic renal disease
  - Metabolic disease (hypokalemia, hypercalcemia)
  - Drugs (lithium, demeclocycline)
  - Osmotic diuresis.

Histiocytosis X accounts for almost 40% of diabetes insipidus in some pediatric series. The treatment of choice for this condition is cranial irradiation along with Desmopressin as a therapeutic measure. The other choices include melphalan and prednisolone. With lytic lesion in the skull, mulitple myeloma is an important differential diagnosis. However, in multiple myeloma, the bone scans usually do not show an increased uptake in the lytic lesions. Moreover multiple myeloma has not been associated with central diabetes insipidus.[1,2]

REFERENCES

1. Nezelof C, Frileux-Herbet F, Cronier-Sachot J. Disseminated histiocytosis X: analysis of prognostic factors based on a retrospective study of 50 cases. Cancer. 1979;44(5): 1824-38.
2. Ahmed M, Sureka J, Koshy C, et al. Langerhans cell histiocytosis of the clivus: An unusual cause of a destructive central skull base mass in a child. Neurol India. 2012;60(3):346.

CASE 43

A 49-year-old man presented with bilateral proptosis of 2 years' duration. He also complained of generalized bone pain, polyuria, and polydipsia. A physical examination was unremarkable except for bilateral proptosis—right eye 28 mm and left eye 26 mm (normal level, ≤20 mm) (Fig. 1). His eye movements were normal as were both fundi and his intraocular pressures. The thyroid gland was not enlarged and his baseline biochemical evaluation was normal. A water deprivation test confirmed that he had central diabetes insipidus and his bone scan showed multiple areas of increased uptake (Fig. 2). A biopsy of his retro-orbital region revealed sheets and aggregates of foamy macrophages (Fig. 3) with occasional "Touton type" giant cells (Fig. 4).

WHAT IS THE LIKELY DIAGNOSIS?

In our patient, 99mTc-methylene diphosphonate bone scintigraphy showed multiple areas of increased uptake in the left orbit and nasomaxillary region. There was bilateral symmetrical tracer uptake in the diaphyseal regions of both humerii, the metadiaphyseal regions of both femorii and foci of increased uptake were also seen in both greater trochanteric regions and in the tibiae with epiphyseal sparing (Fig. 2). The points that clinch the diagnosis are the histology and immunohistochemistry of these tumors. In our patient, a biopsy of his retro-orbital region revealed sheets and aggregates of foamy macrophages (Fig. 3) with occasional "Touton type" giant cells (Fig. 3). These macrophages were positive for KP1 and negative for S-100 and CD-1a. Thus the patient had Erdheim-Chester disease.

Our patient was started on interferon α2b, 3 million units subcutaneously thrice weekly along with the prednisolone 20 mg once daily. The prednisolone was tapered off and stopped entirely after 2 months. After 3 months there was an improvement in his proptosis-exophthalmometry of the right eye was 26 mm and the left eye 24 mm. The repeat bone scintigraphy showed a marked decrease in tracer uptake compared to the pretreatment Bone scan (Fig. 2). We decided to continue treating him with interferon α2b at the same dose and review him again after 3 months. However, he succumbed to his illness subsequently.

DISCUSSION

Histiocytosis is a group of disorders characterized by the infiltration of monocytes, macrophages and dendritic cells into the affected tissues. It is divided into two varieties: Langerhans' cell histiocytosis and non-Langerhans' cell

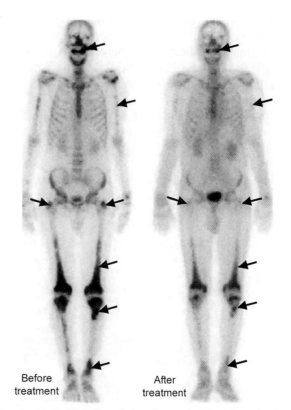

Before treatment   After treatment

Fig. 2: 99mTc-methylene diphosphonate bone scintigraphy showing an increased tracer uptake (shown with the arrows) (Left side picture -before treatment with interferon) and a marked decrease in tracer uptake (after treatment with interferon).

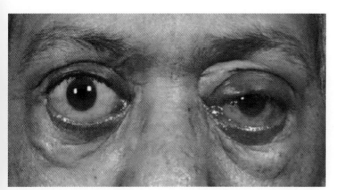

Fig. 1: Bilateral proptosis.

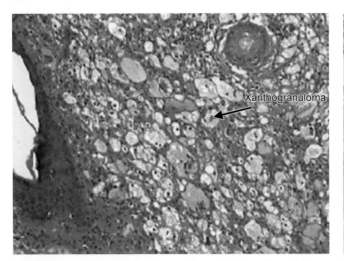

Fig. 3: Biopsy showing foamy macrophages (shown with arrow).

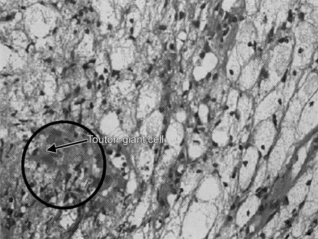

Fig. 4: Photomicrograph showing 'Touton type' giant cells (shown with a circle).

histiocytosis. Langerhans' cell histiocytosis is further classified into: (1) Letter- Sieve disease, (2) Hand-Schuller-Christian disease, (3) eosinophilic granuloma, and (4) congenital self-healing reticulohistiocytosis. Erdheim-Chester disease (ECD) is a rare non-Langerhans histiocytic disorder most commonly characterized by multifocal osteosclerotic lesions of the long bones demonstrating sheets of foamy histiocytes on biopsy with or without histiocytic infiltration of extra-skeletal tissues which was first described by Jacob Erdheim and William Chester in 1930.

The most common clinical presentations are bone pain (26 percent), neurologic features (23 percent), diabetes insipidus (22 percent) and constitutional symptoms (20 percent).

Langerhans' cell histiocytosis is characterized by aggregates of pathological Langerhans' cells, macrophages and giant histiocytes having a nuclei with irregular margins. They are positive for S-100 + CD-1a on immune-histochemisty and show Birbeck granules on the electron microscopy. This disease is an uncommon disorder and there is no consensus on therapy. Various modalities including steroid therapy, immunomodulatory therapy, and radiotherapy have been unsuccessful.

ECD is diagnosed based upon the pathologic evaluation of involved tissue interpreted within the clinical context. ECD can be difficult to diagnose since it is a very rare disease that can affect many organ systems. A biopsy of an osteosclerotic bone lesion is generally preferred, when possible.

Most of these patients do not survive beyond 32 months from the time of diagnosis. There are case reports of interferon α2b been used as the treatment for ECD.[1,2]

REFERENCES

1. Koshy G, Thomas N, Rajaratnam S, et al. Proptosis and polyuria. Hong Kong Med J. 2009;15(6):494–5.
2. Gabrielli GB, Stanzial AM, Moretti L, et al. Erdheim-Chester disease: normal skeletal radiography in a patient with extensive bone involvement. Recenti Prog Med. 2005; 96(12):604–8.

CASE 44

A 28-year-old, Mrs P presented with chief complaints of generalized increase in skin pigmentation all over the body for last 2 months (Figs. 1A and B). Historically, she had a history of sudden onset of headache with right third nerve palsy in 2002. The hormonal evaluation at that time showed a basal serum 8 am cortisol of 28.6 ug%, Human growth hormone (HGH) of 0.8, with normal thyroid functions and normal potassium. She had been amenorrheic following her first child birth. She did not have clinical evidence of Cushing's or Acromegaly. A magnetic resonance imaging (MRI) brain done at that time showed a Hardy's grade C tumor. A clinical diagnosis of non-functioning pituitary adenoma was made and she underwent a transnasal trans-sphenoidal partial excision of the tumor. The biopsy was reported as pituitary apoplexy. Following surgery there was a partial recovery of 3rd nerve palsy. On follow-up, a Computed Tomography (CT) scan of the brain was done, which did not show any lesion and basal cortisol was 17.1 μg% with normal thyroid functions. In the following year, she presented with headache and left VI cranial nerve palsy. The Imaging of the brain showed residual tumor in the left cavernous sinus. She received radiotherapy for the same (Fig. 3). She continued to have amenorrhea and was advised ethinyl estradiol and progesterone. Subsequently 2-years later she presented with weight gain and excessive pigmentation. And she was found to have diabetes mellitus which required twice daily premixed insulin for adequate control of the plasma glucose levels. Her basal 8 am serum cortisol was 26.5 ug% and post 1 mg and 8 mg dexamethasone cortisol were 16.2ug% and 3.3ug% respectively with basal 24-hour urine free cortisol of 925 ug/day. Her thyroid function tests were normal. The serum Adrenocorticotropic Hormone (ACTH) level was also markedly elevated at that time. The MRI of the brain showed the same residual mass in left cavernous sinus which was noted earlier. So she was diagnosed to have ACTH dependent Cushing's syndrome. So she underwent bilateral adrenalectomy for Cushing's syndrome. Following the surgery she was put on replacement doses of Prednisolone, Fludrocortisone and for control of sugars she required only Metformin. She has been on follow-up since then.

WHAT IS THE DIAGNOSIS?

At present she had developed Nelson's syndrome which was evident by progressive hyperpigmentation of the skin and an elevated ACTH level. Initially the patient had history of apoplexy which well could have masked the biochemical finding of Cushings syndrome at that time. On examination, she has generalized hyperpigmentation present. Gingival and nail pigmentation was also visible (Fig. 2A to D).

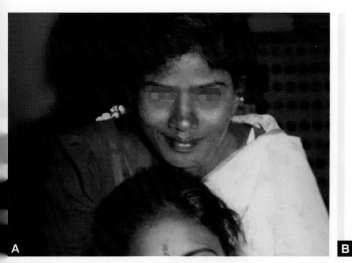
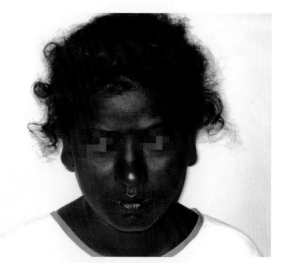

Figs. 1A and B: (A) Before development of any symptoms, (B) present picture after she was incompliant with medications for more than 2–3 months.

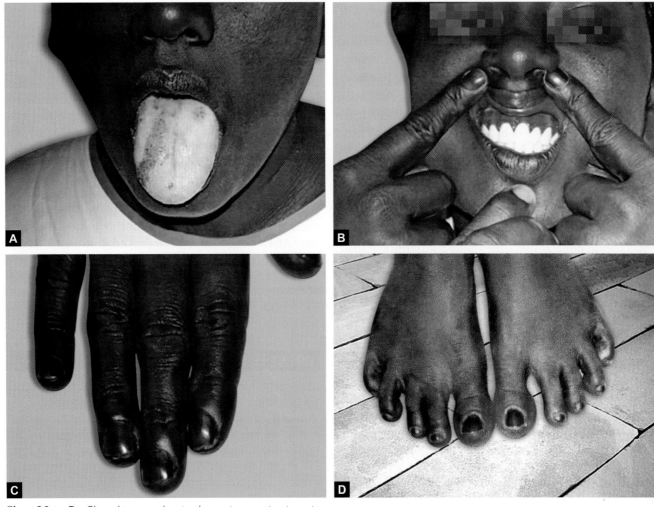

Figs. 2A to D: Clinical images showing hyperpigmentation in various areas.

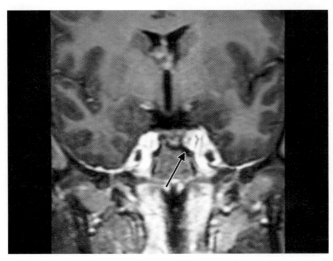

Fig. 3: MRI of the brain showing a residual tumor in the parasellar region (shown with arrow).

Magnetic resonance imaging (MRI) of the brain done recently showed a residual mass lesion in the parasellar region bilaterally, with encasement of the ICA, more on left with reduced enhancement, suggestive of a residual pituitary adenoma (Fig. 3). She did not have field defects or any other new neurological deficits. Subsequently she had developed hypothyroidism and was started on thyroxine replacement.

In summary the pituitary tumor survived apoplexy, surgery and radiotherapy and continues to secrete ACTH. Due to the parasellar extension of the tumor, surgery was not considered. She at present is on prednisolone, fludrocortisone and oral contraceptive pills in addition to the thyroxine as replacement.

DISCUSSION

Nelsons syndrome happens, whereby the ACTH is elevated following bilateral adrenalectomy for either a pituitary or less commonly an ectopic Cushings syndrome. Over the past several decades, various treatment modalities including surgical, radiotherapy, and medical have been proposed for nelsons syndrome. Selective resection of a corticotrophin secreting tumor by trans-sphenoidal approach is currently the procedure of choice for most pituitary tumors. Bilateral adrenalectomy is also a useful treatment modality in patients who have recurrence following a pituitary tumor excision and in patients where the source of ACTH is not identifiable or a moribund cushings disease.

In 1958, Don Nelson et al. described the first case of the eponymous syndrome in a 33-year-old woman who had under gone total bilateral adrenalectomy for the treatment of refractory Cushing's disease. The sellar mass was a pituitary corticotrophinoma, and its surgical removal led to symptom resolution.[1,2]

REFERENCES

1. Barber TM, Adams E, Ansorge O, Byrne JV, Karavitaki N, Wass JA. Nelson's syndrome. Eur J Endocrinol. 2010;163(4):495-507.
2. Gil-Cárdenas A, Herrera MF, Díaz-Polanco A, Rios JM, Pantoja JP. Nelson's syndrome after bilateral adrenalectomy for Cushing's disease. Surgery. 2007;141(2):147-51.

MULTIPLE CHOICE QUESTIONS

1. A 22-year-old gentleman presents with enlargement of the hands and feet. He has been on treatment for hypertension and diabetes for 3 years. His Growth hormone levels after 100 grams of glucose are 25 ng/dL at 2 hours. Which of the following may be *false*?
   A. With a low Insulin Like Growth Factor -1 measurement, this could be liver disease.
   B. The patient may have Carney's complex.
   C. Response to Octreotide is unlikely to occur.
   D. The patient may have MEN-1.

2. A 50-year-old gentleman has headache and visual deterioration for the last 6 months.

   His vision on in the right eye is 10/60 and optic atrophy on the right side with temporal hemianopia on the left side. Which of the following is likely to be *false*?
   A. He is unlikely to have hyperprolactinemia
   B. He may have a Hardy's grade E tumor
   C. He is unlikely to have pituitary carcinoma
   D. Transnasal -Transsphenoidal surgery is possible.

3. A 27-year-old lady presents with weight loss, of 6 kgs over 4 months. She has low grade fever and joint pains and a urine output of 7 liters a day. Detailed evaluation shows normal blood sugars, calcium, hemoglobin. Her 8.00 am cortisol is 2 µg/dL (Normal 8-23 µg/dL). T4 is 6.0 µg/dL (4.5-11.5 µg/dL). The sodium level is 153 mmol/l (Normal 135-144 mmol/L). Which of the following are most likely to be *false*:
   A. She is unlikely to have a pituitary adenoma
   B. She may have sarcoidosis
   C. She may have lymphocytic hypophysitis
   D. She may have pituitary carcinoma.

4. A 60-year-old gentleman presents with headache off and on for 2 years. Examination reveals bilateral papilledema with normal visual acuity and fields. MRI pituitary shows a Hardy's grade B tumor. Your most likely possibility is:
   A. Estrogen excess
   B. Growth hormone excess
   C. Cortisol excess
   D. Diabetes insipidus

5. A 35-year-old lady presents with lack of menstruation for 2 years. She complains of tiredness. On examination, the pubic and axillary hair is sparse. Her T4 is 2.0 µg/dL (Normal 4.5-11 µg/dL) and her TSH is 2.0 mIU/ml (Normal 0.5-4.5 mIU/ml). 8 am Cortisol levels are 4.0 µg/dL (Normal 8-23 µg/dL). She mentions that she has lost 8 kg after her last delivery 5 years ago, after which she did not lactate. Her prolactin level is 60 ng/dL. Which of the following is probably *false*?
   A. She may have an empty sellar on the MRI pituitary
   B. She has a macroprolactinoma.
   C. She has a total cholesterol of 350 mg/dL
   D. Her serum sodium is 128 mmol/L.

6. An 18-year-old girl presents with decline in scholastic performance over 1 year. Her visual examination reveals optic atrophy in the left eye and hemianopia in the right eye. She is 140 cm tall and has not menstruated. Which of the following are likely to be *false*:
   A. Her FSH is 26 mIU/mL
   B. Her MRI shows a cystic lesion with calcification- 2 cm in size in the sellar lesion.
   C. She has a sodium of 154 mmol/l
   D. Her PROP-1 mutation screen is negative.

7. A 10-year-old boy presents with short stature less than minus 2.5 SDS for age. He is a known case of bronchial asthma on regular inhaled steroids, his Hypothalamo-pituitary adrenal axis is normal. His thyroid functions are normal. The liver function test shows an albumin of 4.5 g/l (Normal 3.5-4.5 gm/dL) and the creatinine is normal. All other biochemical parameters are normal. Testicular volume is normal. What would you do next?
   A. Check the height again in 6 months
   B. Do an insulin tolerance test to assess growth hormone
   C. Do an MRI brain
   D. Do a clonidine stimulation test for growth hormone.

8. A 25-year-old man presented with polyuria and a sodium of 155 mmol/L (Normal 135–144 mmol/L) The symptoms have been gradually worsening over the last 6 years. His weight and appetite are stable. Which of the following is probably *false*:
   A. He may have 2 uncles with exactly the same problem.
   B. He may have had a head injury 7 years ago.
   C. He may have an elevated angiotensin converting enzyme elevation.
   D. He may have a pituitary adenoma.

9. A 27-year-old lady presents with weight loss and low grade fever with recurrent headaches. An MRI

of the pituitary shows a suprasellar lesion which is 2 cm in size bright on a T1-weighted image. Hormonal evaluation is normal. Which of the following tests may help in giving the precise diagnosis?

A. ESR
B. CSF Beta-HCG level
C. ACE level
D. FSH level

10. Gonadotropins are heterodimer made of two peptide subunits called alpha and beta subunits. The alpha subunits of human LH, FSH, thyroid-stimulating hormone (TSH), and human chorionic gonadotropin (hCG) have an identical polypeptide structure. Which of the following glycoprotein has longest half (t1/2) life?

A. FSH
B. LH
C. TSH
D. hCG

11. Gonadotropin releasing hormone (GnRH) is a decapeptide. The GnRH neurons are primarily located in the arcuate nucleus of the medial basal hypothalamus and the preoptic area of the anterior hypothalamus. The half-life of GnRH is short (2 to 4) minutes. Gonadotropin-releasing hormone analogs are useful in all of the following clinical conditions, *EXCEPT*

A. GnRH-dependent precocious puberty
B. Breast malignancy
C. Endometriosis
D. Prostate cancer

12. Anovulation of hypothalamic in origin usually manifests as amenorrhea. The most commonly observed form of hypothalamic anovulation is not associated with a demonstrable neuroanatomical finding. This common form of amenorrhea is called as functional hypothalamic amenorrhea. Clinical conditions associated with functional hypothalamic amenorrhea are all *EXCEPT*.

A. Bulimia Nervosa
B. Anorexia Nervosa
C. Pituitary isolation syndrome
D. Stress related

13. Which genetic testing is indicated in premature ovarian failure?

A. 21–hydroxylase gene mutation
B. FMR1 premutation
C. LH–R mutation
D. AIRE pre mutation

14. A 7-year-old male child presented with head nodding, abnormal gait, abnormalities of visual fields with features suggestive of precocious puberty (penile size of 7 cm, testes of 10 mL B/L Sexual Maturity rating -P4). X-ray of pituitary fossa showed erosion and J shaped enlargement of the sella turcica.

A. Hamartoma of the tuber cinereum
B. Arachnoid cysts
C. Craniopharyngioma
D. Germ cell tumor of CNS

15. A 6-year-old girl presented with history of intermittent menstrual bleeding since 3 months. She also had bony deformity of the both lower limbs noticed since 2 years of age and had fracture of shaft of right femur due to trivial trauma at 5 years of age. The family history was not significant. On examination she had café au lait spot in right back and her SMR (Sexual Maturity Rating) was B2P1. Her clinical findings are suggestive of McCune Albright syndrome Say *True* or *False*.

A. Precocious puberty is GnRH independent
B. The distortion of the shape of long bone also known as Shepherd's crook deformity
C. She may be short statured
D. She could develop acromegaly.

CHAPTER 5

Bountiful Bone
(Bone and Parathyroid Disease)

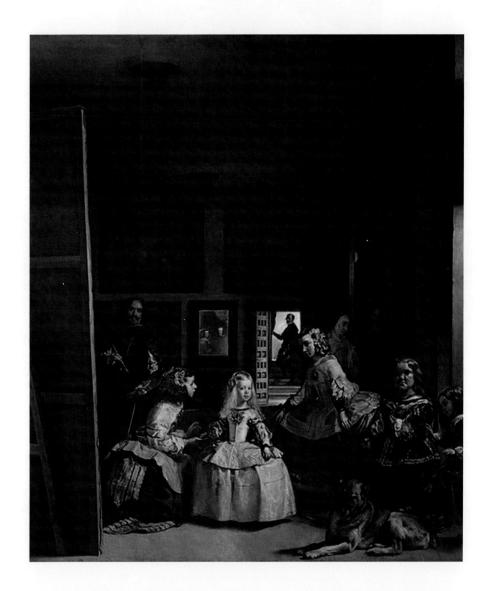

*Diego Velázquez's masterpiece (1656), Las Meninas (The Maids of Honour),
features an achondroplastic dwarf, Maria Barbola, among its subjects*

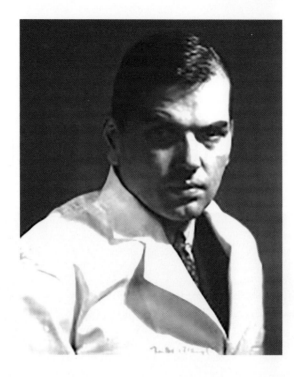

Dr Fuller Albright (FA) was born on January 12th, 1900 in Buffalo, New York, USA. In 1920, FA entered the Harvard Medical School, and graduated in 1924. His interest towards the parathyroid glands and calcium metabolism when he worked as an intern at the Massachusetts General Hospital (MGH). In 1927 and 1928, at Johns Hopkins Hospital in Baltimore, Albright together with Dr R Ellsworth studied and published a case of idiopathic hypoparathyroidism, the first in the bibliography. In the total of 111 publications with his collaborators, the main subject was parathyroid glands, bones and stones. In 1942, he published his research on pseudohypoparathyroidism, the Seabright-Bantam syndrome and in 1952, he discovered pseudo-pseudohypoparathyroidism.

It was Fuller Albright (FA) who, in 1947, invented the end organ unresponsiveness on pseudohypoparathyroidism. He writes *"We thought the primary disturbance was a failure of response to some hormone by the end organ. Another probable example of failure of the end organ to respond is met within patients with low basal metabolic rate without other evidence of hypothyroidism ... still another example is the absence of a beard in the American Indians"*.

At least eight previously unknown diseases or syndromes were discovered and described by FA.

Albright had his interest in the area of gonads too where, together with H Klinefelter and ES Reifenstein, he described the homonymous syndrome characterized by gynecomastia, aspermatogenesis without aleydism in 1941. In 1940, he worked on postmenopausal osteoporosis and its treatment with oestrogens as well as on Paget's disease.

FA never used statistics saying *"Statistic are important, but I don't trust them"*.

In 1936, FA developed the symptoms of Parkinson's disease and he lived with his disease for 20 years. In 1956 he had a brain surgery and following that he remained in a vegetative condition for 13 years until his death on December 8th, 1969.

CASE 1

A 45-year-old woman presented with a 6-week history of progressive increase in pain and stiffness of the left shoulder joint which limited her movement and normal daily activities. She attributed her symptoms to a history of a minor fall onto her left side 4 weeks prior to the onset of pain. Examination revealed a tender left shoulder joint associated with restriction of movement in all directions. Conventional radiology of the left shoulder joint revealed the features shown in Figures 1A to C.

WHAT IS THE DIAGNOSIS?

Laboratory studies showed normal renal functions along with normal serum corrected calcium and phosphate levels. The patient denied having any previous episodes of joint pains or any similar disorders in the family. The findings on radiography of the shoulder joint were consistent with Tumoral calcinosis (TC). The patient was started initially on Alendronate 70 mg once weekly which was later changed over to yearly Zoledronic acid. She is on regular follow-up, with her pain being reduced and limited improvement of the movement of the shoulder joint.

DISCUSSION

Tumoral calcinosis (TC) is a rare clinical and histopathological syndrome characterized by calcium salt deposition in different peri-articular soft tissue regions. It mainly manifests in childhood or adolescence as painless, firm, tumor-like masses around the joints that may lead to limitation of joint movements. The region most commonly involved include the soft tissues of peri-articular upper limb (shoulder and elbow) and hip regions. TC was first mentioned as the so-called progressive lipocalcinogranulomatosis by Teutschlaender in 1935. Inclan et al used the term "tumoral calcinosis" in 1943 for a disease characterized by large juxta-articular lobular calcified masses without visceral or skin calcifications in patients with normal serum calcium and phosphorus levels. Diagnosis of TC relies on typical radiographic features (on plain radiographs and computed tomography) and the biochemical profile. Magnetic resonance imaging can be done in difficult cases, and scintigraphy reflects the disease activity. The management of TC is either medical or surgical. Bisphosphonates have been tried successfully for the treatment of TC. Bisphosphonates have multiple effects on the osteoclast cells, including the following: (1) direct inhibition of osteoclast activity, (2) decrease in the recruitment of osteoclasts, and (3) reduction of the survival of osteoclasts by apoptosis. The characteristic histopathological features of TC are the presence of multiple cysts filled with calcified deposits lined by histiocytes, giant cells, and xanthomatous histiocytes. A similar action on these giant cells as on normal osteoclasts has been postulated in forming the basis of the therapeutic role of bisphosphonates in TC.[1,2]

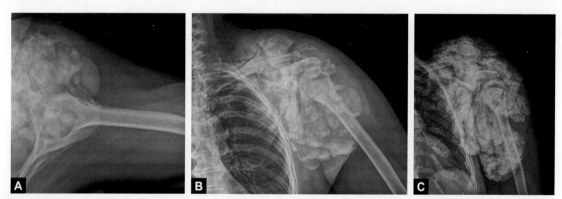

Figs. 1A to C: Chunky calcification adjacent to the lateral margin of the left shoulder joint with no underlying destruction of bone, periosteal resorption, or soft tissue swelling.

REFERENCES

1. Fathi I, Sakr M. Review of tumoral calcinosis: A rare clinico-pathological entity. World J Clin Cases. 2014;2(9):409–14.

2. Jacob JJ, Thomas N, Seshadri MS. Tumoral Calcinosis of the scalp: An Unusual site for a rare tumor. *Laryngoscope.* 2006;117:179-80.

CASE 2

A 15-year-old boy, Master R presented with complaints of swelling followed by pain in the right hip joint for 8 months and swelling in the left elbow and the right ankle joint for 5 months duration. Examination of the joints revealed ill-defined swellings with no inflammation or sinuses around the joints, and restriction of the movements of the right hip, right elbow and the right ankle joints. The X-rays of the elbow joint, ankle joint and the hip joints are shown in Figures 1 to 3.

WHAT IS THE DIAGNOSIS?

Laboratory studies revealed normal renal functions and also normal serum corrected calcium and phosphate levels with normal alkaline phosphatase levels. The findings on radiography of the joints were consistent with Tumoral calcinosis (TC). In view of the extensive involvement of the hip joint he underwent an excision of the TC. The immediate and 6-month postoperative images are shown in the Figures 4 and 5 respectively. He is under regular follow-up with no restriction of hip joint movements and is planned for the excision of TC in the other joints.

DISCUSSION

The main clinical signs of TC are calcium deposits in the soft tissues around the joints, often at multiple sites but not always concomitantly, with an asymptomatic increase in size. The symptoms are usually related to functional impairment or mechanical neural irritation caused by calcification. A careful attention to the plain radiographic features of amorphous calcification should alert the physicians to the possibility of TC. In a subset of cases in which the imaging studies are not diagnostic, a biopsy is necessary. According to the presence or absence of an underlying calcifying disease process, TC can be divided into primary and secondary varieties. Two subtypes of the primary variety exist; (1) a hyperphosphatemic type with familial basis represented by mutations in GalNAc transferase 3 gene (*GALNT3), KLOTHO* or Fibroblast growth factor 23 (*FGF23*) genes, and (2) a normo-phosphatemic type with growing evidence of an underlying familial basis represented by mutation in *SAMD9 (sterile alpha motif domain containing 9)* gene. The secondary variety is mainly associated with chronic renal failure and the resulting

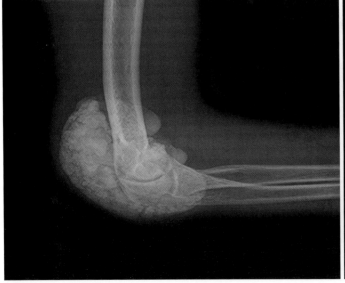
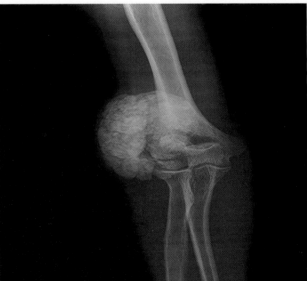

Fig. 1: Chunky calcifications around the left elbow joint.

secondary or tertiary hyperparathyroidism. Treatment is mainly surgical for the primary variety; however, a stage-oriented conservative approach using phosphate binders, phosphate restricted diets and acetazolamide are tried before surgical approach is pursued due to the high rate of recurrences and complications after surgical intervention. Medical treatment is the mainstay of therapy for the secondary variety, with failure warranting subtotal or total parathyroidectomy. Surgical intervention in these patients should be kept as a last resort.[1,2]

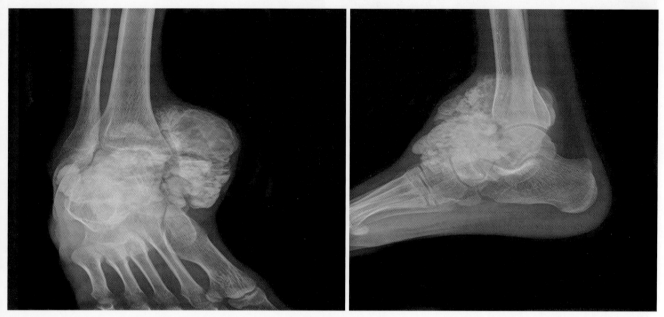

Fig. 2: X-ray of the right ankle joint with similar calcification that of the elbow joint.

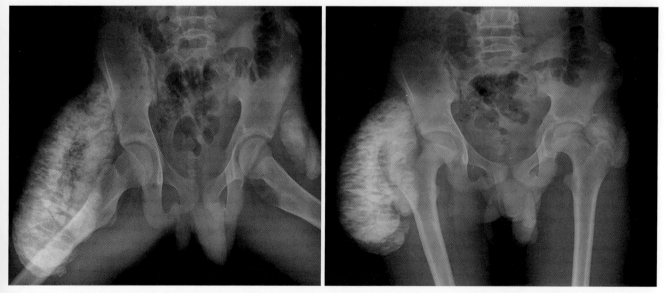

Fig. 3: X-ray of the pelvis showing calcification on the lateral aspect of both the hip joint sparing the joints space and the bones.

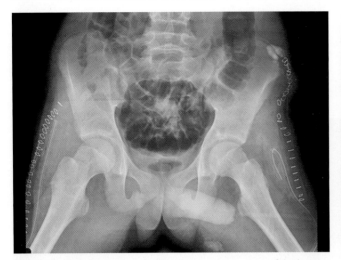

Fig. 4: Postoperative X-ray of pelvis showing no remnant of the lesions, as described before.

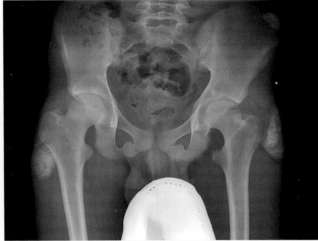

Fig. 5: Six monthly postoperative period X-ray image showing a regrowth of the chunky calcification around both the hip joints.

REFERENCES

1. Jacob JJ, Thomas N, Seshadri MS. Tumoral Calcinosis of the scalp: An Unusual site for a rare tumor. *Laryngoscope.* 2006;117:179-80.

2. Jacob JJ, Mathew K, Thomas N. Idiopathic Sporadic tumoral Calcinosis of the hip; successful oral Bisphosphonate therapy. *Endocrine Practice.* 2007;13:182-86.

CASE 3

A 25-year-old lady presented with complaints of whole body pain with difficulty to stand after squatting. She also complained of pain in the left thigh since the past few days. X-rays of left femur and the left tibia are shown in the Figures 1A and B.

WHAT IS THE DIAGNOSIS?

The "pseudo-fractures" (shown with arrow in Figures 1A and B) are typically transverse zones of rarefaction, varying in width from 1 mm to 1 cm. They are multiple and, in general, symmetrical in distribution, and often occur in apparently normal bone. According to Mondor and Leger (1947) their distribution is mainly as follows: ischiopubis, iliopubis, femur, tibia, radius, fibula, iliac bone. Other common sites are the lower ribs and the infraglenoid region of the scapula. It is also called Milkman's fracture or looser's zones.

DISCUSSION

Pseudofractures correspond with the location of main blood vessels which lie on the bones. It is suggested that the mechanical stress caused by the vessels may result in small breaks in the cortex with subsequent laying down of callus which, in osteomalacia, is uncalcified. This mechanism explains the symmetrical appearance of the pseudofractures in otherwise normal appearing bone and their location at sites not usually subjected to other mechanical stresses.

Differential diagnoses for pseudofractures are (a) fatigue fracture (b) the increment fracture of Paget's disease (c) cough fractures of the ribs.

Fatigue fractures are neither multiple nor symmetrical, but may occur in both the tibiae. They produce normal callus within a few weeks, and this increases rapidly. The radiolucent zone in the developed "pseudofracture" is generally wider than the zone of porosis seen in a fatigue fracture. The zone of condensation above and below a "pseudofracture" is denser, narrower, and better defined than that of the fatigue fracture.

The increment fracture of Paget's disease of bone is usually on the convex surface, is of a finely angled triangular shape with slightly irregular surfaces, and always occurs in areas of bone where the disease process shows definite pathological appearances and the bones are often sclerotic.

"Cough fractures" have all the appearances of ordinary fractures, with fairly sharp irregular edges, and on healing there is more callus than in "pseudofractures". If multiple "pseudofractures" are seen radiologically the presence of osteomalacia can be presumed; no more can be inferred, and it remains for clinical and biochemical examinations to discover the cause of the osteomalacia.

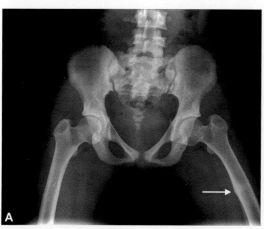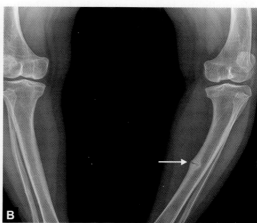

Figs. 1A and B: Breach in the femoral and tibial cortex (shown with arrow).

REFERENCES

1. Stanley Nowell, P. R. C. Evans, F. Kurrein. Multiple Spontaneous "Pseudofractures" of Bone (Milkman's Syndrome) Br Med J. 1951; 2(4723): 91–4.

2. M. Le May, J. W. Blunt, Jr. A factor determining the location of pseudofractures in osteomalacia. J Clin Invest. 1949;28(3): 521–25.

CASE 4

A 30-year-old lady presented with history of repeated fracture of both femurs, following a trivial trauma. She had 2 siblings with dysmorphic facies who had died immediately after delivery. Her paternal uncle was short statured and had a similar history of recurrent fractures in the past. She had blue sclerae but no hearing loss. The X-ray of her lower limbs showed a pencil line cortex with multiple fractures (Fig. 1).

WHAT IS THE DIAGNOSIS?

With the history of recurrent fractures since birth, blue sclera and pencil thin cortices on the radiographs, she was diagnosed to have Osteogenesis Imperfecta. She is at present on yearly Zoledronic acid.

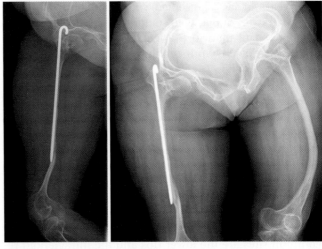

Fig. 1: Femur with "pencil line" cortices.

DISCUSSION

Osteogenesis Imperfecta (OI), brittle bone disease, or "Lobstein syndrome" is a congenital bone disorder characterized by brittle bones that are prone for fractures even with trivial trauma or injury. These patients have a tendency for recurrent fractures due to deficiency of Type-1 collagen which is required for the stability of bones. The stability of bones is compromised due to the amino acid substitution of glycine with bulkier amino acids in the collagen triple helix. Normally the body responds by hydrolyzing these abnormal collagen molecules. In the event of the body not destroying the abnormal collagen, an imbalance between the collagen fibrils and hydroxyapatite crystals occur, leading to the formation of brittle bones. Till date around eight types of OI have been distinguished. Mutations in the *COL1A1* and *COL1A2* genes are the commonest cause for OI. The important differential diagnoses of OI are battered baby syndrome, child abuse as both may present with multiple fractures in various stages of healing, rickets, and osteomalacia.

Classical Skull radiographs and features of OI are intrasutural (wormian) bones and Dentinogenesis Imperfecta.

The X-ray of the chest shows superior rib notching. The X-rays of the limbs may show any of the following features– thin and under-tubulated gracile bones which are normal in length or shortened with thickened or deformed bones (due to multiple fractures)—"Banana fractures". Angiograms may show carotid and vertebral artery dissection. There is no definite treatment for OI. Treatment is aimed at increasing overall bone strength to prevent fracture and maintain mobility. Bisphosphonates may increase bone mass, and reduce bone pain and fractures.[1,2]

REFERENCES

1. Rauch F, Glorieux FH. "Osteogenesis imperfecta". Lancet. 2004;363(9418):1377–85.
2. Chevrel G, Schott AM, Fontanges E, et al. "Effects of oral alendronate on BMD in adult patients with osteogenesis imperfecta: a 3-year randomized placebo-controlled trial". J. Bone Miner. Res. 2006;21(2):300–6.

CASE 5

A 35-year-old lady presented with history of brownish discolouration of the teeth even at the best of her oral hygiene with similar complaints in her family members too (Figs. 1A and B). A diligent physician examined her eyes which are shown in Figures 2A and B. Similar findings were also seen in her youngest daughter and her father (Fig. 3). The X-ray of the teeth of her sister is shown in Figure 4.

WHAT IS THE DIAGNOSIS?

With a clinical and family history of dentition and scleral involvement, the patient was diagnosed to have Dentinogenesis Imperfecta Type 2.

DISCUSSION

Dentinogenesis Imperfecta (DI) or hereditary opalescent dentin, was first described in the late 19th century. DI, an autosomal dominant disease is a localized mesodermal dysplasia affecting both the primary and the permanent dentition. There are three types of Dentinogenesis Imperfecta: (1) DI type 1 is associated with Osteogenesis Imperfecta. (2) DI type 2 has essentially the same clinical radio-graphic and histological features as DI type 1 but without Osteogenesis Imperfecta; (3) DI type 3 is rare and is only found in the triracial Brandywine population of Maryland.[1]

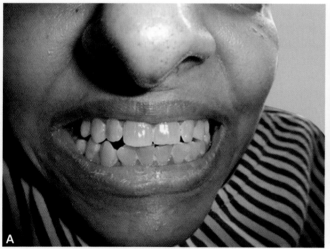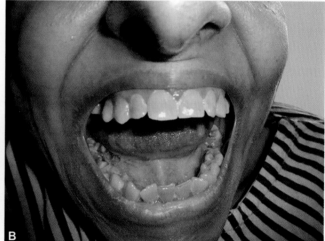

Figs. 1A and B: Brownish discolouration of the teeth.

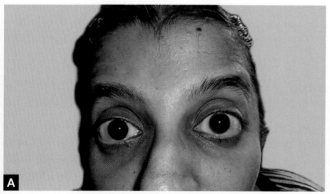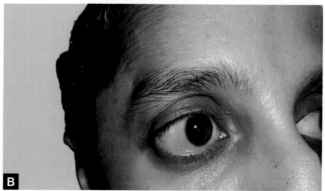

Figs. 2A and B: Blue sclera.

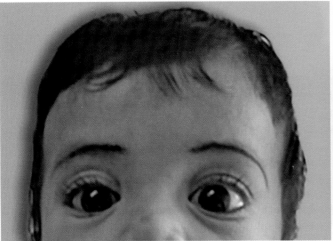 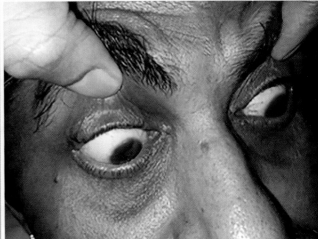

Fig. 3: Patient's daughter and her father's image showing blue sclera.

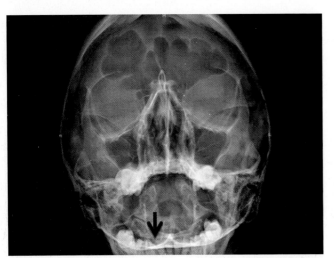

Fig. 4: Radiography of the teeth showing bulbous crown-shaped teeth and constricted short roots.

Clinically, the color of the teeth varies from brown to blue, sometimes described as amber or gray, with an opalescent sheen. The enamel shows a hypoplastic or hypocalcified defects in about one-third of the patients and, in an affected patient, tends to crack away from the defective dentin with early and rapid attrition. Radiographically, the teeth have bulbous crowns with constricted short roots resembling "shell teeth". With restorative treatment, glass ionomers with fluoride-releasing and chemically attaching materials are recommended for occlusally non-stressed areas. An acrylic overlay denture, resting over the remnants of crowns and roots of the primary dentition, has been used successfully.[2]

REFERENCES

1. Beattie ML, Kim J-W, Gong S-G, et al. Phenotypic Variation in Dentinogenesis Imperfecta/Dentin Dysplasia Linked to 4q21. J Dent Res. 2006;85(4):329–33.
2. Barron MJ, McDonnell ST, MacKie I, et al. Hereditary dentine disorders: dentinogenesis imperfecta and dentine dysplasia. Orphanet J Rare Dis. 2008;3(1):31.

CASE 6

A 42-year-old lady presented with progressive stiffness of the neck for the past 15 years with history of low back ache since the past 4 months. Her family members used groundwater for drinking. Clinical examination showed stiffness of the neck joints with restricted movement and her teeth displayed mild mottling (Fig. 1). A similar dental finding was noted in her brother too. His X-rays of the vertebrae (Fig. 2) and bones of the forearm (Fig. 3) revealed diffuse sclerosis. Bone mineral density confirmed a sclerotic bone (Figs. 4A to C).

WHAT IS THE DIAGNOSIS?

Differential diagnoses considered for osteosclerosis were skeletal Fluorosis, Paget's disease, metastases, renal tubular acidosis or renal osteodystrophy. The X-ray of her lumbar

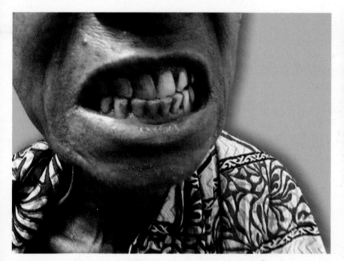

Fig. 1: Mottling of the teeth.

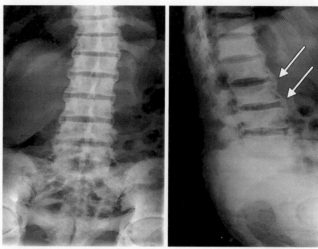

Fig. 2: Extensive sclerosis of the bone with calcification of the anterior spinal ligaments (indicated with the arrows).

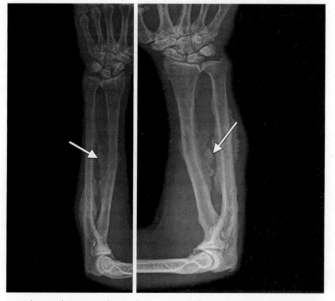

Fig. 3: X-ray of forearm showing osteosclerotic bones and membranous calcification (shown with arrow).

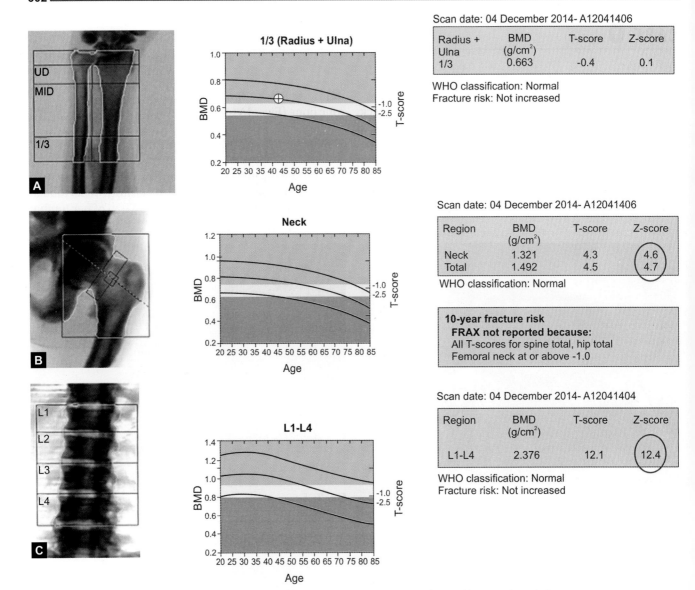

Scan date: 04 December 2014- A12041406

Radius + Ulna	BMD (g/cm²)	T-score	Z-score
1/3	0.663	-0.4	0.1

WHO classification: Normal
Fracture risk: Not increased

Scan date: 04 December 2014- A12041406

Region	BMD (g/cm²)	T-score	Z-score
Neck	1.321	4.3	4.6
Total	1.492	4.5	4.7

WHO classification: Normal

10-year fracture risk
FRAX not reported because:
All T-scores for spine total, hip total
Femoral neck at or above -1.0

Scan date: 04 December 2014- A12041404

Region	BMD (g/cm²)	T-score	Z-score
L1-L4	2.376	12.1	12.4

WHO classification: Normal
Fracture risk: Not increased

Figs. 4A to C: Bone mineral density showing increased bone mass suggesting osteosclerosis (shown with circles).

spine was significant for calcification of the anterior spinal ligament (rugger-jersey appearance) and that of her forearm for inter-osseous membrane calcification - features that were suggestive of skeletal fluorosis. She had elevated 24-hour urinary fluoride levels (>15PPM). Skeletal scintigraphy revealed a picture similar to metabolic "superscan" i.e. increased tracer uptake in axial and appendicular skeleton, reduced soft tissue uptake, poor or absent renal images, and the "tie" sign in the sternum (Fig. 5).

DISCUSSION

Chronic fluoride intoxication (fluorosis) is endemic in areas where the fluoride content is high in drinking water. Endemic skeletal fluorosis is widely prevalent in India, China, and many countries around the world. Cases of endemic skeletal fluorosis have been reported primarily from Southern Rajasthan, Andhra Pradesh, and Kanpur district of Uttar Pradesh in India. The primary manifestations of fluorosis are mottling of teeth, osteosclerosis, soft tissue calcification, and marginal bony overgrowth. The secondary effects include damage to the nervous system.

The optimum safe upper limit for fluoride intake is not more than 6 mg per day. The possible predisposing factors include: (a) continued high fluoride exposure through water and food; (b) strenuous physical activity; (c) malnutrition with deranged renal function and (d) abnormal concentrations of certain trace elements.

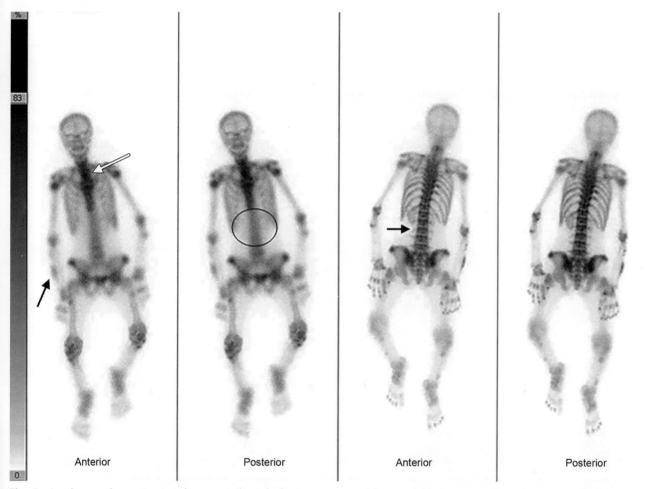

| Anterior | Posterior | Anterior | Posterior |

Fig. 5: A technetium bone scan revealing an uptake in the ligamentous areas (shown with black arrow) with an absent renal uptake (shown with circle) and a "tie" sign in the sternum (shown with white arrow).

Fluorosis in humans have predominantly dental and skeletal manifestations. Dental fluorosis is an early and sensitive manifestation in children presenting as white chalky opacities or pitting on the enamel. In the early stage of fluorosis, patients are asymptomatic or gastrointestinal symptoms may be present. In the advanced stages, skeletal fluorosis causes crippling deformities and neurological complications. Neurological complications occur in 5–10% and are due to compression of the spinal cord and nerve roots. These features usually develop after exposure to a high fluoride content (greater than 4 parts per million [PPM]) for longer than 10 years. Spinal cord involvement is mainly due to compression of the spinal cord and nerve roots by the protruding osteophytes, thickening of the posterior longitudinal ligament, and thickening of the ligamentum flavum resulting in compressive myeloradiculopathy, compressive myelopathy, and/or compressive

radiculopathy. Prevention of the disease should be the aim bearing in mind the pathogenesis of fluorosis.

In skeletal fluorosis, technetium-labeled methylene diphosphonate (^{99m}Tc-MDP) bone scanning shows mostly a superscan appearance with a diffuse linear tracer activity along the ligamentous attachments (Fig. 5). Treatment consists of protection from fluoride exposure, and if osteomalacia is present, calcium supplementation to mineralize the excess osteoid.[1,2]

REFERENCES

1. Kumar P, Gupta A, Sood S, et al. Fluorotic cervical compressive myelopathy, 20 years after laminectomy: A rare event. Surg Neurol Int. 2011;2:11.
2. Kakumanu N, Rao SD. Skeletal Fluorosis Due to Excessive Tea Drinking. N Engl J Med. 2013;368(12):1140.

CASE 7

A 26-year-old male born of a non-consanguineous marriage presented with history of multiple joint pains, associated with early morning stiffness since 4 years of age. He also had history of progressive decrease in height and deformity of hands. He was known to have hypothyroidism and was on Levothyroxine supplements for the same. Physical examination revealed short stature (Height-141 cm with Height centile <3rd centile). His forearm was 2 cm longer than his arm. Also, he had a short neck with enlargement of proximal and distal interphalangeal joints. His hip flexion, knee extension and wrist extension were restricted bilaterally. His skeletal survey is demonstrated in Figures 1A to D.

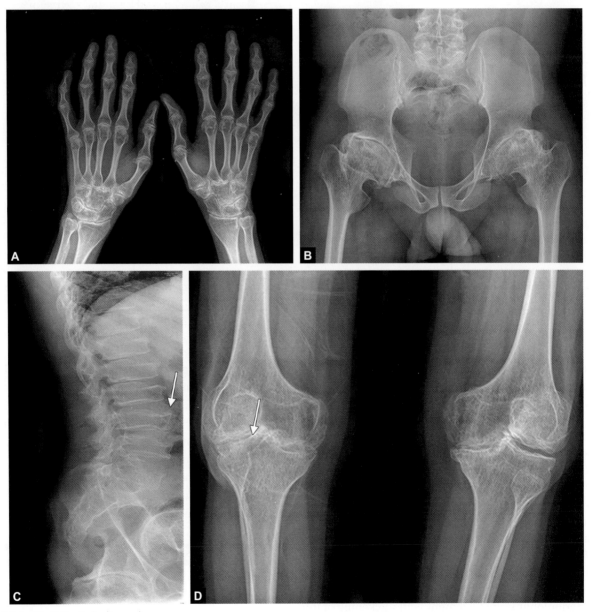

Figs. 1A to D: Patient's Radiographs.

WHAT IS THE DIAGNOSIS?

Radiography of the hand showed decreased joint space in the interphalangeal joints and poor differentiation of the carpal bones. The X-ray of both knee joints showed a reduction in joint space with expanded epiphyses. The thoraco-lumbar spine revealed decreased height of vertebrae (flattened vertebrae) with anterior beaking (Figs. 1A to D, shown with arrow). The X-ray of the Pelvis showed decreased and destroyed joint space suggesting bilateral hip joints arthritis.

The differential diagnoses for the anterior beaking of vertebrae considered were Morquio syndrome (only middle one third), Hurler syndrome, spondylodysplasia, achondroplasia, pseudoachondroplasia, cretinism, and Down syndrome.

In view of his age, disproportionate short stature, flattened vertebrae and destroyed femoral epiphysis with early arthritis of the other joints, spondyloepiphyseal dysplasia was also considered as a diagnosis. He was given genetic counselling and physiotherapy.

DISCUSSION

Spondyloepiphyseal dysplasia (SED) refers to a heterogeneous group of disorders with primary involvement of vertebrae and epiphyseal centres of long bones. Three major types of SED are recognized (1) SED congenita, (2) pseudoachondroplasia SED, and (3) SED tarda. SED was first described in 1966 by Spranger and Wiedemann and is now also known as Wiedemann-Spranger syndrome. Clinically, SED is characterized by short stature (120 to 140 cm), often significant lordosis, pectus carinatum and may have associated features of myopia, retinal detachment, deafness, cleft lip cleft palate, and muscular hypotonia.

SED congenita is a specific skeletal dysplasia inherited as an autosomal dominant disorder which is evident at birth. A cleft palate is common and over half of the patients have high grade myopia or retinal detachment. SED tarda is the term that is used for the X-linked recessive disorder; however an autosomal dominant and recessive form have also been described.

The most consistent radiologic findings in the SED are flattened vertebrae with anterior beaking, and small and deformed (femoral) epiphyses and dysplastic odontoid process. In the cervical spine of children with SED congenita, atlantoaxial instability is the most commonly encountered and most dangerous problem, found in approximately 30–40%. The major clinical characteristics of SED tarda are pain, stiffness, and limitation of movements of the lumbar spine and multiple joints combined with a waddling gait. Progressive symptomatic osteoarthritis of the hips and knees are commonly seen. Scoliosis or thoracic kyphosis with exaggerated pain in the back and hips with limitation of motion in these joints are frequent by the teens. Treatment of SED includes support and compensation for the disabilities. A frequent eye check is also mandatory as these patients can have early cataract which requires surgical intervention. Recurrent middle ear infections should be treated to prevent hearing impairment. Hip joint defects and arthrosis sometimes require surgical intervention. Spinal defects are treated with a corset brace but may require surgery.[1, 2]

REFERENCES

1. Harper JR, Macgregor ME. Pseudoachondroplastic type of Spondyloepiphyseal dysplasia (type Maroteaux-Lamy). Proc R Soc Med. 1968;61(12):1262-3.
2. Singhal A, Singhal P, Gupta R, et al. True Generalized Microdontia and Hypodontia with Spondyloepiphyseal Dysplasia. Case Rep Dent. 2013;2013:e685781.

CASE 8

A 25-year-old gentleman presented with history of progressive deformity of the long bones for over 10 years (Fig. 1). His investigations demonstrated an elevated creatinine with raised alkaline phosphatase and parathyroid hormone (PTH). His X-ray revealed osteosclerosis (Fig. 2). The ultrasound of the abdomen showed bilateral contracted kidneys (Fig. 3).

WHAT IS THE DIAGNOSIS?

He had normal serum calcium with elevated phosphate levels. The differential diagnoses considered for the osteosclerosis were renal osteodystrophy, renal tubular acidosis, skeletal fluorosis, Paget's disease or metastases. This patient had renal dysfunction and secondary hyperparathyroidism (raised PTH and alkaline phosphatase). Thus, in this scenario osteosclerosis of the bone was due to renal osteodystrophy. He was started on oral activated Vitamin D and calcium acetate.

DISCUSSION

The kidneys play a central role in the bone mineral metabolism. The most frequent form of osteodystrophy in renal failure is due to the decreased capacity to synthesize 1, 25 $(OH)_2$ vitamin D and to excrete phosphate. The impairment of calcium absorption in the intestine, and the loss of the feedback inhibitory effect of 1, 25 (OH) 2 Vitamin D levels on PTH production produces severe secondary hyperparathyroidism and ultimately leads to osteitis fibrosis cystica and finally tertiary hyperparathyroidism.

Renal osteodystrophy causes growth retardation and skeletal deformities in children. Both children and adults have bone pain and muscle weakness. Soft issue calcification also occurs as a sequelae of osteodystrophy and produces calciphylaxis leading onto ischemia and gangrene. Calcification is due to the high calcium-phosphorus product and vessel wall changes secondary to renal failure or to direct effects of PTH. To prevent calcification, it is

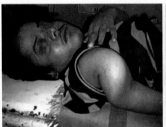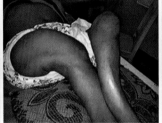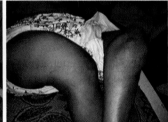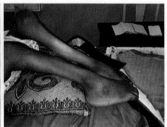

Fig. 1: Deformity of the long bones.

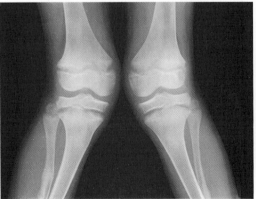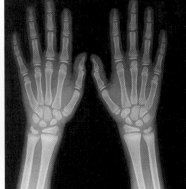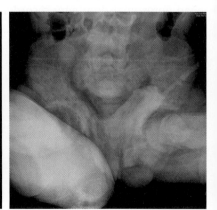

Fig. 2: X-ray done at the age of 15 years showing osteosclerosis of the bones.

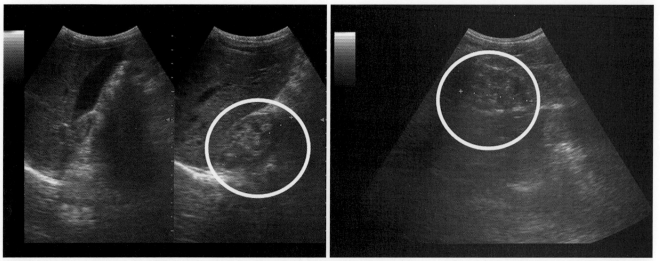

Fig. 3: USG of abdomen showing bilateral contracted kidneys (Right-6 cms and left 5.3 cms) and absent cortico-medullary differentiation (shown with a circle).

important to avoid a high serum calcium-phosphorus ion product and to minimize secondary hyperparathyroidism. The diagnosis of a specific form of renal osteodystrophy can often be made on biochemical grounds. Levels of PTH are high in patients with severe secondary hyperparathyroidism.

A bone biopsy is seldom if ever needed to clarify the pathogenesis of renal osteodystrophy. Using double tetracycline labelling technique, it is possible to determine whether mineralization is impaired. Sections that have not been decalcified show the extent of osteoid seams and resorption surfaces.

The treatment of renal osteodystrophy can be highly successful if done correctly. The goal is to maintain a normal serum calcium and phosphorus levels. Phosphate restriction by administering phosphate binders such as calcium salts, sevelamer, or lanthanum should be instituted relatively early in the renal failure. Early in renal failure, the modest supplementation with vitamin D may be sufficient to maintain 1, 25 $(OH)_2$ vitamin D levels, but eventually calcitriol itself should be administered when the renal failure progresses. Low doses (0.25–0.5 µg/day are usually well tolerated, but higher doses may lead to hypercalcemia and hypercalciuria.

In some cases, a three and half gland parathyroidectomy may be required when the patient has persistent hypercalcemia in patients with renal failure, intractable pruritus, extracellular calcifications, and severe skeletal lesions. However, parathyroidectomy should be avoided in patients with adynamic bone disease because symptoms may be worsened. Renal transplantation corrects many of the biochemical disturbances that lead to renal osteodystrophy; however the bone disease may progress.[1,2]

REFERENCES

1. Slatopolsky E, Gonzalez E, Martin K. Pathogenesis and treatment of renal osteodystrophy. Blood Purif. 2003;21 (4-5):318–26.
2. Narula A, Jairam A, Baliga K, et al. Pathogenesis and management of renal osteodystrophy. Indian J Nephrol. 2007;17(4):150.

CASE 9

A 34-year-old lady was admitted with complaints of recurrent quadriparesis requiring repeated parenteral fluid therapy. She also revealed that she had dry eyes and dry mouth with no history of joint pains. The investigations showed low serum potassium and bicarbonate levels. The skeletal survey is shown in Figure 1. The ultrasonography (USG) of the abdomen demonstrated bilateral nephrocalcinosis.

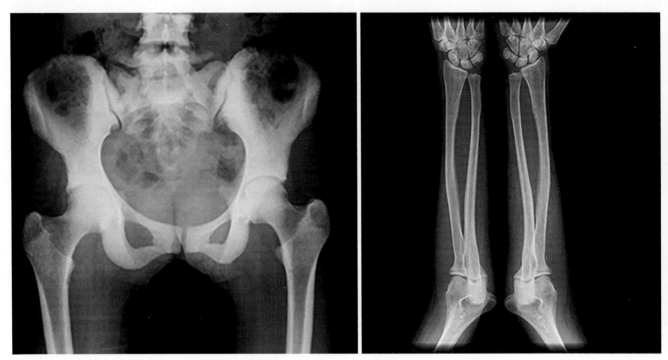

Fig. 1: Patchy osteosclerosis of the bones with no interosseous membrane calcification.

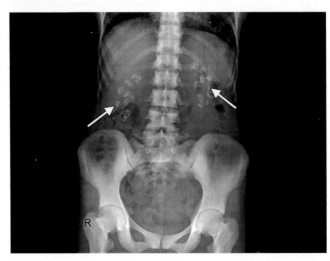

Fig. 2: X-ray erect Abdomen with bilateral nephrocalcinosis (shown with the arrows) with no ligamental calcification of the spine.

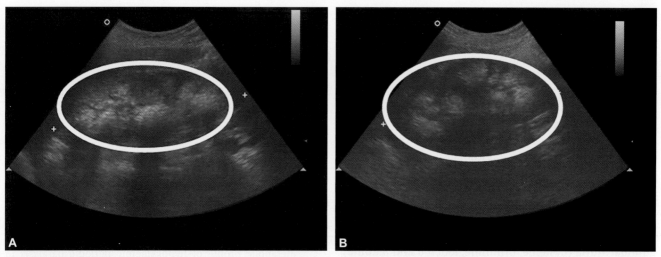

Figs. 3A and B: Ultrasonography of the abdomen showing bilateral medullary nephrocalcinosis (shown with a circle).

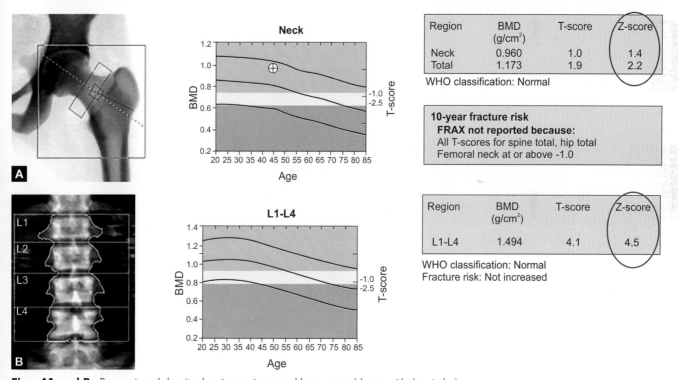

Figs. 4A and B: Bone mineral density showing an increased bone mass (shown with the circles).

WHAT IS THE DIAGNOSIS?

The other blood investigations showed normal calcium and fasting phosphate levels. The fasting urinary pH was 7.1. The lip biopsy showed chronic lymphocytic infiltrate, consistent with Sjögren's syndrome. Her ultrasonography of the abdomen revealed bilateral medullary nephrocalcinosis (Fig. 3A and B). The bone mineral density revealed an increased bone mass (Figs. 4A and B). Thus, a diagnosis of renal tubular acidosis of distal type was made and she was started on oral potassium with bicarbonate. Following therapy with potassium and bicarbonate she did not have paraparesis or quadriparesis.

DISCUSSION

Renal tubular acidosis is characterised by a normal anionic gap hyperchloremic metabolic acidosis. Type 1 or distal renal tubular acidosis is due to the acid secretion failure in the distal tubules of the kidneys. Thus, the kidneys are unable to acidify urine to a pH value of less than 5.5 in the presence of systemic metabolic acidosis, or following acid loading (ammonium chloride loading test). Type 2 or proximal renal tubular acidosis is a result of impaired bicarbonate re-absorption in the proximal tubules, which is the primary area of bicarbonate re-absorption. They also have hypophosphatemia with phosphaturia, hypokalemia, renal glycosuria (glycosuria in the presence of normal plasma glucose concentration) and aminoaciduria (cysteine, ornithine, leucine and alanine). Renal tubular acidosis may be a result of cystinosis, tyrosinaemia, hereditary fructose intolerance, galactosaemia, glycogen storage disease Type 1 or Wilson's disease, or it may be due to heavy metal poisoning such as lead, copper or mercury poisoning. In adults one of the common causes for distal renal tubular acidosis is an underlying connective tissue disorder or Sjögren's syndrome. The management of distal renal tubular acidosis includes alkali therapy and replacement with potassium supplements.[1,2]

REFERENCES

1. Jebasingh F, Paul TV, Spurgeon R, et al. Klinefelter's syndrome with renal tubular acidosis: impact on height. Singapore Med J. 2010;51(2):e24–6.
2. Rao N, John M, Thomas N, et al. Aetiological, clinical and metabolic profile of hypokalaemic periodic paralysis in adults: a single-centre experience. Natl Med J India. 2006; 19(5):246–9.

CASE 10

A 15-year-old 10th Standard student was seen in the endocrinology OPD for complaints of short stature, and delay in the eruption of permanent teeth. His height was 155 cms at the 10th centile on the growth chart, with a mid-parenteral height of 165.5 cms. He had a triangular face and hypertelorism with lower part of the face being hypoplastic (Fig. 1). His oral examination revealed persistent temporary milk teeth. He had normal secondary sexual characters. He was able to shrug his shoulders and approximate them due to hypoplastic clavicles (Fig. 2). X-ray image is demonstrated in Figure 3.

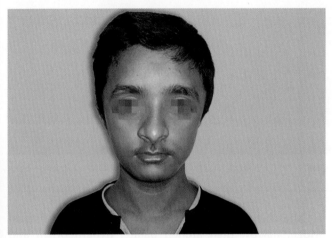

Fig. 1: Triangular face with hypoplastic lower half and hypertelorism, an "Arnold's" face.

WHAT IS THE DIAGNOSIS?

The patient was diagnosed to have Cleidocranial dysostosis in view of the open anterior and posterior fontanelle, hypoplastic maxillae, low set ears and ability to shrug shoulders and approximate them due to hypoplastic clavicles (Figs. 1 to 5) with unerupted permanent teeth. He had normal serum calcium and phosphorus levels without supplements. He was found to have Vitamin D insufficiency and was started on supplements.

DISCUSSION

Cleidocranial dysostosis(CCD) is a rare autosomal dominant disorder which is characterized by a persistently open anterior fontanelle and skull sutures, hypoplastic or aplastic clavicles, supernumerary teeth, delayed eruption of permanent dentition, short stature, a wide pubic symphysis and a variety of other skeletal changes. A major finding of CCD is hypoplasia or aplasia of clavicular bones resulting in the ability of the patient to approximate the shoulders.

CCD primarily affects bones that undergo intramembranous ossification. It is also known as Marie and Sainton disease, Scheuthauer-Marie-Sainton syndrome, mutational dysostosis and Cleidocranial dysplasia. The classical pathognomic triad of CCD includes multiple supernumerary teeth, partial or complete absence of the clavicles and open sagittal sutures and fontanelles. The skull base

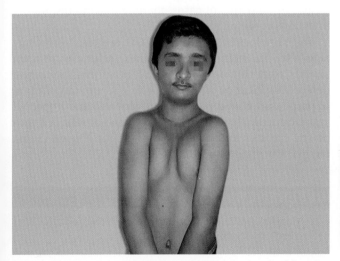

Fig. 2: The Patient has been able to approximate his shoulders due to hypoplastic clavicles.

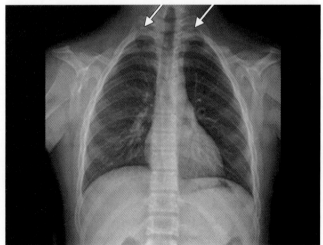

Fig. 3: X-ray of chest showing hypoplastic clavicles (shown with the arrows).

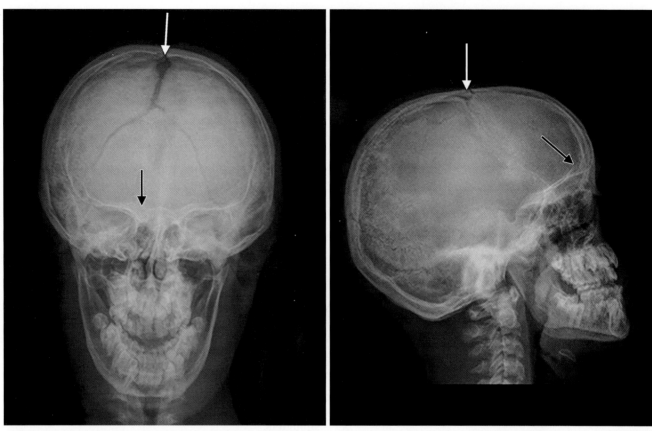

Fig. 4: X-ray of skull showing a persistent opening of the anterior and posterior fontanelles (indicated with white arrow) and an absent frontal sinuses (indicated with black arrow).

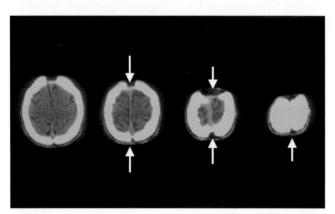

Fig. 5: CT images showing an open anterior and posterior fontanelles (indicated with the arrows).

is also dysplastic and the growth is retarded, which results in increased skull width leading on to brachycephaly and hypertelorism. Delayed closure of anterior fontanelle and metopic sutures result in frontal bossing. Bossing of the frontal, occipital and parietal regions give the skull a large globular shape with a small face which is also referred to as "Arnold's head".

Other facial features are broad and depressed nasal bridge, narrow high arched palate, hypertelorism and absent paranasal sinuses due to underdeveloped maxilla. The thoracic cage is small with short ribs, and underdeveloped clavicles to varying degrees. Clavicles are completely absent in upto 10% of cases, thereby making respiratory infections common in CCD.

The radiological features of CCD are also very characteristic. The cranial abnormalities include wide-open sutures, patent fontanelles, presence of wormian bones and delayed ossification of skull, decreased pneumatization of paranasal, frontal and mastoid sinuses, and impacted supernumerary teeth. Chest X-ray shows absent or hypoplastic clavicles and scapulae with a cone shaped thorax and narrow upper thoracic diameter.[1,2]

REFERENCES

1. Mundlos S. Cleidocranial dysplasia: clinical and molecular genetics. J Med Genet. 1999;36(3):177–82.
2. Bhargava P, Khan S, Sharma R, et al. Cleidocranial Dysplasia with Autosomal Dominant Inheritance Pattern. Ann Med Health Sci Res. 2014;4(Suppl 2):S152–4.

CASE 11

A 22-year-old gentleman presented with complaints of pain and deformity of the right lower limb for 15 years. His chest X-ray and bone scan images are displayed in Figures 1 and 2.

WHAT IS THE DIAGNOSIS?

The blood investigation revealed normal renal function and normal serum calcium and phosphate levels. With the radiological and the bone scan findings, she was diagnosed to have fibrous dysplasia and was started on oral Bisphosphonates, namely Alendronate. She has been on regular follow-up since then.

DISCUSSION

Fibrous dysplasia (FD) is a benign skeletal disorder, described by Lichtenstein in 1938 and Lichtenstein and Jaffe

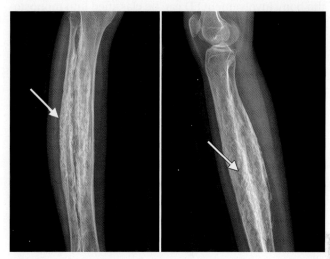

Fig. 1: X-ray showing mixed sclerotic and lytic lesions on the tibia and fibula.

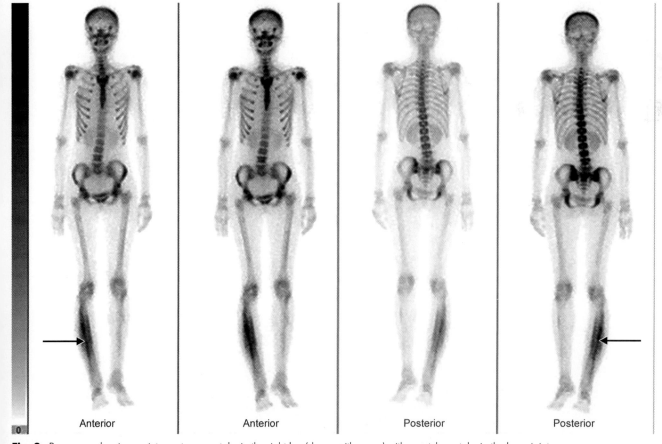

| Anterior | Anterior | Posterior | Posterior |

Fig. 2: Bone scan showing an intense tracer uptake in the right leg (shown with arrow) with a patchy uptake in the large joints.

in 1942. It accounts for 0.8% of primary and 7% of benign bone tumors. Fibrous dysplasia is an uncommon and debilitating skeletal disorder resulting in fracture, deformity, functional impairment, and pain. Depending upon the bony involvement FD can be classified into monostotic FD (which affects one bone) or polyostotic FD (which affects many bones). FD can occur with extraskeletal features, most commonly café-au-lait macules and also certain hyperfunctioning endocrinopathies like precocious puberty, hyperthyroidism, growth hormone excess, hypercortisolism, and FGF 23-mediated hypophosphatemia. FD when occurs with one or more of these extraskeletal features is termed as the McCune-Albright syndrome (MAS).[1]

Osteogenic cells derived from the progenitors are functionally impaired, leading to abnormal bone matrix deposition and formation of subsequent bone that is morphologically and structurally unstable. The most commonly involved sites include the ribs (28%), proximal femur (23%), and craniofacial bones (20%). The course of both monostotic and polyostotic fibrous dysplasia are variable. Surgery is indicated only for confirmatory biopsy, correction of deformities, failure of nonsurgical therapy, prevention of pathologic changes, and eradication of symptomatic lesions. Careful assessment of the endocrine system in such is mandatory in ruling out the McCune-Albright syndrome as early intervention can prevent irreversible changes especially in case of precocious puberty. The bone lesions usually respond to bisphosphonate. Treatment with 1,25 (OH) Vitamin D may reduce PTHrP production and decrease activity of the bone lesions.[2]

REFERENCES

1. Shetty S, Varghese RT, Shanthly N, et al . Toxic Thyroid Adenoma in McCune-Albright Syndrome. J Clin Diagn Res [Internet]. 2014:2 281–2.
2. John AM, Behera KK, Mathai T,et al. Mazabraud syndrome. Indian J Endocrinol Metab. 2013;17(4):740–2.

CASE **12**

A 26-year-old lady presented with complaints of pain in both the legs for the past 3 years which was predominantly more during the night time. She had normal hematological parameters. She had her bone scan done which revealed an increased uptake in both the tibiae.

WHAT IS THE DIAGNOSIS?

In view of the age of the patient with bilateral symmetrical pain in both the tibiae, and a symmetrical (Figs. 1A and B) tracer uptake in the diaphyseal region in the bone scan the patient was diagnosed to have Camurati-Engelmann disease. Subsequently she was started on Alendronate 70 mg once a week and later changed to twice a week. Her pain subsided and she is on regular follow-up since then.

DISCUSSION

Camurati-Engelmann disease (CED) or progressive diaphyseal dysplasia is an autosomal dominant condition that belongs to the group of craniotubular hyperostoses. Cockayne described the disorder in 1920, but in 1922, Camurati discovered the hereditary nature of the disease. In 1929, Engelmann reported a single case of CED. The initial name of progressive diaphyseal dysplasia was given with an emphasis on the progressive nature of the hyperostosis and the involvement of the diaphysis. However currently, the eponym Camurati-Engelmann disease is widely being used.

The onset of the disease is generally during childhood and almost always before the age of 30. Most patients present with limb pain, muscular weakness, a waddling gait, and easy fatigability. Systemic manifestation such as anaemia, leukopenia, and hepatosplenomegaly occasionally occur due to bone marrow suppression and extramedullary erythropoiesis. The hallmark of the disorder is cortical thickening of the diaphyses of the long bones. Hyperostosis is usually bilateral and symmetrical and usually starts at the diaphyses of the femur and tibiae, expanding to the fibulae, humerii, ulnae, and radii. As the disease progresses, the metaphyses is also affected, however the epiphyses are spared. CED usually responds to glucocorticoids showing diminution of bone pain when oral prednisone is given on alternate days. The improvement of CED with glucocorticoid therapy indicates that CED is an inflammatory connective tissue disease. Various Bisphosphonates may help in reducing pain, but there are reports suggestive of exacerbation of the symptoms too.[1,2]

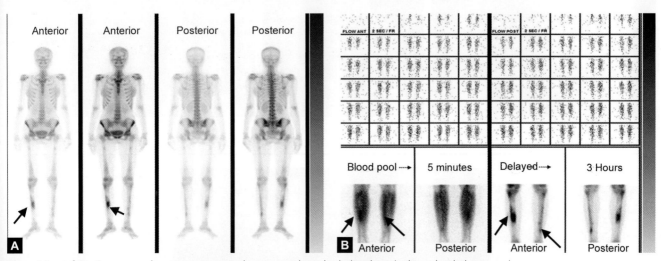

Figs. 1A and B: Bone scan showing an increased tracer uptake in both the tibiae (indicated with the arrows).

REFERENCES

1. Janssens K, Vanhoenacker F, Bonduelle M, et al. Camurati-Engelmann disease: review of the clinical, radiological, and molecular data of 24 families and implications for diagnosis and treatment. J Med Genet. 2006;43(1):1–11.

2. Whyte MP, Totty WG, Novack DV, et al. Camurati-Engelmann Disease: Unique Variant Featuring a Novel Mutation in TGFβ1 Encoding Transforming Growth Factor Beta 1 and a Missense Change in TNFSF11 Encoding RANK Ligand. J Bone Miner Res. 2011;26(5):920–33.

CASE 13

A 17-year-old boy presented with the history of fracture of the left humerus which he sustained following trivial trauma (Fig. 1A). He also gave history of similar multiple episodes of pathological fractures followed by deformities since childhood. Physical examination revealed a dark brown hyperpigmented lesion over the upper back with irregular borders (Fig. 2). A skeletal survey of the long bones is demonstrated in Figures 1B and C.

WHAT IS THE DIAGNOSIS?

His investigations revealed a normal calcium and phosphate levels with slightly elevated alkaline phosphatase levels. With the radiographic findings of polyostotic fibrous dysplasia and café au laite spots, he was diagnosed to have McCune-Albright syndrome. He was started on once a year pamidronate and is on regular follow-up.

DISCUSSION

Fibrous dysplasia is a skeletal developmental anomaly of the bone-forming mesenchyme; with a significant defect in the osteoblastic differentiation and maturation, and thereby a progressive replacement of normal bone with immature woven bone. McCune- Albright syndrome (MAS) is a sporadic genetic disorder which is defined by

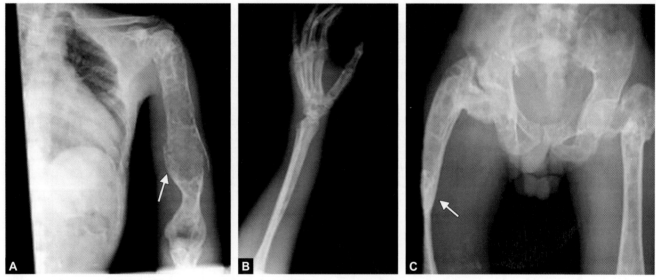

Figs. 1A to C: The radiographs showing multiple lucent lesions in the metaphysis of the long bones, with endosteal scalloping and bone expansion (shown with arrow).

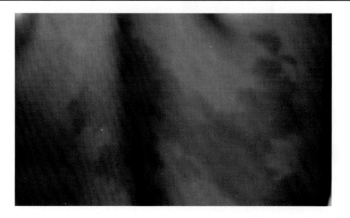

Fig. 2: Café au lait spot.

the presence of polyostotic fibrous dysplasia, café au lait cutaneous spots and hyperfunctioning endocrinopathies. The typical endocrinopathies that have been described are central precocious puberty, hyperthyroidism, growth hormone excess, hyperprolactinemia, and hypercortisolism. MAS is characterized by post-zygotic mutation of the gene GNAS1, which is involved in the G-protein signaling pathway of G protein coupled receptors. In its classic form the triad includes autonomous endocrine hyperfunction in addition to the above two lesions. The presence of any two features among the three warrants a diagnosis of MAS.[1,2]

REFERENCES

1. Natarajan MS, Prabhu K, Chacko G, et al. Endoscopic transsphenoidal excision of a GH-PRL-secreting pituitary macroadenoma in a patient with McCune-Albright syndrome. Br J Neurosurg. 2012;26(1):104–6.
2. Shetty S, Varghese RT, Shanthly N, et al. Toxic Thyroid Adenoma in McCune-Albright Syndrome. J Clin Diagn Res JCDR. 2014;8(2):281–2.

CASE 14

A 25-year-old lady presented with progressive swelling and pain in the left thigh since 7 years duration without any cachexic symptoms. Examination of the left thigh revealed bowing of the left femur and a soft tissue swelling not attached to the bone which was mobile and mildly tender. She did not have any bony deformity or café au lait spots. The X-rays of pelvis and hip showed expansile bony swelling with cortical thinning of both the tibiae shown in Figure 1. Magnetic resonance imaging (MRI) of the left thigh showed a well-defined intramuscular mass lesion (Fig. 2). Bone scan is demonstrated in Figure 3.

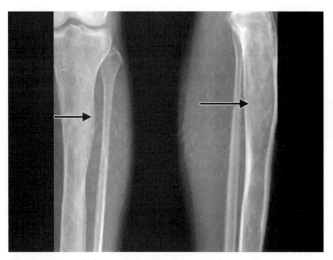

Fig. 1: Expansile lesion in the tibia (shown with arrow).

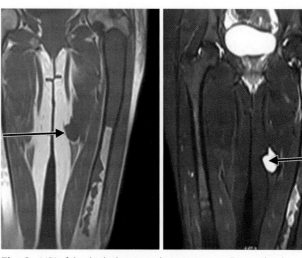

Fig. 2: MRI of the thigh showing a hypointense on T1 weighted image and hyperintense on T2W lesion (shown with arrow).

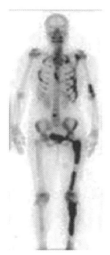

Fig. 3: Bone scan with an abnormal, irregularly increased tracer activity in left scapula, left tibia, left femur, pubis and left sacroiliac joints, L5 vertebra, left distal humerus and multiple ribs.

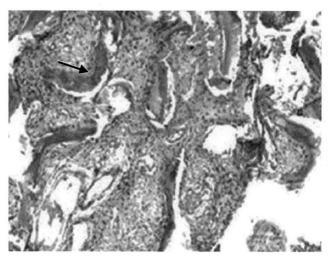

Fig. 4: Bone biopsy showing irregular trabeculae of woven bone lacking osteoblastic rimming set in a fibrous stroma. (Hematoxylin & Eosin stain, 10 x magnification) (demonstrated with arrow).

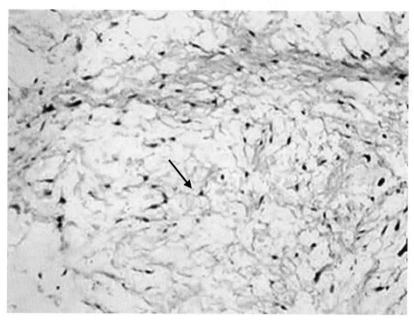

Fig. 5: Biopsy of the intramuscular myxoma showing loosely arranged haphazard fascicles of spindle to stellate shaped cells embedded in a hypovascular myxoid stroma (H&E stain at 10x magnification).

WHAT IS THE PROBABLE DIAGNOSIS?

On biochemical evaluation she had a normal alkaline phosphatase, normal serum calcium, phosphorous and 24 hrs urine calcium, phosphorous and creatinine. She had a low level of 25 hydroxy vitamin D of 4.85 ng/mL (20.0–32.0 ng/mL). She underwent a bone scan which was suggestive of polyostotic fibrous dysplasia. There was a partly exophytic lesion in the thigh which is shown in Figure 3. A bone biopsy (Fig. 4) from the left femur revealed fibrous dysplasia. The biopsy of the soft tissue mass from left thigh confirmed an intramuscular myxoma (Fig. 5).

DISCUSSION

Polyostotic fibrous dysplasia in association with intramuscular myxomas is a rare condition. This association is known as the Mazabraud syndrome. Intramuscular myxomas associated with polyostotic fibrous dysplasia occur in multiple sites in adulthood while fibrous dysplasia occurs at a younger age. Most patients present with minimal symptoms thereby delaying the diagnosis. Intramuscular myxomas are usually benign though local recurrence can occur if incompletely excised. Myxomas in this syndrome are exclusively intramuscular and usually affect middle-aged women. Most common location is the thigh. A malignant transformation of fibrous dysplasia can also occur as part of the Mazabraud syndrome.[1,2]

REFERENCES

1. Paul T, John A, Behera K,et al. Mazabraud syndrome. Indian J Endocrinol Metab. 2013;17(4):740.
2. Szendrói M, Rahóty P, Antal I,et al. Fibrous dysplasia associated with intramuscular myxoma (Mazabraud's syndrome): a long-term follow-up of three cases. J Cancer Res Clin Oncol. 1998;124(7):401–6.

CASE 15

A 16-year-old boy presented with progressive proximal myopathy for 3 years with bony aches and pains. His clinical picture is shown in Figure 1. The Technetium Bisphosphonate scan revealed a "super scan" (Fig. 2) with multiple increased uptakes in the bones. Histopathological details are shown in Figure 3.

WHAT IS THE DIAGNOSIS?

The diagnosis is Osteitis fibrosa cystica (OFC) which is also known as osteitis fibrosa, osteodystrophia fibrosa, Von Recklinghausen's Disease of Bone. A typical OFC histopathology shows Howship's lacunae and multinucleated osteoclasts lining the space in bone-destructive lesions regardless of the cause. The histopathology of the bone biopsy (Shown with arrow) revealed that the bone is undergoing a regenerative process even as it undergoes concomitant destruction.

DISCUSSION

Osteitis fibrosa cystica is the result of unchecked hyperparathyroidism, or the over-activity of the parathyroid glands, which results in an overproduction of parathyroid hormone (PTH). Parathyroid hormone causes the release of calcium from the bones into the blood, and the reabsorption of calcium in the kidney. Thus, excess PTH in hyper-

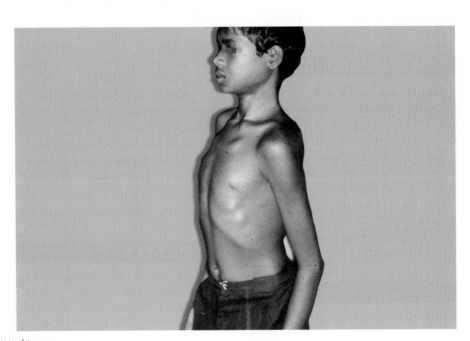

Fig. 1: Patient's clinical image.

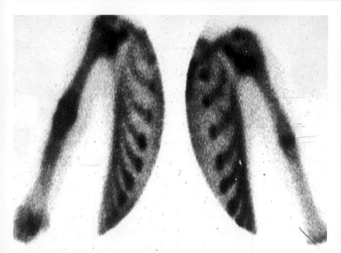

Fig. 2: Super scan showing an increased uptake in the costochondral junction.

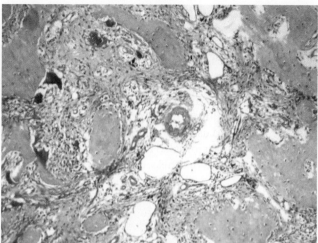

Fig. 3: Histopathological specimen from the Bone.

parathyroidism causes elevated blood calcium levels, or hypercalcemia.

Osteitis fibrosa cystica (OFC) is a common presentation of renal osteodystrophy, which is a term used to refer to the skeletal complications of end stage renal disease (ESRD). Osteitis fibrosa cystica occurs in approximately 50% of patients with ESRD. Generally, the first bones to be affected are the fingers, facial bones, ribs, and pelvis.

Medical management of OFC consists of active Vitamin D treatment, generally with 1-alfacalcidol or calcitriol. In patients with hyperparathyroidism, parathyroid adenoma removal is the treatment of choice.[1,2]

REFERENCES

1. Rubin, MR. "Tc99m-Sestamibi Uptake in Osteitis Fibrosa Cystica Simulating Metastatic Bone Disease". *Journal of Clinical Endocrinology & Metabolism*. 2001;86(11):5138-4.
2. Eubanks, PJ; Stabile, BE. "Osteitis Fibrosa Cystica with Renal Parathyroid Hormone Resistance: A Review of Pseudohypoparathyroidism with Insight into Calcium Homeostasis". *Archives of Surgery*. 1998;133(6):673-6.

CASE 16

A 9-year-old girl, born of a non-consanguineous marriage presented with pain in the left leg for 6 months with recent exacerbation during the last one month especially at night. She also had associated low grade fever during this period. Examination revealed that she had an antalgic gait with swelling and tenderness over the left mid-shaft of the tibia. Radiograph of the tibia is shown in Figure 1. The Technetium bone scintigraphy is shown in Figure 2. She presented again four months later with pain in the right leg with similar characteristics as mentioned before. The radiographs (Fig. 3), blood investigations and bone scintigraphy (Fig. 4) were similar.

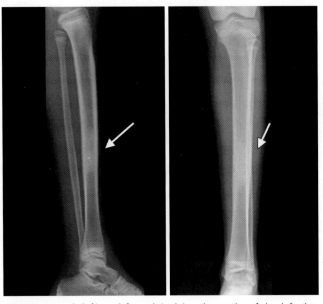

Fig. 1: Lateral (left) and frontal (right) radiographs of the left tibia showing sclerosis of mid-diaphysis with a periosteal reaction (shown with the arrows).

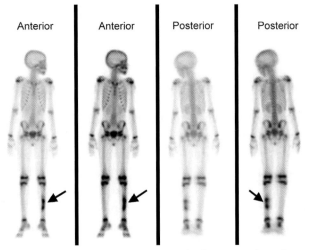

Fig. 2: Bone scintigraphy shows a markedly increased uptake over the mid-shaft of the left tibia (shown with arrow).

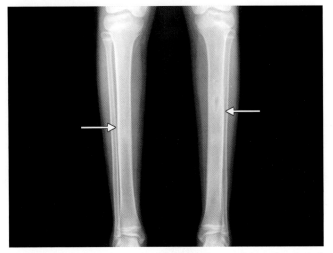

Fig. 3: Repeat X-ray done after 4 months showing bilateral mid-shaft sclerosis (shown with arrow) which was seen prior.

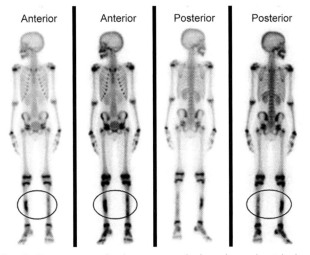

Fig. 4: Bone scintigraphy showing a marked uptake on the right than the left side tibia, compared to the previous scan (circled).

WHAT IS THE DIFFERENTIAL DIAGNOSIS?

The differential diagnoses considered were osteomyelitis, sickle cell crisis, malignant bone tumor, juvenile Paget's disease and osteonecrosis. Her other investigations are as follows: total leucocyte count of 7,600/mm^3 (normal 4,000–11,000/mm^3), hemoglobin of 13 g/dL (13–15 g/dL), serum calcium 9.9 mg/dL (8.3–10.4 mg/dL), fasting serum phosphorus 8.3 mg/dL (2.5–4.6 mg/dL), serum alkaline phosphatase 159 u/L (50–125 u/L), sickle cell preparation was negative, and serum creatinine was 0.8 mg/dL (0.8–1.2 mg/dL).

X-ray of the tibia showed patchy sclerosis involving the medulla in the mid third of the tibial diaphysis (Figs. 1 and 3) with periosteal reaction in the initial and the subsequent radiograph. Bone scan also showed an isolated marked increased uptake in the left tibia (Figs. 2 and 4). She underwent an open biopsy which showed abundant new bone formation and chronic inflammation. Subsequently she had excellent pain relief without any treatment.

With the history, clinical and radiological finding, the diagnosis of Hyperostosis-hyperphosphatemia syndrome (HHS) was made. The patient was treated for her symptoms with analgesics. The patient fulfilled all the criteria for this syndrome; these were recurrent episodes of painful swelling of the long bones, normal renal function, vitamin D and parathormone levels, and increased renal reabsorption of phosphates.

DISCUSSION

Hyperostosis-hyperphosphatemia syndrome (HHS) was first described in 1970 and is predominantly seen in girls. Though the presentation of this condition mimics osteomyelitis and bone neoplasms, the elevated serum phosphate level along with other normal parameters help in the diagnosis of this condition. This syndrome should be considered as part of the differential diagnosis for osteomyelitis, neoplasms and vaso-occlusive crises such as sickle cell anaemia. In conclusion, HHS should be considered in patients between 6 and 16 years of age, who present with a painful swelling of the long bones involving the diaphysis and an isolated hyperphosphatemia. The early and accurate diagnosis will help in avoiding multiple invasive investigations. The painful episodes can recur in HHS and surgical decompression is an option when conservative measures fail.[1,2]

REFERENCES

1. Nithyananth M, Cherian VM, Paul TV, et al. Hyperostosis and hyperphosphataemia syndrome: a diagnostic dilemma. Singapore Med J. 2008;49(12):e350-2.
2. Talab YA, Mallouh A. Hyperostosis with hyperphosphatemia: a case report and review of the literature. J Pediatr Orthop 1988;8:338-41.

CASE 17

A 4-year-old boy presented with delay in developmental milestones and aggressive behavior with mentally challenged state. An axial computed tomography (CT) scan of the brain was done (Fig. 1). Subsequent evaluation revealed a normal serum calcium and inorganic phosphorus values with an elevated serum alkaline phosphatase. His arterial blood gas analysis was suggestive of metabolic acidosis with anionic gap of minus 15.1. His skeletal X-rays were done (Figs. 2A and B).

WHAT IS YOUR DIAGNOSIS?

Carbonic anhydrase II (CA II) deficiency is an autosomal recessive disorder in which CA-II enzyme activity is lost. CA II deficiency syndrome produces cerebral calcification (Fig. 1), osteosclerosis (Figs. 2A and B) and renal tubular acidosis.

DISCUSSION

The anion gap is the difference in the measured cations and the measured anions in serum. If the gap is greater than normal, then high anion gap metabolic acidosis is diagnosed. The normal anion gap is < 11 mEq/L. Over 90% of patients with this disorder may have a mentally challenged state. Cerebral calcifications appear early in life by 2–5 years of age, and are more pronounced in childhood. Carbonic anhydrase II (CA-II) enzyme activity is necessary for osteoclast-mediated bone resorption. Skeletal diseases in CA-II deficiencies resemble certain forms of osteopetrosis and are associated with multiple pathological fractures. In the kidney, this enzyme is necessary for bicarbonate reabsorption. Therefore the patient with CA II deficiency present with hyperchloremic metabolic acidosis with a high urine pH and osteosclerosis. There is no established medical treatment for CA-II

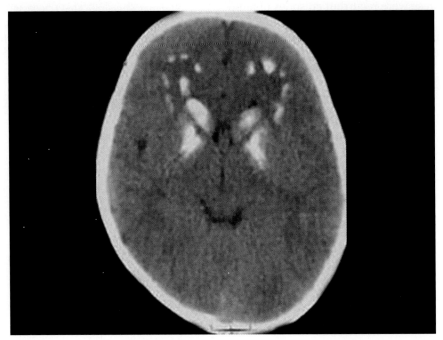

Fig. 1: Cerebral calcifications.

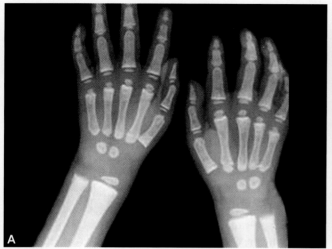 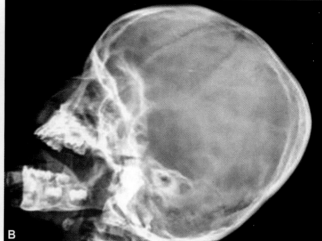

Figs. 2A and B: X-ray of the hand and the skull showing osteosclerosis.

deficiency. In malignant form of osteopetrosis, bone marrow transplantation from a human leukocyte antigen (HLA)-identical donor is an accepted form of therapy.[1,2]

REFERENCES

1. Prabhu S, Jacob JJ, Thomas N. Medical image. Dense bones and brain stones. Carbonic anhydrase-II (CA-II) deficiency. N Z Med J. 2007;120(1262):U2731.

2. Shah GN, Bonapace G, Hu PY, et al. Carbonic anhydrase II deficiency syndrome (osteopetrosis with renal tubular acidosis and brain calcification): novel mutations in CA2 identified by direct sequencing expand the opportunity for genotype-phenotype correlation. Hum Mutat. 2004;24 (3):272.

CASE 18

A 68-year-old gentleman presented with a history of sudden onset of low back pain radiating to both the lower limbs. He denied history of prostatic or respiratory symptoms. A diagnosis of osteoporotic collapse of D5, D7 and L1 was made and the patient was advised further evaluation (Fig. 1). A biopsy from the thoracic vertebrae had shown only changes of chronic inflammation. A bone scan done is shown in Figures 2A and B.

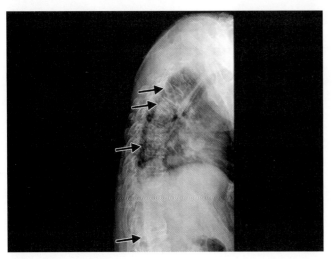

Fig. 1: X-ray of spine showing multiple compressions in the thoracic and lumbar vertebrae (shown with the arrows).

WHAT IS THE PROBABLE DIAGNOSIS?

His investigations revealed a normal serum electrophoresis. Other investigations done to rule out metastasis were normal except for a high alkaline phosphatase (221 U/L). Bone scan demonstrated an increased tracer activity in both the scapulae, right humeral head, sternum, left rib -posteriorly, and in multiple thoracic and lumbar vertebrae with the axial and appendicular skeleton demonstrating a normal tracer uptake. Considering the age and multiple compression fractures with asymmetrical tracer uptake in the bone scintigraphy a possible osseous metastatic disease was diagnosed. He was started on parenteral Zoledronic acid after which he had minimal pain relief.

DISCUSSION

Bone scintigraphy is more sensitive than radiography for detection of bony metastases. The tracer accumulates in the new reactive bone that is formed in response to the metastases. In addition, the amount of accumulation is sensitive to the level of blood flow to the particular bone. Often, a diffuse tracer uptake is seen throughout the skeleton due to disseminated disease and may lead to an erroneous diagnosis of a normal scan. However the bone scan suffers from a lack of specificity, because the tracer accumulation may occur in any skeletal site with an elevated

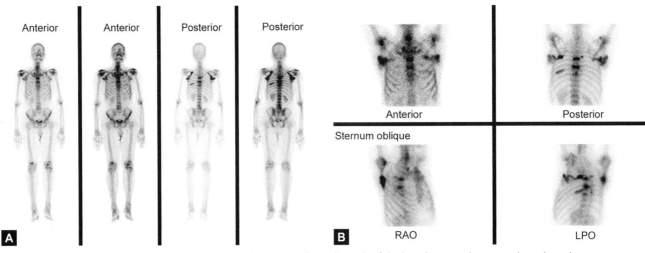

Figs. 2A and B: Bone scan showing an asymmetrical tracer uptake at the ends of the long bones with a normal renal uptake.

rate of bone turn-over due to trauma, infection or arthropathy. In a patient with foci of asymmetrical increased uptake and a known primary tumor, the scan strongly suggests metastases. Even a small number (less than 4 areas of uptake) of abnormalities is more likely to represent metastatic disease, in the presence of rib lesions. However, at this point of time FDG –PET has superseded the bone scan in diagnosing metastasis.[1,2]

REFERENCES

1. Cheran SK, Herndon JE, Patz EF. Comparison of whole-body FDG-PET to bone scans for detection of bone metastases in patients with a new diagnosis of lung cancer. Lung Cancer Amst Neth. 2004;44(3):317–25.
2. Houssami N, Costelloe CM. Imaging bone metastases in breast cancer: evidence on comparative test accuracy. Ann Oncol. 2011;mdr397.

CASE 19

A 66-year-old post-menopausal lady presented with right breast enlargement, for which she was investigated and found to have a malignant spindle cell tumor. A bone scan done to rule out osseous metastasis showed tracer uptake, as shown in Figure 1. A subsequent radiograph of the pelvis is demonstrated in Figure 2.

WHAT IS THE DIAGNOSIS?

Her investigations revealed an elevated alkaline phosphatase level and normal serum calcium and phosphate levels. The differential diagnoses considered were concurrent Paget's disease with breast cancer or osteoblastic metastasis from breast cancer. The biopsy from the left ileum was suggestive of metastatic breast cancer and the patient was advised parenteral Zoledronic acid. Later on she was referred to Department of radiotherapy for further management.

DISCUSSION

Osteosclerotic or blastic bone metastases can arise from malignancies such as prostate carcinoma (most common), breast carcinoma (usually post therapy tumors), transitional cell carcinoma (TCC), carcinoid, medulloblastoma, neuroblastoma, mucinous adenocarcinoma of the gastrointestinal tract (e.g. colon carcinoma) and lymphoma. Invasion of the bone compartment by cancer

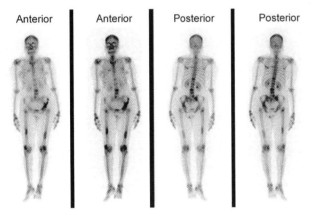

Fig. 1: Bone scan with an asymmetrical increased tracer in ribs, lower thoracic and lumbar vertebrae, right humerus, left ilium, right sacroiliac region, shaft of both femorii and right proximal femur.

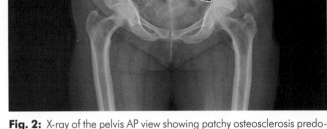

Fig. 2: X-ray of the pelvis AP view showing patchy osteosclerosis predominantly in the left ileo-pectinal line -indicated by an arrow.

cells causes an imbalance in the osteoclastic and osteoblastic activities. It therefore results in predominantly bone lysing or bone forming phenotypes depending on the imbalance. Therapies that can restore the balance including Bisphosphonates and Denusomab mainly aims at pain relief and in the stabilisation of the bones in patients with metastasis.[1,2]

REFERENCES

1. Guise TA, Mohammad KS, Clines G, et al. Basic Mechanisms Responsible for Osteolytic and Osteoblastic Bone Metastases. Clin Cancer Res. 2006;12(20):6213s–6216s.
2. Ortiz A, Lin S-H. Osteolytic and osteoblastic bone metastases: two extremes of the same spectrum? Recent Results Cancer Res. 2012;192:225–33.

CASE 20

A 62-year-old male presented initially with severe tooth ache and headache. On evaluation he was found to have bilateral mixed hearing loss (Figs. 1A and B). His clinical picture is displayed in Figures 1A and B. He had a head circumference of 58 cms. He was also noted to have an elevated alkaline phosphatase level of 1214 U/L (40–125 U/L). His skeletal survey images are displayed in Figures 2A to D. A bone scan was ordered after noticing the findings on the X-ray (shown in Fig. 3).

WHAT IS THE DIAGNOSIS?

He was diagnosed with Paget's disease and was started on Alendronate 70 mg weekly since 2002. Initially his alkaline phosphatase values were in the normal range.

Analysis of the radiological images demonstrated a patchy increased thickening and sclerosis of all the involved bones with underlying lytic lesions. The X-ray of the skull showed the typical cotton wool appearance seen in Paget's disease. The bone scan demonstrated an intense tracer activity in the skull and the iliac region which was suggestive of Paget's disease (Fig. 3). He was initially treated with twice weekly oral alendronate with which the alkaline phosphatase levels normalised. The therapy was subsequently changed over to twice yearly Zoledronic acid and he is under regular follow up.

DISCUSSION

Paget's disease of bone is a fairly common finding in aging bone, with estimates ranging from 2.3% to 9% in older patients within affected populations; it is most often asymptomatic with onset typically after age 55, with a slight predominance towards male gender. There are three stages classically described (1) lytic (incipient active): predominated by osteoclastic activity, (2) mixed (active): osteoblastic as well as osteoclastic activity, (3) sclerotic/blastic (late inactive). These patients have elevated serum alkaline phosphatase (ALP) and urine Hydroxyproline levels. In X-ray the early phase features osteolytic (lucent) region which is later followed by coarsened trabeculae and bony enlargement. Sclerotic changes occur much later in the disease process. The skull X-ray shows osteoporosis circumscripta: large well defined lytic lesion, cotton wool appearance: mixed lytic and sclerotic lesions of skull or a diploic widening: when both inner and outer calvarial tables are involved. X-ray of the spine shows classically described signs such as the picture frame sign, squaring of vertebra or vertical trabecular thickening. In the pelvis the involvement of cortical thickening and sclerosis of the ileo-pectinal and ischiopubic lines is more suggestive of Paget's disease. Other minor findings in pelvis X-ray are acetabular protrusio and the enlargement of the pubic and the ischial rami.

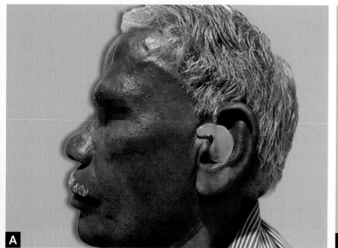
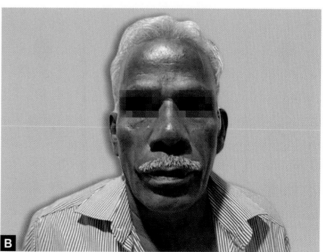

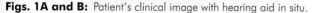

Figs. 1A and B: Patient's clinical image with hearing aid in situ.

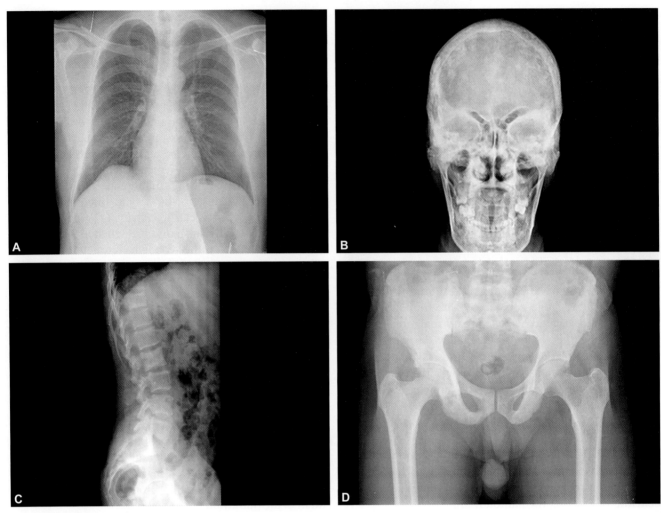

Figs. 2A to D: X-rays of the patient.

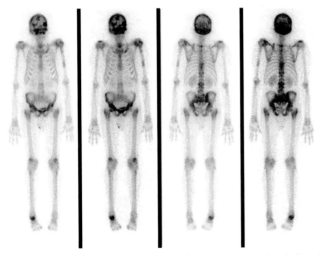

Fig. 3: Bone scan showing an increased tracer activity in the skull and illiac bones and also in the right ankle joint.

The other features in the long bones are blade of grass appearance, candle flame sign or zig-zag saw bones or a mosaic appearance of the long bones. Though bone scintigraphy is not highly specific it is a good tool in diagnosing patients with Paget's disease of bone. The main aim of treatment is to prevent fractures and complications that pertain to Paget's disease. The main stay of treatment is Bisphosphonates. Calcitonin has also been tried with limited success.[1,2]

REFERENCES

1. Anjali, Thomas N, Rajaratnam S, et al. Paget's disease of Bone: Experience from a Centre in Southern India. J Assoc Phys Ind. 2006;54:525-29.
2. Paul TV, Gurdasani D, Spurgeon R. Visual vignette. Paget disease of bone. Endocr Pract. 2008;14(2):255.

CASE 21

A 58-year-old gentleman presented with insidious onset of non radiating low back ache since the past 3-years. He was a reformed smoker. He did not have any other addictions or clinical or biochemical features to suggest hypogonadism. His X-ray spine showed compression fractures of the lumbar vertebrae L4 and L5 (Fig. 1). His bone scan is shown in Figure 2. Subsequently a bone biopsy from the L4 vertebra was done, and is demonstrated in Figure 3.

WHAT IS THE DIAGNOSIS?

His biochemical investigations revealed a normal serum calcium, phosphorus, 25-hydroxy vitamin D, parathyroid hormone (PTH), testosterone, prostate specific antigen and serum electrophoresis. His alkaline phosphatase level was elevated (557 U/L (40–125). The bone scan showed an intense abnormal activity in the entire skull, lower thoracic and lumbar vertebrae and pelvic bones (Fig. 2).

The differential diagnoses considered were multiple myeloma, metastasis, lymphoma, osteosarcoma and PD. The Biopsy from the L4 vertebra showed trabeculae of cortical and cancellous bone with intervening fibrotic marrow. The cancellous bone appeared thickened with prominent irregular cement lines, resembling jigsaw pattern and increase in osteoclastic and osteoblastic activity

with new bone formation, which was consistent with Paget's disease. (Fig. 3) He was initiated on bisphosphonate therapy with which there was significant clinical improvement and regression in the levels of alkaline phosphatase.

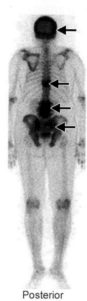

Fig. 2: Bone scan with an increased tracer uptakes in the skull, spine and pelvic region (shown with the arrows).

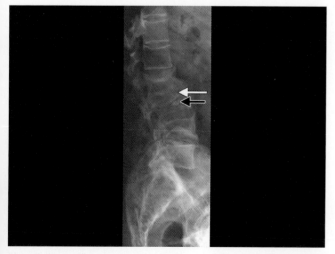

Fig. 1: X-ray of spine showing L4,5 compression fractures (shown with the arrows).

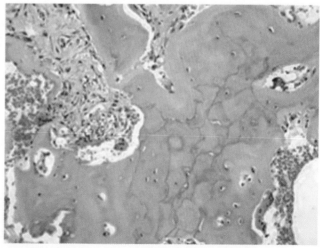

Fig. 3: Histopathological picture of the bone biopsy from the L4 vertebra.

DISCUSSION

Coexistence of Paget's disease and carcinoma of breast is rare and only a few case reports have been published. Bone scan is more sensitive than plain radiography for the identification of Paget's lesions and is often helpful in the diagnosis because of the characteristic distribution patterns and scintigraphy findings. These findings can guide the clinician in deciding the appropriate management. However, if there is an associated malignancy, it may be difficult to distinguish Paget's disease from metastasis, and a bone biopsy may be necessary for the diagnosis.

In Paget's disease, the tracer uptake on scintigraphy is often intense, well demarcated and evenly distributed in the affected skeleton. In contrast, metastatic disease usually presents with random asymmetric spotty lesions or patchy dense tracer uptake.[1,2]

REFERENCES

1. Shetty S, Kapoor N, Prabhu AJ, et al. Paget's disease: a unique case snippet. BMJ Case Rep. 2014;2014.
2. Sonoda LI, Balan KK. Co-existent Paget 's disease of the Bone, Prostate Carcinoma Skeletal Metastases and Fracture on Skeletal Scintigraphy-Lessons to be Learned. Mol Imaging Radionuclide Ther. 2013;22(2):63–5.

CASE 22

A 25-year-old man was referred for the evaluation of hypothyroidism and progressive difficulty in walking since the past 15 years. He gave history of snake bite 15 years back requiring three sessions of hemodialysis due to renal failure (Fig. 1). He appeared lethargic with absent facial hair and slow ankle reflexes (Fig. 2). His X-ray pelvis is shown in Figure 2.

WHAT IS THE PROBABLE DIAGNOSIS?

Clinical examination showed central obesity, a scar in the right ankle joint (due to prior snake bite) (Fig. 1), and a waddling gait. His height was 153 cm with a mid-parental height of 166.5 cms. He had a testicular volume of 10 mL bilaterally with tanner 1 pubic hair and absent

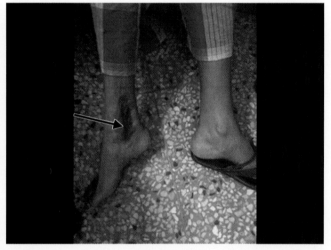

Fig. 1: Patient's image with a scar in the right leg due to a prior snake bite (shown with arrow).

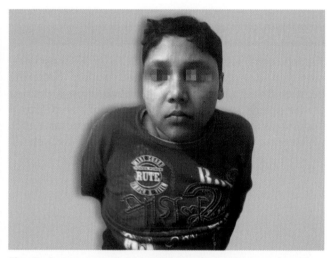

Fig. 2: Patients image having a lethargic look with absent facial hair.

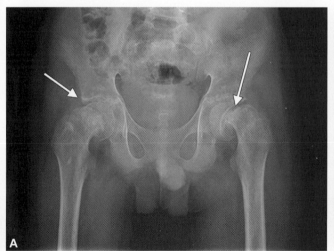

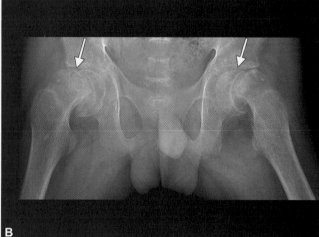

Figs. 3A and B: X-ray of the pelvis showing bilateral femoral head epiphyses slipped posteriorly and medially (shown with the arrows).

facial and axillary hair (_see_ Fig. 2). Laboratory studies showed low free T4 (0.5 ng/dL; normal 0.7–2.0), slightly elevated TSH (7.97 μIU/mL; normal 0.5–5.0), 8 am Cortisol-0.86 mcg/dL, FSH 1.11mIU/mL and testosterone <20 ng/dL. X-ray of pelvis AP view and the frog leg position showed a slipped femoral head, and a Candle drip appearance (_see_ Figs. 3A and B). So from the clinical, laboratory and radiological features, panhypopituitarism due to snake bite leading on to a slipped capital femoral epiphysis (SCFE) was diagnosed. He was started on oral prednisolone, thyroxine and parenteral testosterone. He was planned for fixation of the SCFE after 6 weeks of hormonal replacements.

DISCUSSION

Slipped capital femoral epiphysis (SCFE) is the most common hip disorder in adolescents, usually occurring between 8 and 15 years of age. The condition is defined as the posterior and inferior slippage of the proximal femoral epiphysis on the metaphysis (femoral neck), which occurs through the epiphyseal plate (growth plate).

Slipped capital femoral epiphysis occurs during young adolescence, especially during the growth spurt. Overweight children during pubertal growth spurt (between age 9 and 16 years) are generally considered to be at highest risk. Etiological factors suggested for SCFE are local trauma, obesity, endocrine disorders (such as hypothyroidism, hypopituitarism, hyperparathyroidism, growth hormone deficiency and during course of growth hormone (GH) therapy) and genetic factors. The potential complications include avascular necrosis of the femoral head, chondrolysis- acute cartilage necrosis, deformity, long-term degenerative osteoarthritis and limb length discrepancy. So, the treatment must be aimed at minimising AVN and chondrolysis by pinning the slipped epiphysis.[1,2]

REFERENCES

1. Jacob J, Paul T. A boy with a limp. Slipped capital femoral epiphysis. N Z Med J. 2007;120(1250):U2447.
2. Hu M-H, Jian Y-M, Hsueh Y-T, Lin W-H, Yang R-S. Slipped capital femoral epiphysis in an adult with panhypopituitarism. Orthopedics. 2011;34(3):222.

CASE 23

A 41-year-old man presented with the history of progressive diminution of bilateral vision since the past 2 years. He also had history of decreased hearing in both ears for the past 1-year. He had history of bifrontal headache since the same duration. Examination demonstrated a dolichocephaly with head circumference of 58 cms (Fig. 1) a left facial nerve palsy, mandibular enlargement, pectus carinatum and clubbing. All his biochemical parameters were normal. X-ray skull showed thickened skull bones (hyperostosis) (Figs. 2A to C) and Bone Mineral Density (BMD) testing showed a high normal bone mass (Fig. 3).

WHAT IS THE PROBABLE DIAGNOSIS?

The differential diagnoses considered were Von Buchem's disease or sclerostosis. With the presence of nerve involvement-facial palsy, decreased hearing and hyperostosis,

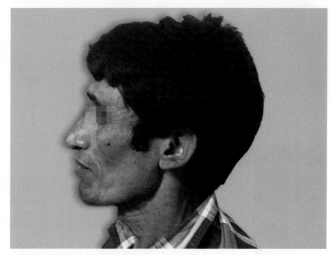

Fig. 1: Clinical image.

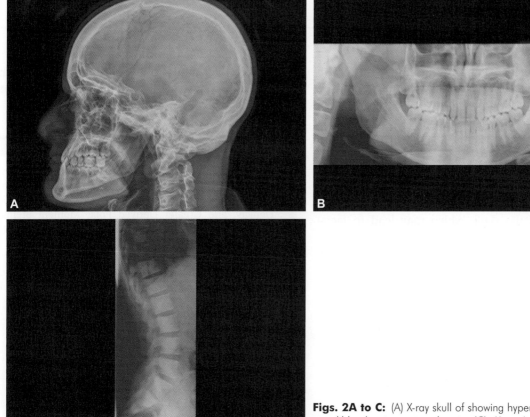

Figs. 2A to C: (A) X-ray skull of showing hyperostosis. (B): X-ray mandible showing osteosclerosis. (C): X-ray Lumbosacral spine showing diffuse osteosclerosis of the vertebrae.

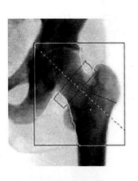

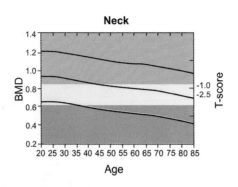

Neck

Region	BMD (g/cm²)	T-score	Z-score
Neck	0.933	0.0	0.5
Total	1.142	0.7	0.9

WHO classification: Normal

10-year fracture risk
FRAX not reported because:
Man under age 50
All T-scores for spine total, hip total
Femoral neck at or above -1.0

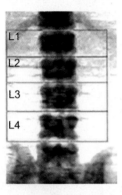

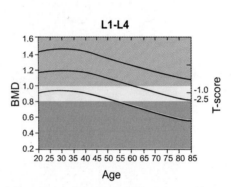

L1-L4

Region	BMD (g/cm²)	T-score	Z-score
L1-L4	1.299	1.9	2.0

WHO classification: Normal
Fracture risk: Not increased

Fig. 3: Bone mineral density of the patient with high normal bone mass (shown with the circles).

and the absence of syndactyly and facial distortion, the patient was diagnosed to have endosteal generalised hyperostosis-probable Van Buchem's disease.

may explain their milder phenotype compared to that of patients with sclerosteosis, in whom the serum sclerostin is undetectable.[1,2]

DISCUSSION

Van Buchem's disease is an autosomal recessive disease characterized by overgrowth of the skeleton. The most striking clinical features are the enlargement of the jaw and thickening of the skull, which may lead to facial nerve palsy, hearing loss, and optic atrophy. Increased formation, by osteoblasts, of qualitatively normal bone has been proposed as the underlying pathological mechanism, but the molecular defect is unknown. The small amounts of sclerostin produced by patients with VBD

REFERENCES

1. Wergedal JE, Veskovic K, Hellan M, et al. Patients with Van Buchem Disease, an Osteosclerotic Genetic Disease, Have Elevated Bone Formation Markers, Higher Bone Density, and Greater Derived Polar Moment of Inertia than Normal. J Clin Endocrinol Metab. 2003;88(12): 5778–83.
2. Van Lierop AH, Hamdy NAT, van Egmond ME,et al. Van Buchem disease: clinical, biochemical, and densitometric features of patients and disease carriers. J Bone Miner Res. 2013;28(4):848–54.

CASE 24

A 42-year-old lady was admitted in 2005 with complaints of non pulsatile swelling in the lateral aspect of the skull. The bone scintigraphy done at that time is shown in Figures 1A and B. The biopsy from the lesion in the skull showed tumor composed of large cells with grooved nuclei and eosinophilic cytoplasm, which were CD1a positive. She was given chemotherapy and was on regular follow-up since then. In 2007 she complained of head-ache and a computed tomography (CT) scan of the brain revealed a lytic lesion in the sphenoid sinus (Fig. 2). In

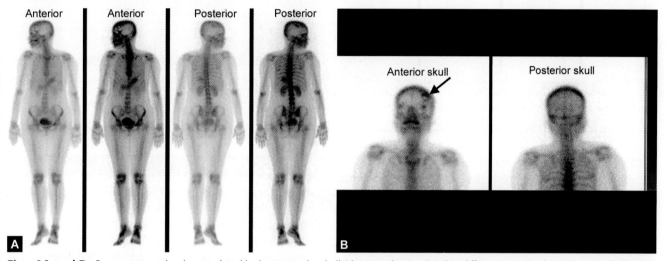

Figs. 1A and B: Bone scintigraphy showing lytic like lesions in the skull (shown with arrow) with a diffuse tracer uptake in the rest of the skull.

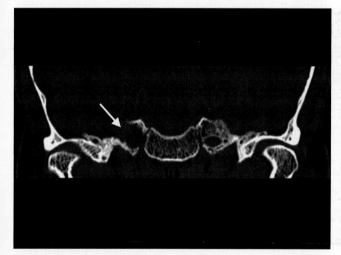

Fig. 2: CT scan of the brain showing a lytic lesion and an erosion of the right sphenoid bone (shown with arrow).

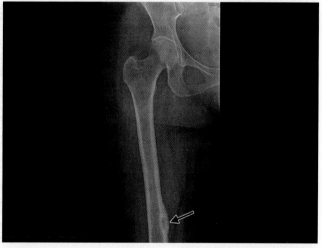

Fig. 3: X-ray of right femur with a lytic lesion in the mid shaft (shown with arrow).

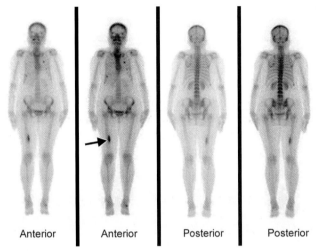

Anterior   Anterior   Posterior   Posterior

Fig. 4: Bone scintigraphy showing an increased tracer uptake in the right mid shaft femur (shown with arrow). Also showing a focal increased tracer activity in the left side of the skull, multiple ribs (not seen in the bone scan done initially).

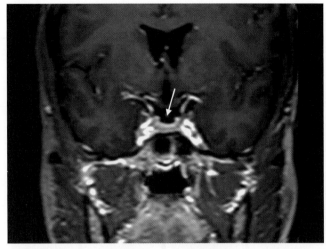

Fig. 5: Magnetic Resonance Imaging (MRI) showing a partially empty sella (shown with arrow).

2013 she again presented with the complaints of pain in the right femur and also polyuria since the past 6 months duration. X-ray femur also showed a lytic lesion in the right mid shaft (Fig. 3) Bone scintigraphy done in 2014, is demonstrated in Figure 4. She was also known to have hypothyroidism with secondary amenorrhoea since the past 2 years.

WHAT IS THE PROBABLE DIAGNOSIS?

With the involvement of the bones and the biopsy revealing the cell immunochemistry positive for CD1a, she was diagnosed to have Langerhans cell Histiocytosis (LCH). In 2013 she was investigated for complaints of polyuria and secondary amenorrhoea. Investigations revealed low normal 8 am cortisol-6.96 mcg/dL and overnight water deprivation revealed serum sodium of 148 meq/dL with a urine osmolarity of 148 mosm/kg suggesting diabetes insipidus. Her magnetic resonance imaging (MRI) pituitary showed a partial empty sella (Fig. 5). She was diagnosed to have Langerhans Cell Histiocytosis with partial hypopituitarism with Central Diabetes Insipidus. She is at present on thyroxine and carbamazepine with hydrocortisone for stress. She was referred to Department of Hematology for management for active LCH.

DISCUSSION

The skeletal system is the most commonly involved organ system in LCH. There is proliferation of Langerhans cells with an abundance of eosinophils, lymphocytes and neutrophils. These cells produce prostaglandins which result in medullary bone resorption. In the long bones LCH mainly involves diaphysis and, endosteal scalloping, periosteal reaction, cortical thinning and intracortical tunnelling are also seen. The prognosis is excellent when disease is confined to the skeleton, especially if it is a solitary lesion, with the majority of such lesions spontaneously resolving by fibrosis. Hypothalamic pituitary adrenal axis is commonly involved in LCH. Diabetes insipidus is the most common manifestation and sometimes other anterior pituitary hormone deficiency may also occur.[1,2]

REFERENCES

1. Ahmed M, Sureka J, Koshy C, et al. Langerhans cell histiocytosis of the clivus: An unusual cause of a destructive central skull base mass in a child. Neurol India. 2012;60(3):346.
2. Howarth DM, Mullan BP, Wiseman GA, et al. Bone Scintigraphy Evaluated in Diagnosing and Staging Langerhans' Cell Histiocytosis and Related Disorders. J Nucl Med. 1996; 37(9):1456–60.

CASE **25**

A 36-year-old lady was investigated for pain in the left femur since the past 3 years. X-ray and a bone scintigraphy done are shown in Figures 1 and 2. A bone biopsy from the left femur showed histiocytes positive for CD1a. She did not have any other lesions.

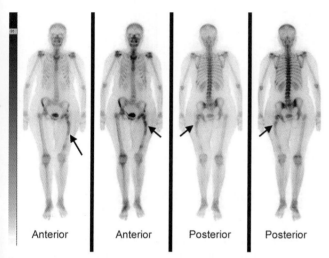

| Anterior | Anterior | Posterior | Posterior |

Fig. 1: Bone scintigraphy showed an increased tracer uptake, in the proximal left femur (shown with arrow).

WHAT IS THE DIAGNOSIS?

In view of the isolated bony lesion with biopsy showing cells positive for CD1a, a diagnosis of eosinophilic granuloma (EG). was made. A repeat bone scan after 2 years of the treatment also revealed a persistent lesion in the left femur (Fig. 3). She was referred to radiotherapy for further management. The differential diagnoses of eosinophilic granuloma include aneurysmal bone cyst, bone infarct and bone metastases, fibrous dysplasia and osteosarcoma.

DISCUSSION

Localized Langerhans-cell histiocytosis of bone is a benign tumour-like condition. The clinical spectrum of Langerhans-cell histiocytosis (LCH) is wide, ranging from a potentially lethal leukaemia-like disorder to a solitary lytic lesion of bone. Localised LCH of bone is a benign tumor-like condition which is characterised by a clonal proliferation of Langerhans-type histiocytes, and is commonly referred to as eosinophilic granuloma. The bones which are the most commonly involved are the skull, the pelvis, and the diaphysis of long bones. The second form of LCH is the Hand-Schuller-Christian disease with a triad

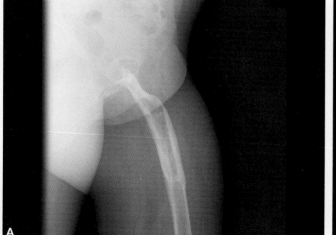

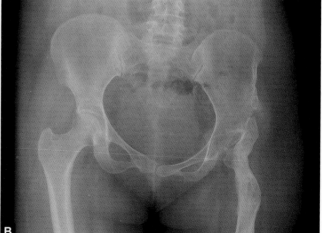

Figs. 2A and B: X-ray showing a lytic and sclerotic lesion in the proximal end of left femur.

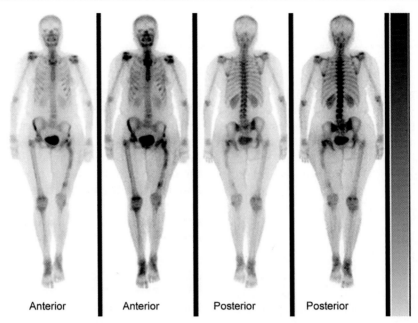

| Anterior | Anterior | Posterior | Posterior |

Fig. 3: Bone scintigraphy showing a similar tracer uptake, comparing the 2 years prior scan.

of exophthalmos, diabetes insipidus and osteolytic lesions of the skull. The Letterer-Siwe disease is also a type of histiocytosis with hepatosplenomegaly, lymphadenopathy, skin rash, fever, anemia and thrombocytopenia. Different forms of treatment have been reported to give satisfactory results for EG. For EG the treatment includes enucleation with or without radiotherapy. Of late radiofrequency ablation of the local lesion is also being tried.[1,2]

REFERENCES

1. Ardekian L, Peled M, Rosen D, et al. Clinical and radiographic features of eosinophilic granuloma in the jaws. Oral Surg Oral Med Oral Pathol Oral Radiol Endod. 1999; 87(2):238–42.
2. Corby RR, Stacy GS, Peabody TD, et al. Radiofrequency ablation of solitary eosinophilic granuloma of bone. Am J Roentgenol. 2008;190(6):1492–4.

CASE **26**

A 6-year-old girl of non-consanguineous parentage, presented with the concern of decreased vision in the left eye since the last 1½ years. On physical examination she had head circumferance of 50 cm; ICD-3 cm; bluish sclera, overcrowding of teeth and frontal bone prominence. Her left eye had absent direct with normal consensual light reflex. She also had liver enlarged 5 cms below the right costal margin. X-rays done are displayed in Figure 1.

WHAT IS THE DIAGNOSIS?

Investigations revealed anemia with normal serum creatinine and calcium levels. Her fundoscopy and the visual evoked potentials (VEPs) were suggestive of bilateral optic atrophy. With these clinical and radiological findings the patient was dignosed to have osteopetrosis with bilateral optic atrophy.

The alternative diagnoses to be considered include fluorosis; berylliosis, lead and bismuth poisoning; myelofibrosis; Paget's disease (sclerosing form); and malignancies (lymphoma, osteoblastic cancer metastases).

DISCUSSION

Osteopetrosis is a family of bone diseases mainly characterized by osteoclast failure thereby causing impaired bone resorption. It was first identified by Albers-Schönberg and is also described as "marble bone disease"due to

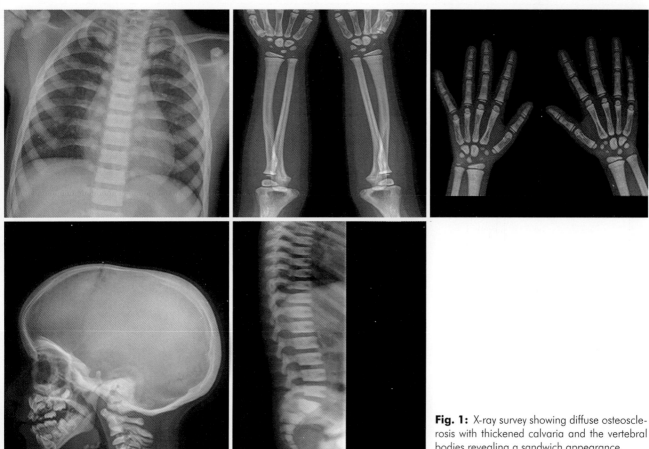

Fig. 1: X-ray survey showing diffuse osteosclerosis with thickened calvaria and the vertebral bodies revealing a sandwich appearance.

intense sclerosis of the skeleton. The most common and frequent form of osteopetrosis has Autosomal Dominant (ADO) inheritance. It has a milder course and is frequently observed in adults and is called Albers-Schönberg disease or ADO type II. In children it is the autosomal recessive form, which is common and has a fatal outcome.

The wide spread clinical manifestations include increased bone density, diffuse and focal sclerosis of varying severity, modeling defects at metaphyses, pathological fractures, osteomyelitis, dental abnormalities: tooth eruption defects and dental caries. However it is not easy to diagnose this condition in neonates in view of the neonatal bones being denser than in normal children or adults. At present, no effective medical treatment for osteopetrosis exists. Treatment is largely supportive and is aimed at providing multidisciplinary surveillance and symptomatic management of complications.[1,2]

REFERENCES

1. Stark Z, Savarirayan R. Osteopetrosis. Orphanet J Rare Dis. 2009;4(1):5.
2. Sobacchi C, Schulz A, Coxon FP, et al. Osteopetrosis: genetics, treatment and new insights into osteoclast function. Nat Rev Endocrinol. 2013;9(9):522–36.

CASE 27

A 26-year-old gentleman from Ranchi was referred to the Endocrine service for the evaluation of progressive proximal muscle weakness since the past 5 years. His investigations revealed hypophosphatemia with normal serum corrected calcium and parathyroid hormone (PTH). His renal phosphate threshold was low (Tmp/GFR 2.0) suggesting renal phosphate wasting. His vitamin D levels were high and the alkaline phosphate levels were also raised. He also had evidence of Hypercalciuria (24-hour urine calcium >6 mg/kg). He however did not have any evidence of metabolic acidosis on Arterial Blood Gas or hypokalemia. His brother also had similar complaints with similar biochemical findings. The X-ray Pelvis with both the hip joints is displayed in Figure 1. His Bone scan is shown in Figure 2.

WHAT ARE THE PROBABLE DIFFERENTIAL DIAGNOSES?

Based on the history, clinical features and biochemical parameters, differentials considered were: Hereditary Hypophosphatemic osteomalacia with Hypercalciuria-due to *NPT2c/2a* gene, mutation, and Primary renal tubular dysfunction with an acquired Fanconi's like presentation, Hypophosphatemic osteomalacia like oncogenic osteomalacia and X-linked Hypophosphatemic osteomalacia.

But the most likely diagnosis in this clinical and biochemical scenario is Hereditary Hypophosphatemic osteomalacia with Hypercalciuria—due to *NPT2c/2a* gene mutation. However the genetic confirmation could not be done. He was given oral neutral phosphate and hydrochlorothiazide.

DISCUSSION

Hereditary hypophosphatemic rickets with hypercalciuria (HHRH), a renal phosphate (Pi) wasting disease, is characterized by hypophosphatemia, elevated serum 1,25-dihydroxyvitamin D levels, hypercalciuria, rickets, and osteomalacia. These biochemical abnormalities are associated with bone pain, muscle weakness, growth retardation,

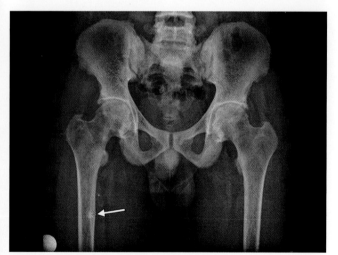

Fig. 1: X-ray of pelvis showing a patchy osteosclerosis with a looser zone in the right mid-femur (shown with arrow).

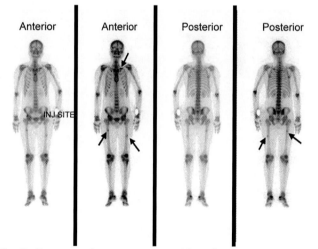

Fig. 2: Bone scan showing an increased foci of tracer concentrations in left clavicle and shaft of femorii (shown with the arrows) with the axial and appendicular skeleton revealing an enhanced activity.

and evidence of rickets and osteomalacia. The high serum $1,25(OH)_2D$ concentration and hypercalciuria distinguish HHRH from Mendelian renal Pi wasting disorders, such as X-linked hypophosphatemia and autosomal dominant hypophosphatemic rickets. Treatment of HHRH is accomplished by oral Pi supplementation. It increases growth rate, corrects the rickets and osteomalacia, and normalizes all biochemical abnormalities, with the exception of renal Pi wasting.[1,2]

REFERENCES

1. Tieder M, Arie R, Bab I, et al. A new kindred with hereditary hypophosphatemic rickets with hypercalciuria: implications for correct diagnosis and treatment. Nephron. 1992;62(2):176–81.
2. Jones AO, Tzenova J, Frappier D, et al. Hereditary hypophosphatemic rickets with hypercalciuria is not caused by mutations in the Na/Pi cotransporter npt2 gene. j am soc nephrol. 2001;12(3):507–14.

CASE **28**

A 20-year-old lady was admitted with history of bony pains, bony deformities and proximal muscle weakness for the past 4 years which had caused her to be confined to bed for the last 2 years. She was diagnosed to have congenital ichthyosis since 2 months of age. She did not have chronic diarrhea or polyuria. Examination revealed dry, scaly ichthyotic skin with bony tenderness and deformities in the form of kyphoscoliosis, pectus carinatum and flexion deformity of both hip and knee joints. Her X-rays are displayed in Figures 1 to 3.

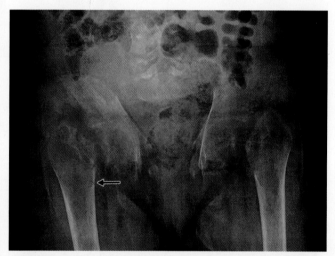

Fig. 1: X-ray of pelvis with osteopenia and resorption of the bilateral femoral neck and a triradiate like pelvis and a looser zone (shown with arrow).

WHAT IS THE DIFFERENTIAL DIAGNOSIS?

The various differentials considered in this patient were Congenital ichthyosis with vitamin D deficiency and osteomalacia, Malabsorption with vitamin D deficiency and osteomalacia, and hypophosphatemia due to renal tubular acidosis.

Investigations revealed normal electrolyte levels with no metabolic acidosis on ABG analysis. Her fasting urine pH was 8. She was found to have corrected serum calcium of 6.88 mg/dL with phosphate of 2.4 mg%. Her alkaline phosphatase level was 937 U/l and elevated PTH (Parathyroid hormone)-1321.9 pg/mL. Her hemoglobin was 16.1 gm% with normal albumin levels, of 4.8 gm% suggesting that there was no malabsorption. The serum 25 (OH) vitamin D level was <3 ng/dL. X-ray pelvis showed osteopenia with triradiate type pelvis and resorption of the bones. Bone scan was also suggestive of metabolic bone disease in view of the poor renal uptake (Fig. 4). She was started on oral calcium carbonate and parenteral vitamin D (6, 00,000 units). It was planned to continue her on parenteral Vitamin D once in 6 months for one year followed by once a year dose.

DISCUSSION

Osteomalacia is an impairment of bone mineralization, which is not as common as osteoporosis. The most common

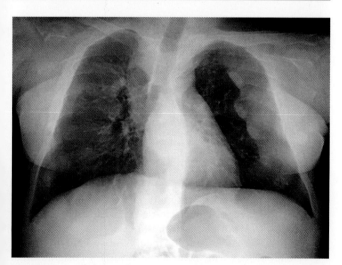

Fig. 2: X-ray of chest with osteopenic ribs and multiple rib fractures.

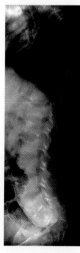

Fig. 3: X-ray of spine with kyphoscoliosis and decreased vertebral bodies height.

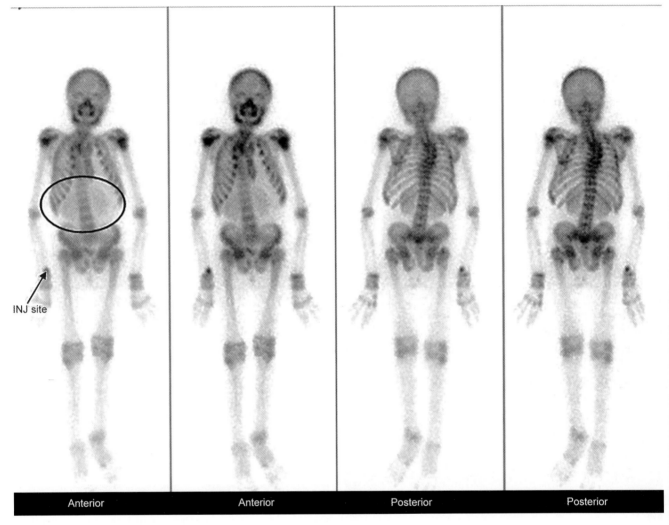

| Anterior | Anterior | Posterior | Posterior |

Fig. 4: Bone scintigraphy showing a poor renal uptake (shown with a circle).

cause of osteomalacia in older adults is vitamin-D deficiency as a result of inadequate intake or poor sunlight exposure. The excessive use of phosphate-binding antacids, chronic use of anticonvulsants, chronic renal failure, hepatobiliary disease, and malabsorption syndrome also result in osteomalacia. Patient complains of diffuse bone pain and proximal muscle weakness. A characteristic waddling gait may result from the hip pain and thigh weakness. Laboratory studies typically demonstrate an elevated alkaline phosphatase and parathormone levels, low phosphate, low or normal calcium, and low 25 (OH) Vitamin D levels. Plain radiographic films may show osteopenia or characteristic pseudofractures, most commonly seen in the proximal femur and in severe cases. Osteomalacia is managed by treating the underlying cause. If vitamin-D deficiency is diagnosed, repletion can be accomplished with oral vitamin D, 60000IU for a week for 6–8 weeks followed by once a month. If there is severe vitamin D deficiency, parenteral therapy may be given in view of better bio-availability. Osteomalacia due to hepatobiliary disease or chronic renal failure is managed with supplemental 25 (OH) D and 1, 25 (OH)$_2$ D, respectively.[1,2]

REFERENCES

1. Hazzazi M, Alzeer I, Tamimi W, et al. Clinical presentation and etiology of osteomalacia/rickets in adolescents. Saudi J Kidney Dis Transplant. 2013;24(5):938.
2. Sathish Kumar T, Scott X, Simon A, et al. Vitamin D deficiency rickets with Lamellar ichthyosis. J Postgrad Med. 2007;53(3):215.

CASE 29

A 20-year-old Mr S was referred to the Metabolic Bone disease clinic with the complaints of pain in the lower back since the past 10 months without any significant past history of trauma prior to the event. It was a generalized pain all over the spine with no localized tenderness. There was no history of fractures in the past. X-ray spine showed osteopenia, and is displayed in Figure 1. Bone Mineral Density (BMD) is shown in Figure 2.

WHAT IS THE DIAGNOSIS?

A further examination showed, that he did not have blue sclera or any bony deformity. His clinical features were suggestive of marfanoid habitus. However he did not have other major features to suggest Marfan syndrome. He had normal secondary sexual characters too. His investigations revealed a normal serum calcium and Vitamin D insufficiency with normal LH, FSH and serum testosterone levels. His Bone Mineral Density revealed a low bone mass with Vertebral Fracture Assessment (VFA)

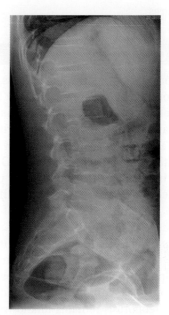

Fig. 1: X-ray of spine showing an osteopenic picture.

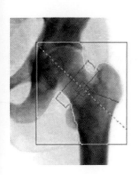
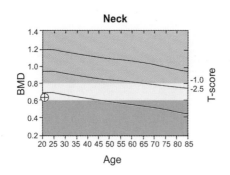

Region	BMD (g/cm²)	T-score	Z-score
Neck	0.612	-2.3	-2.3
Total	0.692	-2.3	-2.3

WHO classification: Osteopenia

10-year fracture risk
  FRAX not reported because:
  Man under age 50
  Some T-scores for spine total or hip total or
  Femoral neck at or above -2.5

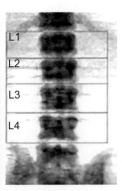
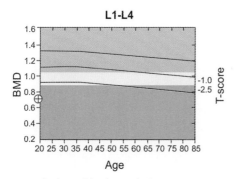

Region	BMD (g/cm²)	T-score	Z-score
L1-L4	0.494	-5.4	-5.4

WHO classification: Osteoporosis
Fracture risk: High

Fig. 2: BMD showing low bone mass (Indicated by the circles).

showing a low risk of vertebral fracture. He was diagnosed to have Idiopathic juvenile osteoporosis and was supplemented with oral calcium and vitamin D and once a week 70 mg alendronate. He was instructed to follow fall preventive measures.

DISCUSSION

In BMD, Z-score is used in individuals of less than 50 years of age and more than 75 years of age. Low bone mineral mass is defined as a Z-score that is less than or equal to −2.0, as compared to that of the same age group. A Z-score between −1.0 and −2.0 is defined as the low range of normalcy. Idiopathic juvenile osteoporosis (IJO) is a primary condition of bone demineralization that presents with pain in the back and extremities, walking difficulties, multiple fractures, and radiological evidence of osteoporosis. The onset is usually in the prepubertal period, between 8 and 12 years of age. The first sign of IJO is usually pain in the lower back, hips and feet. Low bone mineral density, vertebral collapse and metaphyseal compression fractures of the long bones are common. The etiology of idiopathic juvenile osteoporosis remains unknown. Diagnosis is based on clinical presentation, skeletal X-rays and bone density tests (dual-energy X-ray absorptiometry-DEXA and quantitative computed tomography). Osteogenesis Imperfecta is the main differential diagnosis. The management is aimed at protecting the spine and other bones from any future fractures. Physiotherapy and exercise (non- weight-bearing activities), and other supportive measures are mandatory in avoiding the complications. There is no established treatment strategy. However calcium and vitamin D, calcitonin, and bisphosphonates (in severe, long-lasting cases) have been tried in the treatment of IJO. The disease is self-limiting with spontaneous resolution after the onset of puberty. Rarely, in more severe cases, permanent disability (kyphoscoliosis and rib deformity) can develop.[1,2]

REFERENCES

1. Bacchetta J, Wesseling-Perry K, et al. Idiopathic juvenile osteoporosis: a cross-sectional single-centre experience with bone histomorphometry and quantitative computed tomography. Pediatr Rheumatol. 2013;11(1):6.
2. Shaw NJ. Management of osteoporosis in children. Eur J Endocrinol. 2008;159(suppl 1):S33–9.

CASE 30

A 32-year-old housewife was referred to the endocrine clinic for the evaluation of progressive proximal myopathy since the past 1 & 1/2 years. Arterial blood gas did not reveal metabolic acidosis. The serum phosphate was 1.9 mg% with normal corrected serum calcium level. She had normal (25) OH vitamin D level with high alkaline phosphatase (182 U/L). The 24-hour urine calcium, phosphate and creatinine levels were suggestive of low maximal tubular reabsorption of phosphate corrected for glomerular filtration rate Tmpo4/GFR- 1.5 (reference range, 2.5–4.5). Her FGF23 level was more than 1400 RU/mL (21.6–91). The CT scan of the paranasal sinus is displayed in Figure 1.

WHAT IS THE DIAGNOSIS?

Considering the clinical, biochemical and radiological findings she was diagnosed to have adult onset tumor

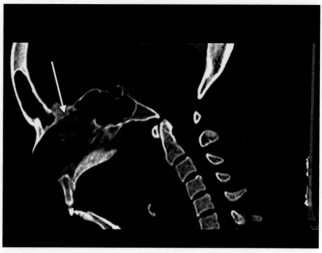

Fig. 1: CT scan showing a pedunculated mass in the sinus (indicated with arrow).

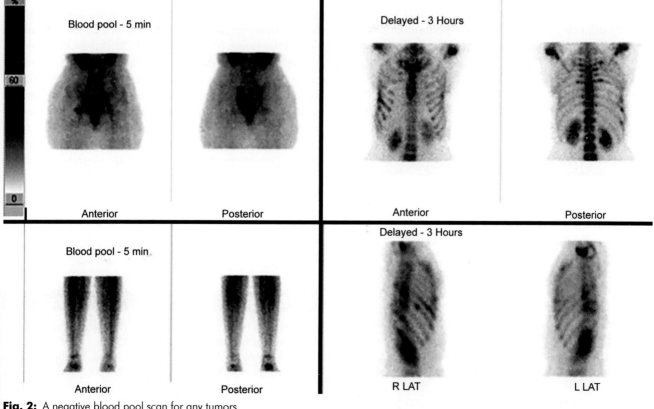

Fig. 2: A negative blood pool scan for any tumors.

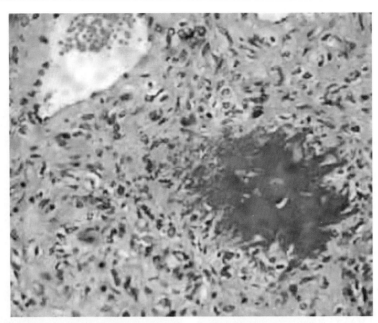

Fig. 3: Histopathological feature of the tumor excised (H&E; original magnification, x 40).

induced osteomalacia due to a probable mesenchymal tumor of the paranasal sinus. She was started on oral neutral phosphate and activated vitamin D following which the serum phosphate normalised. She was subsequently subjected to excision of the pedunculated mass. The histopathology of the tumor showed distinctive grungy pattern of matrix calcification with surrounding bland small round-to-spindle cells suggestive of a phosphaturic mesenchymal tumor (Fig. 3). Postsurgery the serum phosphate normalized and she is off oral phosphate supplements till date.

DISCUSSION

Tumor-induced osteomalacia (also known as oncogenic osteomalacia) is an uncommon condition. Tumors that cause TIO are often small, slow-growing, vascular, and often benign; they are commonly mesenchymal in origin. Hemangiopericytoma is the most dominant histologic diagnosis noted in TIO. Based on their histologic features, they have been sub-divided into 4 types: (i) phosphaturic mesenchymal tumor, mixed connective tissue type (PMTMCT); (ii) osteoblastoma-like tumors; (iii) ossifying fibroma-like tumors; and (iv) nonossifying fibroma-like tumors. Hemangiopericytoma is the subtype of PMTMCT of all tumors associated with TIO which secretes FGF23.

Fibroblast growth factor 23 is of mesenchymal origin, and the measurement of serum FGF-23 facilitates an early diagnosis. The fibroblast growth factor 23 (FGF-23) is a polypeptide secreted by mesenchymal tumors, which causes phosphaturia, resulting in defective mineralization of the bone. In addition, FGF-23 causes suppression of the enzyme 1α-hydroxylase located in the proximal convoluted tubules of kidneys which is responsible for the final activation of vitamin D (from 25-hydroxyvitamin D to 1, 25-dihydroxyvitamin D). So an unexplained generalized bone pain, proximal weakness and fractures must be investigated for calcium and phosphate homeostasis. Detection of renal phosphate wasting indicates the need for further evaluation of possible hereditary or acquired causes of renal phosphate wasting. DOTATATE PET-CT helps in the localization of mesenchymal tumors, as these tumors express somatostatin receptors. Surgery is the treatment modality of choice for patients with TIO.[1,2]

REFERENCES

1. Jacob JJ, Finny P, Thomas N, et al. Oncogenic osteomalacia. J Assoc Physicians India. 2007;55:231–3.
2. Bhatt AA, Mathews SS, Kumari A, et al. Tumour-induced osteomalacia. Hong Kong Med J. 2014;20(4):350.e1–350.e2.

CASE 31

A 40-year-old woman presented with a 3-year history of multiple musculoskeletal complaints with progressive proximal muscle weakness. She had sustained fractures of the left tibia after a trivial trauma. She also complained of having left nasal blockage periodically. However her anterior rhinoscopy was normal. Biochemical evaluation revealed a low serum phosphorus level of 1.2 mg/dL (reference range, 2.5–4.6) in conjunction with an inappropriate phosphaturia and a maximal tubular reabsorption of phosphate corrected for glomerular filtration rate (TmPo4/GFR) of 0.5 mg/dL (reference range, 2.5–4.5). She also had an elevated alkaline phosphatase value of 161 U/l and a parathyroid hormone concentration of 158 pg/mL (reference range, 10–69) in the presence of normocalcemia. Her 25-hydroxyvitamin D level was 29.4 ng/mL (reference range, 20–55). The work-up for renal tubular acidosis was negative. Her X-ray examination of the pelvis is demonstrated in Figure 1. Further evaluation included a computed tomography of the paranasal sinuses (Figs. 2A and B).

WHAT IS THE DIAGNOSIS?

The clinical and biochemical features were suggestive of adult onset hypophosphatemia. The CT paranasal sinus revealed a mass in the left ethmoidal sinus (Figs. 2A and B). She underwent surgical treatment in the form of excision of the ethmoidal mass, after which she had remarkable improvement. During the last follow-up, she was ambulatory, and her serum phosphorus level was 3.0 mg/dL. Histologically, the tumor composed of interlacing fascicles of spindle shaped cells with oval to elongated, mildly pleomorphic nuclei with coarse chromatin and occasional mitotic figures. Scattered amongst these were osteoclast like giant cells. There was prominence of the vasculature including thick walled, hyalinised

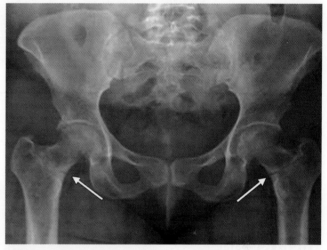

Fig. 1: Pseudo-fractures involving the both proximal femurs (shown with the arrows).

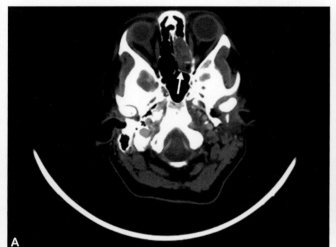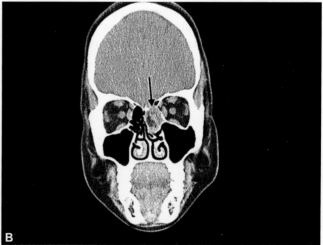

Figs. 2A and B: CT Paranasal sinus showing a mass involving the left ethmoid sinus (shown with arrow).

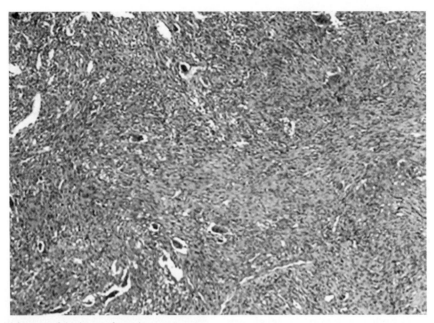

Fig. 3: Histopathological feature of the biopsy from the mass.

and occasional hemangiopericytomatous blood vessels suggestive of phosphaturic mesenchymal tumor (nonossifying fibroma like variant) (Fig. 3).

Thus the patient was diagnosed to have tumor induced osteomalacia due to left ethmoidal sinus phosphaturic mesenchymal tumor (non-ossifying fibroma like variant).

DISCUSSION

Hypophosphatemia is usually due to either decreased intestinal absorption or excessive renal loss of phosphorus. Chronic hypophosphatemia, as in this patient, usually signifies renal tubular wasting. In such cases, TIO should be considered—especially if the onset is in adulthood. Tumor-induced osteomalacia is a rare cause of adult-onset hypophosphatemic osteomalacia associated with tumors of mesenchymal origin. Tumor-derived products, including fibroblast growth factor 23, have been implicated in its pathogenesis. The majority of reported tumors are benign, locally occult lesions, most commonly found in bony or soft tissue sites in the head and neck.[1,2]

REFERENCES

1. R Kurien MTM. Oncogenic osteomalacia in a patient with an ethmoid sinus tumour. J Laryngol Otol. 2009;124(7):799–803.
2. Bhatt AA, Mathews SS, Kumari A, et al. Tumour-induced osteomalacia. Hong Kong Med J. 2014;20(4):350.e1–350.e2.

CASE 32

A 50-year-old woman presented with two episodes of acute abdominal pain within the past one year, and was diagnosed with recurrent pancreatitis. Her medical examination was unremarkable. An ultrasonography of the abdomen showed bilateral renal stones with features of acute pancreatitis. Her corrected serum calcium was 11.5 mg/dL (normal, 8.5–10.2 mg/dL), Phosphate was 1.2 mg/dL and intact parathormone level of 182 pg/mL (normal, 14–74 pg/mL). The rest of the biochemical parameters were within normal limits. Her bone mineral density (BMD) showed osteoporosis with a T-Score of –2.8 at the spine and neck of the femur with -4 at the forearm. She had regular menstrual cycles. The ultrasound of the neck was unremarkable. However, a Sestamibi scan revealed an increased tracer uptake in the mediastinum (Figs. 1 and 2).

WHAT IS THE DIAGNOSIS?

She was found to have phosphaturia with a low TmPo4/GFR of 0.5 mg/dL. Thus, the clinical, biochemical and radiological features were suggestive of ectopic parathyroid adenoma. She underwent an open bilateral neck and mediastinum exploration without sternotomy, and an 1-cm ectopic parathyroid adenoma was excised. Postoperatively her serum calcium and phosphorus levels normalized. The histopathological features confirmed the diagnosis of parathyroid adenoma (Figs. 3 and 4).

DISCUSSION

Primary hyperparathyroidism is a common endocrine disorder that is often missed due to its varied presentation. In the present era, the disorder is detected during an asymptomatic stage in developed countries. Embryonal migration patterns of parathyroid tissue account for different possible sites of ectopic parathyroid adenomas. Precise localization is important to prevent further delay in definitive therapy after biochemical confirmation of the diagnosis. Parathyroid scintigraphy remains an important tool for precise localization. A SPECT scan is an advanced radionuclide study with a three-dimensional (3-D) component. Pre-operative evaluation is helpful in directing the surgeon particularly in recurrent or residual hyperparathyroidism. The parathyroid glands arise in an ectopic site in 1–3% of the cases and can occur anywhere from the angle of the

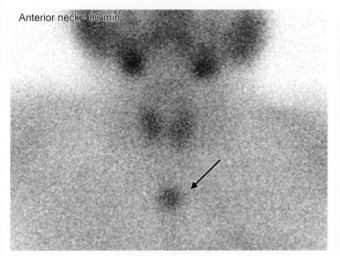

Fig. 1: Sestamibi scan showing a persistent tracer uptake in the mediastinum after 90 minutes (shown with arrow).

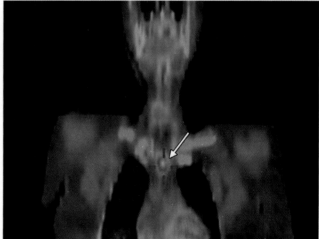

Fig. 2: Single-photon emission computed tomography image indicating an increased uptake in the mediastinum (shown with arrow).

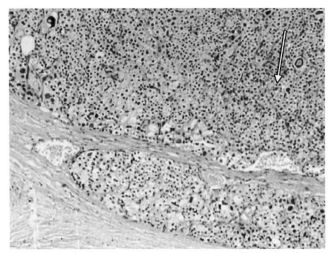

Fig. 3: Histopathology composing of highly cellular sheets of the chief cells (amphophilic or lightly eosinophilic cytoplasm and contain prominent fat droplets), (shown with arrow).

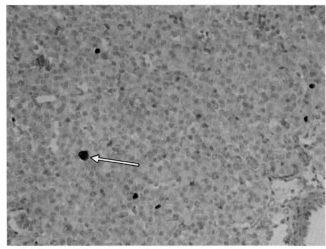

Fig. 4: Parathyroid tissue showing a low MIB-1 index; arrow mark showing MIB-1 immunostaining

jaw to the pericardium. This is a consequence of variability in the glandular tissue migration during embryonic life. The ectopic parathyroid may be in close proximity to or sometimes within the thymus in the anterior mediastinum. A Sestamibi scan is done pre-operatively and the selective uptake of tracer by the adenoma, allows for adequate delineation of glandular anatomy prior to surgery.[1,2]

REFERENCES

1. Naik D, Jebasingh KF, Cherian AJ, et al. Ectopic thymic parathyroid adenoma. Case Rep. 2014;2014(sep25 1): bcr 2014206634.
2. Mruthyunjaya MD, Abraham DT, Oommen R, et al. Visual vignette. Ectopic parathyroid adenoma. Endocr Pract Off. 2013;19(2):383.

CASE **33**

A 21-year-old lady presented with complaints of bony pain and a history of fracture of shaft of the right femur that had been sustained in the fifth month of pregnancy. She had severe proximal muscle weakness with impaired mobility and was bed bound on presentation.

WHAT IS THE DIAGNOSIS?

Investigations showed high serum calcium (10.8 mg) with elevation of serum alkaline phosphatase to 10 times the upper limit of normal and intact parathormone (PTH) level of 1050 pg/mL. Bone Mineral Density (BMD) showed Z Score of less than -2.5 in all the three sites suggestive of low bone mass. Other investigations were negative for syndromes associated with hyperparathyroidism.

X-ray chest showed anterior mediastinal widening (Fig. 1). Corresponding SPECT-CT thorax also showed an expansile lytic lesion in the sternum (Fig. 2). Bone scan showed multiple sites of tracer uptake suggesting multiple brown-tumours (Fig. 3). A Technitium-99 scan showed tracer accumulation in the right lower pole of thyroid in the initial image which persisted in the delayed image at 90 minutes after complete tracer washout from the thyroid gland. A SPECT- CT co-registered images (at 10 minutes)

confirmed the presence of the same lesion, localized to right inferior pole of thyroid gland, a right inferior parathyroid adenoma (Fig. 4).

Ultrasound neck also showed a right parathyroid adenoma which was concordant with the SPECT-CT (Fig. 5). Thus, a diagnosis of primary hyperparathyroidism, right parathyroid adenoma with multiple browns tumor was made. Patient underwent focused parathyroidectomy and her brown tumor regressed after four months (Fig. 6).

DISCUSSION

Hyperparathyroidism (HPT) is classified into primary, secondary and tertiary categories. Primary HPT occurs in the setting of excessive parathyroid hormone (PTH) secretion by an autonomous gland resulting in hypercalcemia and further sequelae. Secondary HPT occurs in the setting of hypocalcemia or vitamin D deficiency or chronic kidney disease, acting as a stimulus for PTH production. Tertiary HPT is associated with renal failure and results from autonomous functioning glands in patients with long-standing secondary HPT. Brown tumors are non-neoplastic lesions resulting from an abnormal bone

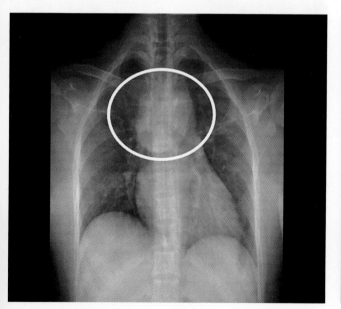

Fig. 1: X-ray of chest AP view showing anterior mediastinal widening (shown with a circle).

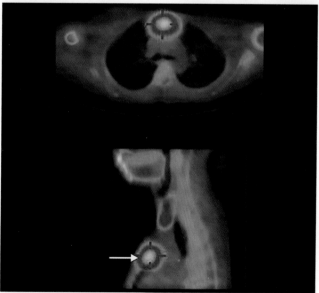

Fig. 2: SPECT-CT image with an increased tracer uptake (shown with arrow) similar to the corresponding region (shown with a circle) in X-ray chest.

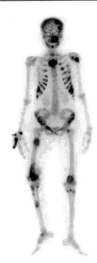

Fig. 3: Bone scintigraphy showing multiple tracer uptakes in multiple area suggesting multiple brown tumors.

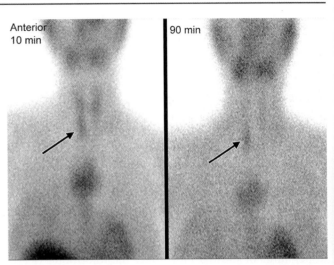

Fig. 4: Parathyroid scintigraphy showing an increased tracer uptake in the right inferior parathyroid region after 10 and 90 minutes wash out (shown with arrow).

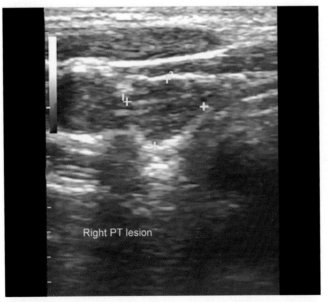

Fig. 5: Ultrasound neck showing a right side parathyroid lesion with a feeding artery, suggestive of right parathyroid adenoma.

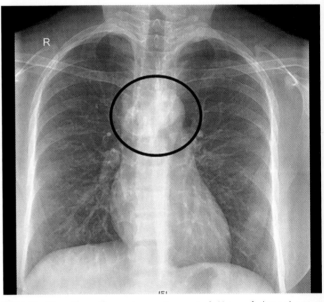

Fig. 6: After 4 months postoperative period, X-ray of chest showing regressed anterior mediastinal mass (shown with a circle).

metabolism in HPT. It represents the terminal stage of the bone remodeling process. The committed brown sites involved in HPT are facial bones, clavicles, ribs, pelvis, and/or femur. In contrast to secondary HPT, jaw bones are commonly affected by brown tumors in primary HPT. The term brown tumor is due to the color of the lesion, which results from vascularity, hemorrhage and deposits of hemosiderin in the tumour. Therefore, the brown tumor is actually a kind of giant cell lesion and often appears as multiple and expansile osteolytic areas of the bone. Usually brown tumors regress after the stimulus, which is the parathyroid adenoma has been removed.[1,2]

REFERENCES

1. Jebasingh F, Jacob JJ, Shah A, et al. Bilateral maxillary brown tumours as the first presentation of primary hyperparathyroidism. Oral Maxillofac Surg. 2008;12(2):97–100.
2. DasGupta R, Shetty S, Keshava SN, et al. Metastatic parathyroid carcinoma treated with radiofrequency ablation: A novel therapeutic modality. Australas Med J. 2014;7(9):372–5.

CASE 34

A 55-year-old male from Bangladesh, was referred to the Endocrine service for the evaluation of recurrent renal stones since the past 18 years. His father had died at the age of 50 years, with a history suggestive of probable hypoglycaemia. He also had renal stones and bone pain before death. He gave history of his brother having been operated for a pituitary tumor as well as for a tumor in the neck that had been associated with high serum calcium levels. Two of his sisters had similar history of bone pain and had been operated for high serum calcium levels. His investigations revealed a high serum calcium level (11.4 mg%) with low TmP/GFR (1.9 mg/dL) and elevated intact PTH with normal serum creatinine. His serum Prolactin was 5.75 ng/mL. His Sestamibi-Parathyroid scintigraphy done is shown in Figure 1.

WHAT IS THE SYNDROMIC DIAGNOSIS?

The parathyroid scinitgraphy showed features suggestive of parathyroid hyperplasia after 90 minutes wash out.

The SPECT-CT done, further confirmed the uptake in bilateral parathyroid gland regions suggestive of bilateral parathyroid gland hyperplasia (Fig. 2). These features, in the background of a strong family history that was suggestive of hyperparathyroidism and hypoglycaemia in first degree relatives, made the diagnosis of multiple endocrine neoplasia (MEN) type 1 very likely. The patient was subjected to 3 and 1/2 gland parathyroidectomy. Postoperatively, his serum calcium levels normalized.

DISCUSSION

Primary hyperparathyroidism may occur as a part of an inherited syndrome in combination with the pancreatic endocrine tumors and/or pituitary adenoma, which is classified as Multiple Endocrine Neoplasia type 1 (MEN-1). Primary hyperparathyroidism is the most frequent clinical presentation of MEN-1, which usually appears in the second decade of life as an asymptomatic hypercalcemia

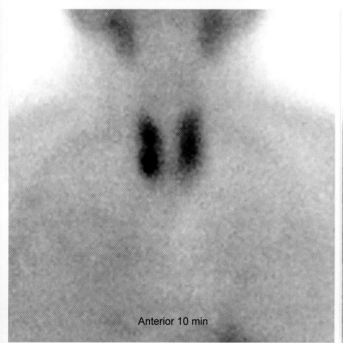
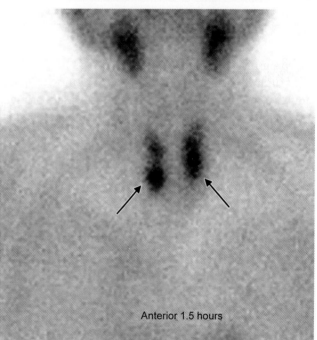

Anterior 10 min

Anterior 1.5 hours

Fig. 1: Sestamibi parathyroid scintigraphy showing uptakes in both sides of the neck after 10 and 90 minutes wash out (shown with the arrows).

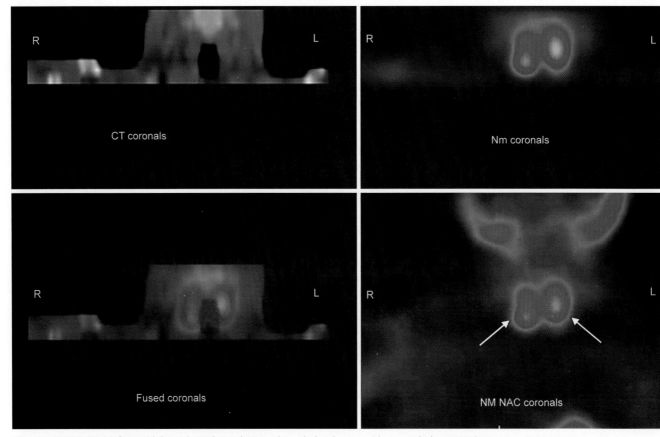

Fig. 2: SPECT-CT confirming bilateral uptake in the parathyroid gland region (shown with the arrows).

and progresses through the next decades. It is seen in 95% of individuals with MEN 1 mutation. The most frequent clinical presentation of the MEN-1-associated primary hyperparathyroidism is bone demineralization and recurrent kidney stones. Most frequently multinodular hyperplasia of parathyroid glands is present; however solitary tumors have also been observed. Parathyroid carcinoma is infrequent in MEN-1 syndrome even though it is due to mutation of MENIN gene which is a tumor suppressor protein. Patients with parathyroid hyperplasia should undergo extensive neck exploration with 3 and ½ gland parathyroidectomy in view of the high chance of recurrence that is observed with focused parathyroidectomy.[1,2]

REFERENCES

1. Kapoor N, Shetty S, Asha HS, et al. An unusual presentation of a patient with multiple endocrine neoplasia- 1. Journal of Clinical and Diagnostic Research [serial online] 2014 December cited: 2014; 8:MJ01-MJ02.
2. Paul TV, Jacob JJ, Vasan SK, Thomas N, Rajarathnam S, Selvan B, et al. Management of insulinomas: analysis from a tertiary care referral center in India. World J Surg. 2008; 32(4):576–82.

CASE 35

A 22-year-old lady presented to the endocrinology out patient department (OPD) with the history of recurrent episodes of seizures since early childhood and progressive decline in eye sight over the past 4 months. A physical examination revealed a short fourth metatarsal bone (Fig. 1). A CT scan of brain done in view of recurrent seizures showed bilateral calcification of the basal ganglia (Fig. 2).

WHAT IS THE DIAGNOSIS?

Latent signs of tetany in the form of positive Chvostek's sign and Trousseau's sign were present during clinical examination. The differential diagnoses for short fourth metatarsal bone are pseudohypoparathyroidism, Albright's syndrome, trisomy 21, Turner syndrome and diastrophic dysplasia. Investigations revealed a serum calcium level of 5.6 mg% and a serum albumin level of 3.9 gm% with high serum phosphate level. She also had high levels of intact parathyroid hormone (PTH) (425 pg/mL). In view of the low serum calcium with high plasma PTH levels a possibility of pseudohypoparathyroidism without Albright

hereditary osteodystrophy phenotype was considered (Type 1B). She was started on oral calcium supplements and activated vitamin D. She is seizure free since the start of her treatment.

DISCUSSION

The causes for basal ganglia calcification are hypoparathyroidism, pseudohypoparathyroidism, Fahr's syndrome, carbon monoxide poisoning, Lead poisoning and Leigh's syndrome. Pseudohypoparathyroidism is a hereditary disorder of clinical hypoparathyroidism without AHO phenotype, characterized by blunted nephrogenous cyclic-AMP (cAMP) response to exogenous parathyroid hormone (PTH). Patients with Albright's hereditary osteodystrophy have short stature, characteristically shortened fourth and fifth metacarpals, rounded faces, and often mild mental retardation. There are three types of pseudohypoparathyrodism. Type1a is an autosomal dominant disorder with Albright's hereditary osteodystrophy and is associated with thyroid stimulating hormone resistance. Type 1b has the same biochemical features as that of 1a

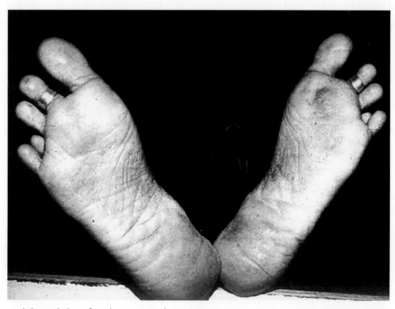

Fig. 1: Clinical image showing bilateral short fourth metatarsals.

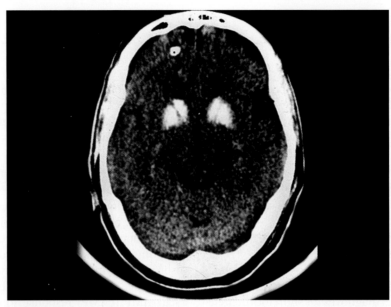

Fig. 2: CT scan brain showing bilateral basal ganglia calcifications.

without Albrights hereditary osteodystrophy. Type 2 lacks the physical appearance of type 1a. Since the biochemical features are same, type 1 and 2 disease may be distinguished by the differing urinary excretion of cyclic AMP in response to exogenous PTH. Biochemically, PHP1b is classically characterized by blunted urinary cAMP and phosphaturic response to PTH, whereas type 2 has normal urinary cAMP excretion and a reduced phosphate excretion.[1,2]

REFERENCES

1. Christopher RHP, David K, Pricilla R. Primary hypoparathyroidism presenting with new adult onset seizures in family practice. J Fam Med Prim Care. 2014;3(3):266.
2. A mentally challenged adult with tonic convulsions, dysmorphic face and sebopsoriasis. J Postgrad Med. 2006;52 (2):145.

CASE 36

A 65-year-old lady was referred to the endocrinology clinic with the complaints of low back ache since the past 3 years. She did not have any significant co-morbidities. X-ray spine is shown in Figure 1. Bone mineral density was done in view of her postmenopausal status and is displayed in Figures 2A and B.

WHAT IS THE DIAGNOSIS?

Her serum (25)OH Vitamin D levels were within normal limits. She was also started on oral calcium carbonate and vitamin D supplements with once a year Zoledronic acid which is to be continued for at least 5 years. She was given calcitonin nasal spray for the low back pain.

DISCUSSION

Osteoporosis is the most common metabolic bone disorder and remains an increasingly significant problem. Osteoporosis is often undertreated and under-recognized,

because it is a clinically silent disease until it manifests with fracture. Bone mineral density can be measured using a DEXA-Dual Energy X-ray Absorptiometry or a Quantitative Computed Tomography. The T-score represents the number of Standard Deviations (SDs) from the normal young adult mean values, whereas The Z-score represents the number of Standard Deviations (SDs) from the normal mean value for age-, race-, and sex-matched control subjects. T score is used for the diagnosis of osteoporosis between the ages 50–75 years. According to the World Health Organization criteria, a T score that is less than minus 2.5 is classified as osteoporosis and a T-score that is between minus 1 to minus 2.5 is called osteopenia. Evidence has shown effectiveness of alendronate, risedronate, Zoledronic acid, Denosumab, and Teriparatide in reducing the risk of non-vertebral fractures. But only alendronate, risedronate, Zoledronic acid, and Denosumab have been shown to reduce the risk of hip Fracture. Hence AACE (American Association of Clinical Endocrinology) recommends alendronate, risedronate, Zoledronic acid, or Denosumab as the first-line agents and Ibandronate as a second-line agent.

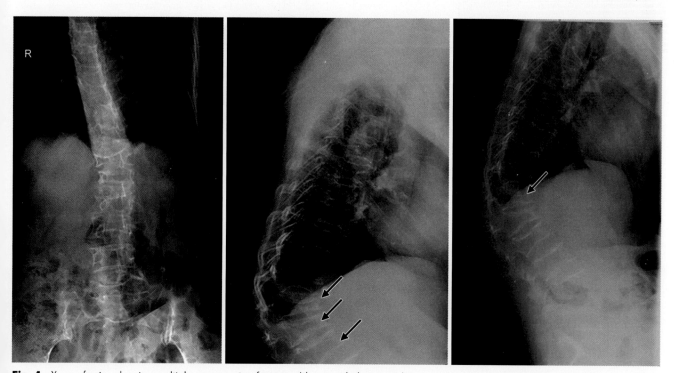

Fig. 1: X-ray of spine showing multiple compression fractures (shown with the arrows).

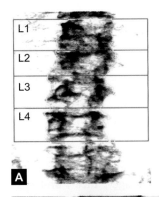

DXA results summary:

Region	Area (cm²)	BMC (g)	BMD (g/cm²)	T-Score	PR (%)	Z-Score	AM (%)
L1	12.58	6.64	0.528	-4.2	53	-3.0	62
L2	11.27	5.48	0.486	-4.9	47	-3.6	55
L3	14.38	6.53	0.454	-5.7	42	-4.3	49
L4	15.44	6.53	0.423	-5.8	40	-4.3	47
Total	53.67	25.17	0.469	-5.3	45	-3.9	53

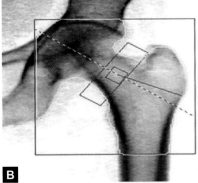

DXA results summary:

Region	Area (cm²)	BMC (g)	BMD (g/cm²)	T-Score	PR (%)	Z-Score	AM (%)
Neck	4.71	2.25	0.541	-2.8	64	-1.5	76
Troch	9.28	3.62	0.390	-3.1	56	-2.2	63
Inter	17.77	11.75	0.662	-2.8	60	-2.1	67
Total	31.76	17.93	0.564	-3.1	60	-2.2	68
Wards	1.04	0.30	0.292	-3.8	40	-1.8	58

Figs. 2A and B: BMD showing T score less than 2.5 suggestive of osteoporosis (shown with the circles).

The selective estrogen receptor modulator (SERM), raloxifene has been recommended as a second or third-line agent and nasal calcitonin as the last resort in the management of osteoporosis. Teriparatide has been shown to reduce the risk of vertebral and non-vertebral fractures. However it is recommended for patients with very high fracture risk or those in whom bisphosphonate therapy has been ineffective.[1,2]

REFERENCES

1. Paul TV. Images in Medicine - Bisphosphonate induced atypical fracture. J Clin Diagn Res [Internet]. 2014 [cited 2014 Dec 24];
2. Shetty S, Kapoor N, Naik D, et al. The impact of the Hologic vs the ICMR database in diagnosis of osteoporosis among South Indian subjects. Clin Endocrinol (Oxf). 2014;81(4):519–22.

CASE 37

A 51-year-old lady was seen in the Medical Oncology out-patient for the management of metastatic breast cancer wherein she was treated with recurrent injections of Zoledronic acid. Subsequently she developed extensive periodontitis and was referred to the dental and endocrine departments. Orthopantomograph images are shown in Figure 1.

WHAT IS THE DIAGNOSIS?

Clinical examination revealed mandibular sequestration and ulceration. With these clinical and radiographic features, the patient was diagnosed to have osteonecrosis of the jaw due to bisphosphonates.

DISCUSSION

In the absence of radiotherapy to the jaw and in patients on bisphosphonate therapy, if there is an exposed bone in the maxillofacial region for more than 8 weeks, the diagnosis of osteonecrosis of the jaw can be confirmed clinically. All patients receiving intravenous bisphosphonate therapy should ensure that they maintain a good oral hygiene. Prior to starting intravenous bisphosphonate therapy in a cancer patient, a detailed examination and panoramic X-ray scans of the oral cavity should be obtained. If an invasive procedure in the oral cavity is necessary while on high-dose intravenous bisphosphonate therapy, the bisphosphonate treatment should be interrupted, if medically possible, and any essential dental work should be completed.[1,2]

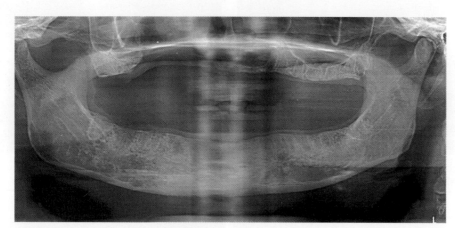

Fig. 1: Orthopantomograph of the patient with osteonecrosis of the jaw.

REFERENCES

1. Khan A. Bisphosphonate-associated osteonecrosis of the jaw. Can Fam Physician. 2008;54(7):1019–21.

2. Morag Y, Morag-Hezroni M, Jamadar DA, et al. Bisphosphonate-related Osteonecrosis of the Jaw: A pictorial review. RadioGraphics. 2009;29(7):1971–84.

CASE 38

A 66-year-old lady was diagnosed to have postmenopausal osteoporosis in 2004 and was started on oral Bisphosphonates. She was known to have diabetes mellitus for which she was on oral antidiabetic agents with good glycemic control. She is also a known patient of Rheumatoid arthritis and has been on methotrexate but has never been on steroids for disease control. X-ray done in 2007 is shown in Figure 1. In 2009 she sustained a fall in the restroom and sustained fracture of the right shaft of femur which required intramedullary nailing (Fig. 2).

In 2013 she slipped in her house and sustained a similar fracture in the left mid shaft of femur which also required invasive surgery (Figs. 3A and B).

WHAT IS THE CAUSE FOR THE RECURRENT FRACTURE?

Her investigations revealed low serum alkaline phosphatase level even prior to starting bisphosphonates. X-ray of

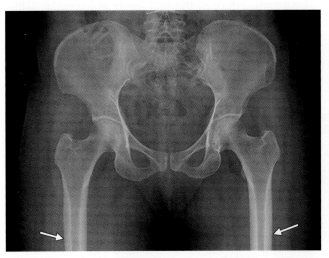

Fig. 1: X-ray of pelvis (2007) showing a thickened femoral cortex (shown with the arrows).

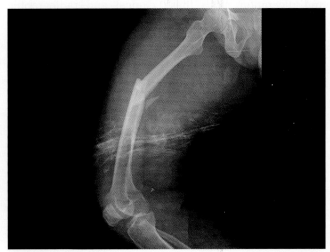

Fig. 2: X-ray of right femur showing an oblique fracture with generalised thickened cortex.

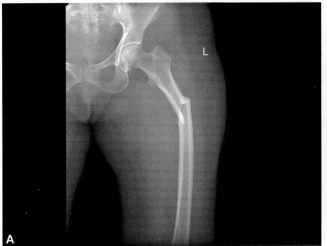

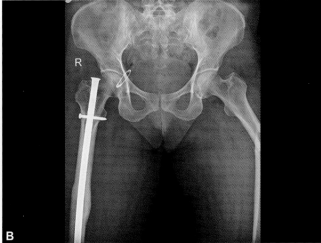

Figs. 3A and B: X-ray of left femur and Pelvis AP view showing a thick femoral cortex and an oblique fracture of the left femur.

pelvis AP view done in 2007 after 3 years of initiation of the bisphosphonates revealed a thickened femoral cortex (Fig. 1). The X-ray done following the minor trauma in 2009 and 2013 showed an oblique femoral fracture with a localized periosteal reaction in the lateral cortex and generalized cortical thickening suggesting an atypical fracture due to bisphosphonates (Figs. 2 and 3). Bisphosphonates were discontinued after the second surgery and she was offered the option of injectable parathyroid hormone therapy.

DISCUSSION

Bisphosphonates are the mainstay of treatment of osteoporosis, and the common side effect is upper gastrointestinal tract irritation. The rare complication of bisphosphonate therapy is an atypical subtrochanteric and femoral shaft fracture. The mechanisms behind the atypical fracture are reduced toughness and increased brittleness of bone following deposition of bisphosphonates in the sites of microfracture repair and increased mineralization of the bones (Usually seen as thickened cortex in the X-rays of the long bones). The other postulated mechanism is that the increased mineralization with alterations in non enzymatic collagen cross linking further augment the fracture risk in patients on prolonged bisphosphonates. The diagnostic hallmarks are generalized cortical thickening with low-energy trauma, non-comminuted, bilateral, transverse or oblique femoral fractures, poor callus formation and a localized periosteal reaction. Treatment includes immediate cessation of bisphosphonate therapy. Intramedullary nailing is still the gold standard treatment for such atypical fractures. There are case reports of using teriparatide with great success.[1,2]

REFERENCES

1. Shetty S, Kapoor N, Thomas N, et al. Response to Teriparatide in a patient with bisphosphonate-induced atypical femur fracture. IBMS BoneKEy [Internet]. 2014 Aug 13 [cited 2014 Dec 24];11.1
2. Paul TV. Images in Medicine - Bisphosphonate Induced Atypical Fracture. J Clin Diagn Res [Internet]. 2014 [cited 2014 Dec 24];

CASE 39

A 48-year-old gentleman, presented with history of recurrent trivial fractures and renal stones, and severe generalized bony pain as well as restricted mobility. His symptoms began 13 years back when he had severe left-sided hip pain and difficulty in movement. The patient gave history of having had a neck surgery 10 years back. Following the surgery, he had clinical and biochemical remission and was asymptomatic for the duration of next 10 years. Investigations revealed: corrected serum calcium of 12.8 mg/dL (8.5–10.0 mg/dL), phosphate of 1.7 mg/dL (2.5–4.0 mg/dL), intact parathormone (PTH) levels of 1,500 pg/mL (8.0–52.0 pg/mL), and creatinine of 0.67 mg/dL (0.6–1.5 mg/dL). His X rays are shown in Figures 1A to D. The CT thorax images are shown in Figure 2.

WHAT IS THE DIAGNOSIS?

With these clinical and biochemical parameters the patient was diagnosed to have primary hyperparathyroidism with multiple Brown tumors. A parathyroid scintigraphy was done for the localization of parathyroid adenoma (Fig. 3). Biopsy from the right pulmonary nodule is shown in

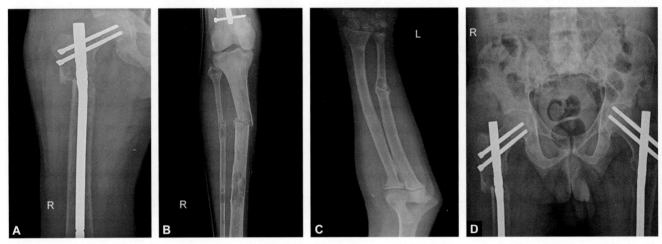

Figs. 1A to D: X-ray of right femur with non union of the shaft of femur fracture and thinned out cortex. (B) X-ray right tibia and fibula with fracture without a callous and multiple lytic lesions suggestive of brown tumors. (C) X-ray of forearm with a fracture radius. (D) X-ray pelvis AP view showing bilateral shaft of femur fracture with an intramedullary nail in situ.

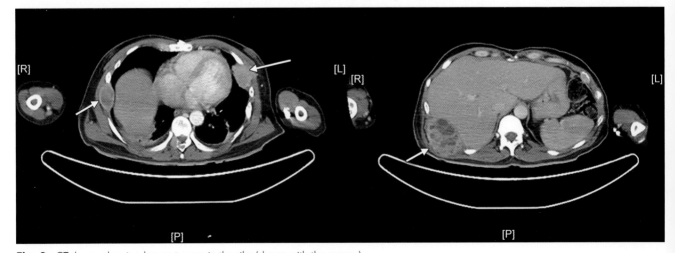

Fig. 2: CT thorax showing brown tumors in the ribs (shown with the arrows).

Figure 4. CT-guided biopsy from the pulmonary lesions was subjected to a histopathological examination along with tissue parathormone (PTH) assay from the biopsy sample (Figs. 5 and 6).

The treatment options that were initially considered were surgical resection of the metastatic lung nodules, radiotherapy to the lung lesions, and chemotherapy. Owing to the extensive metastatic lesions, severe metabolic bone disease, the need for extensive lung resection and cardiac comorbidities (Past history of CABG), none of the existing treatment options were tenable. Hence, radiofrequency ablation of the pulmonary nodules was considered as the most viable alternative after going through the literature. Postradiofrequency ablation the lesion had decreased in size with normalization of serum calcium level. However, there was a rise in serum calcium levels after 1 month of the procedure

DISCUSSION

Parathyroid carcinoma (PCA) is a rare malignant neoplasm accounting for 0.005 percent of all malignancies. Patients with PCA typically have a severe primary hyperparathyroidism (PHPT) with marked hypercalcaemia (14 mg/dL) with a profoundly elevated (three to 10 times normal) parathormone (PTH) levels. They are more prone to have metabolic bone and renal problems than those with benign parathyroid disease. Parathyroid carcinoma with metastasis significantly worsens the overall disease prognosis. *HRPT2* gene mutations play a central role in the pathogenesis of parathyroid carcinoma and are observed both in sporadic as well as in familial cases. The lung metastases from parathyroid carcinoma are very rare. So it is challenging and difficult to treat patients with functioning lung metastases from parathyroid carcinoma.[1,2]

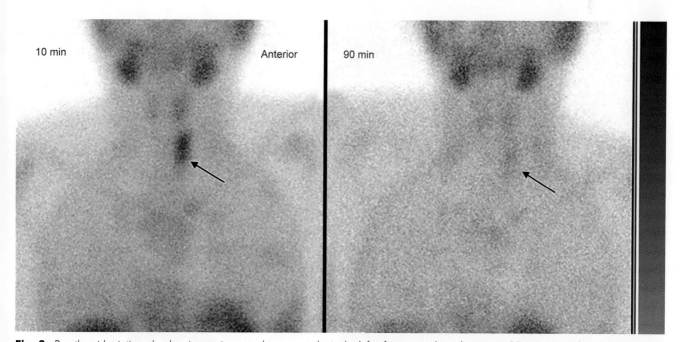

Fig. 3: Parathyroid scintigraphy showing an increased tracer uptake in the left inferior parathyroid region in 90 minutes washout image (shown with arrow).

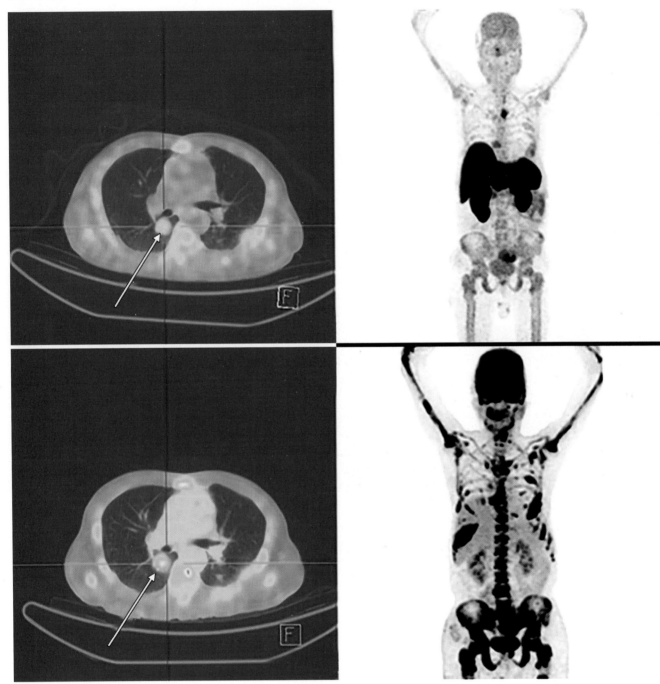

Fig. 4: DOTATATE PET-CT showing an increased tracer uptake in the right lung (shown with arrow) as well in the multiple areas in the bone suggestive of metastasis and brown tumors respectively.

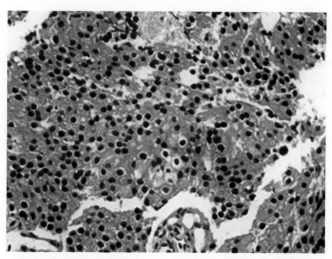

Fig. 5: Biopsy from the right pulmonary nodule showing lung parenchyma with neoplasm suggestive of metastasis from the primary parathyroid carcinoma.

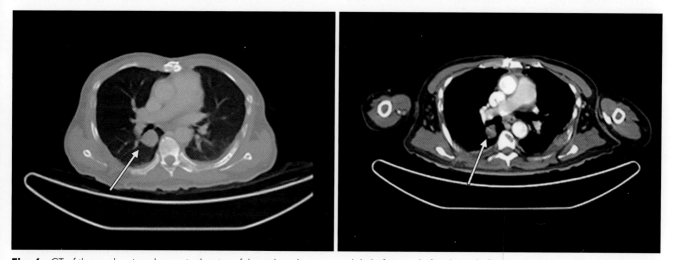

Fig. 6: CT of thorax showing change in the size of the right pulmonary nodule before and after the radiofrequency ablation (shown with arrow).

REFERENCES

1. DasGupta R, Shetty S, Keshava SN, et al. Metastatic para-thyroid carcinoma treated with radiofrequency ablation: A novel therapeutic modality. Australas Med J. 2014;7(9): 372–5.

2. Shane E. Clinical review 122: Parathyroid carcinoma. J Clin Endocrinol Metab. 2001;86(2):485–93.

MULTIPLE CHOICE QUESTIONS

1. A 54-year-old postmenopausal woman is brought with history of difficulty in getting up from squatting position and generalized bone pain. She never had fractures in the past. The first line of investigations should include all the following *EXCEPT:*
   A. Serum calcium
   B. Serum phosphorus
   C. Bone scan
   D. Serum 25 hydroxy vitamin D level

2. A 21-year-old gentleman presented with history of fracture of right hip following a trivial trauma. He was evaluated and found to have—serum phosphorus of 1.3 mg/dL (Normal 2.5–4.5 mg/dL); serum calcium 12.8 mg/dL (Normal 8.3–10.3 mg/dL); alkaline phosphatase 685 IU/l (40-125 IU/l); serum PTH 560 pg/mL (Normal 8–50 pg/mL). Which imaging modality would be best suited for localization.
   A. Tc99m scintigraphy
   B. Sestamibi scan
   C. MIBG scan
   D. FDG PET scan

3. A 40-year-old gentleman is brought with history of severe proximal myopathy and bone pain. He has no family history of similar problems. He is a farmer and works for 5-6 hours outdoor per day. The appropriate first line investigations in this patient include all *EXCEPT:*
   A. Ultrasound neck to locate the enlarged parathyroid
   B. Serum calcium, phosphorus, albumin, alkaline phosphatase and creatinine
   C. Serum creatinine
   D. X-ray pelvis AP view

4. All of the following regarding HRPT2 are true, *EXCEPT:*
   A. HRPT2 mutation has increased risk of parathyroid neoplasms, ossifying fibroma of mandible and maxilla, cystic and hamartomatus lesion of kidney.
   B. Autosomal recessive mutation in HRPT2 mutation causes hyperparathyroidism Jaw tumor syndrome
   C. HRPT2 mutation causes familial isolated hyperparathyroidism
   D. HRPT2 mutation leads to inactivation of protein product "parafibromin"

5. A 30-year-old gentleman is brought with history of bone pain. On evaluation he was found to have serum calcium 13.2 mg/dL, serum phosphorus 1.6 mg/dL and alkaline phosphatase 900 IU/l. He has multiple rounded nodules over the face and trunk. He has a café-au-lait spot with smooth border over the chest.

His mother had renal stones and multiple fractures. What is the diagnosis?
   A. McCune Albright syndrome
   B. Neurofibromatosis
   C. Familial isolated hyperparathyroidism
   D. Hyperparathyroidism jaw tumor syndrome

6. A 18-year-old Ms. A, is brought with history of short stature. She was diagnosed to have Thalassemia major at the age of 3 months and has required multiple transfusions—recently 6 transfusions per year. She has not attained menarche. Her Tanner's stage of breast-2, pubic hair-2. On examination she also has Chevostek's and Trousseau's signs positive. Her serum calcium is 6.8 mg/dL (Normal 8.3–10.3 mg/dL), serum phosphorus 5.9 mg/dL (Normal 2.5–4.5 mg/dL), serum albumin 4 gm/dL (3.5–5.5 gm/dL), FSH 2 mIU/mL, LH 1.8 mIU/mL and TSH 3 µIU/mL. What is the diagnosis for her hypocalcaemia?
   A. Hypogonadism
   B. Pseudohypoparathyroidism
   C. Hypothyroidism
   D. Hypoparathyroidism

7. A 13-year-old boy is brought with history of recurrent fractures. He has decreased hearing and blue sclera. His mother has blue sclera and had three fractures following minimal trauma. What is the diagnosis?
   A. Osteopetrosis
   B. Osteogenesis Imperfecta
   C. Juvenile osteoporosis
   D. McCune Albright syndrome

8. Match the following—The Fracture Intervention Trial aimed to investigate the effect of alendronate on the risk of morphometric as well as clinically evident fractures in postmenopausal women with low bone mass. Women aged 55–81 with low femoral-neck BMD were enrolled in two study groups based on presence or absence of an existing vertebral fracture. Results for women with at least one vertebral fracture at baseline are reported here. 2027 women were randomly assigned placebo (1005) or alendronate (1022) and followed-up for 36 months. The dose of alendronate (initially 5 mg daily) was increased (to 10 mg daily) at 24 months, with maintenance of the double blind. Lateral spine radiography was done at baseline and at 24 and 36 months. New vertebral fractures, the primary endpoint, were defined by morphometry as a decrease of 20% (and at least 4 mm) in at least one

vertebral height between the baseline and latest follow-up radiograph. Follow-up radiographs were obtained. 78 (8.0%) of women in the alendronate group had one or more new morphometric vertebral fractures compared with 145 (15.0%) in the placebo group

A. 7%
B. 14%
C. 28%
D. 48%
E. 72%
F. 10
G. 12
H. 14
I. 16
J. 18

   a. The absolute risk reduction(ARR) with alendronate is
   b. The RRR for any new morphometric fracture with this drug is ----%
   c. The number needed to treat to prevent one new vertebral fracture is

9. Match the Following—A 50-year-old lady has been referred for evaluation of hypercalcemia which was detected during a master health checkup. Use the options below to answer the following questions.

A. Ectopic PTH secretion
B. Primary Hyperparathyroidism
C. Tertiary Hyperparathyroidism
D. Multiple myeloma
E. Osteosarcoma
F. Chronic kidney disease
G. Local osteolytic hypercalcemia
H. Calcitriol induced hypercalcemia
I. PTHrp mediated tumoral hypercalcemia of malignancy
J. Secondary hyperparathyroidism

   a. If this patient on evaluation was found to have a squamous cell carcinoma oesophagus. The cause of hypercalcemia would be.
   b. If this patient also has anemia and deranged renal function you would suspect
   c. If she had breast cancer 5 years ago for which she had undergone surgery followed by local RT. Your likely diagnosis would be.

10. Match the following—A 30-year-old lady is admitted for evaluation of severe proximal myopathy and bone pain. Her fasting serum phosphate 1.8 mg/dL (normal 2.5–4.5 mg/dL), serum creatinine 0.8 mg/dL (normal 0.6–1.3 mg/dL). Match the best possible diagnosis to the different sets of associated clinical and biochemical parameters from the options below. Each option can be used only once

A. Osteomalacia due to vitamin D deficiency
B. Renal tubular acidosis
C. Fluorosis
D. Primary hyperparathyroidism
E. Secondary hyperparathyroidism
F. Adult onset hypophosphatemic osteomalacia
G. Tumor induced osteomalacia
H. Osteogenesis Imperfecta
I. Fibrous dysplasia
J. Paget's Disease

   a. Associated hip fracture, treated for renal stones in the past—serum calcium 11.8 mg/dL (Normal 8.3–10 mg/dL); alkaline phosphatase 800 IU/l (normal 40–125IU/L); TmPO4 / GFR – 2.1.
   b. Asymmetric face bony deformities in the lower limbs café au lait spot over the back and history of two fractures in childhood with trivial trauma-serum calcium 8.6 mg/dL (normal range 8.3–10.3 mg/dL).
   c. History of polyuria was treated for renal calculi 1 year ago. Urine analysis shows glucose++, serum potassium 3 m.mol/l (Normal 3.5–5 m Mol/l) and serum bicarbonate 20 m.mol/l (Normal 23–29 m Mol/l).
   d. Recent onset swelling over the face since 1 year. History of hip fracture with trivial trauma 3 months ago, operated. Serum calcium 9 mg/dL (Normal range 8.3–10.3 mg/dL).; alkaline phosphatase 780 IU/l (Normal 40–125 IU/l); serum PTH 50 pg/mL (8-75 pg/mL); FGF 23—11,000 RU/mL. (Normal mL <180 RU/mL
   e. Patient's younger brother also has bone pain and proximal myopathy. His serum phosphate (fasting) is 2.0 mg/dL (Normal 2.5–4.5 mg/dL) with TmPO4/ GFR – 1.9

CHAPTER 6

Endocrine Miscellany

(Miscellaneous Disorders including Growth, Sexual Differentiation and other Metabolic Disorders)

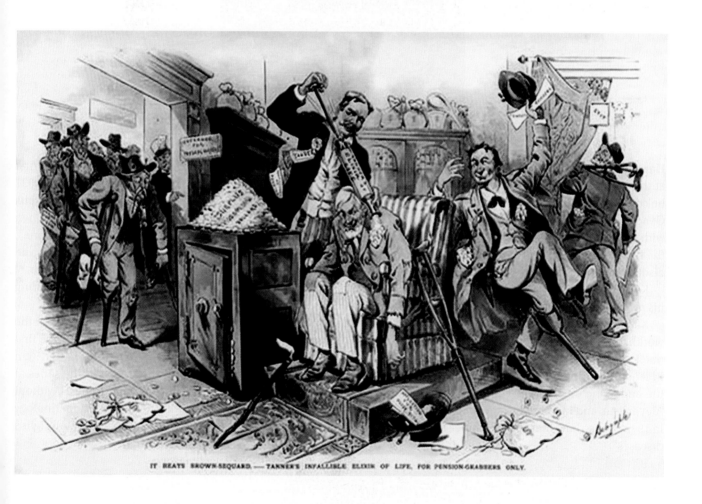

IT BEATS BROWN-SEQUARD. — TANNER'S INFALLIBLE ELIXIR OF LIFE, FOR PENSION-GRABBERS ONLY.

Brown-Sequard's notoriety was demonstrated in this 1896 satirical cartoon---based on a political incident of the time---published in the weekly magazine, "Judge". Brown-Sequard poses with a hypodermic needle at the ready and flasks full of the "elixir of life" on either side.

Brown Sequard used bull's testis extract to treat features of androgen deficiency.

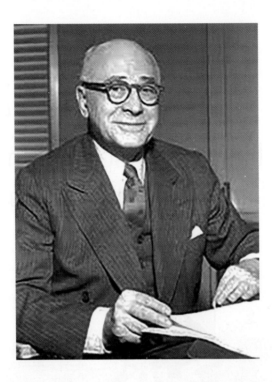

Harry Fitch Klinefelter, Jr. (1912–1990) was an American endocrinologist and rheumatologist. Klinefelter studied first at the University of Virginia, Charlottesville and then at Johns Hopkin's Medical School. After his graduation in 1937 he continued his training in internal medicine at the Johns Hopkins Hospital. Klinefelter worked at the Massachusetts General Hospital in Boston from 1941–1942; under the supervision of Fuller Albright he described a group of nine men with "gynecomastia, aspermatogenesis without aleydigism, and increased excretion of follicle-stimulating hormone", the first description of what would be called the Klinefelter syndrome. Initially he suspected this to be an endocrine disorder and postulated the presence of a second testicular hormone, but later recognized the chromosomal cause.

Klinefelter served in the Armed Forces from 1943–46 and then returned to Johns Hopkins where he remained during his professional life till he retired at the age of 76.

Klinefelter described his findings as follows, "Dr. Albright was the most outstanding clinical endocrinologist in the world...Albright's Saturday morning clinics were famous throughout the Massachusetts General Hospital. At the first one I attended, I saw a tall black boy named George Bland who had gynecomastia and very small testes (1.0–1.5 cm in length). During the rest of the year, we found 8 other patients with this same condition and reported the series at the endocrine meetings in 1942. The title, 'A Syndrome Characterized by Gynecomastia, Aspermatogenesis without Aleydigism, and Increased Excretion of Follicle-Stimulating Hormone,' (Published in Journal of Clinical Endocrinology in 1942) was so long that the syndrome came to be known by my name, though it was really just another of Dr. Albright's diseases".

CASE 1

A 20-year-old lady presented to the endocrinology clinic with complaints of irregular menstrual cycles since menarche. She had a gradual weight gain of 10 kg over the past 5 years. She had noticed darkening of the skin over her neck, face and hands which was progressive in nature. She also complained of an increase in the hair over her face, chin and abdomen. Upon examination, she had a BMI of 31.6 kg/m². Velvety hyperpigmented patches were noted over her neck, axillae and knuckles. She had significant facial hirsutism with hypertrichosis over the rest of the body (Figs. 1A to C). The rest of the systemic examination was unremarkable.

WHAT IS THE SKIN LESION SEEN IN THIS PATIENT? WHAT ARE THE DIFFERENT CLINICAL CONDITIONS ASSOCIATED WITH IT?

Acanthosis nigricans is a common condition characterized by velvety, hyperpigmented plaques on the skin. Intertriginous sites, such as the neck and axillae, are common sites for involvement. Less frequently, acanthosis nigricans appears in other skin sites or on mucosal surfaces. She was diagnosed to have Obesity with Insulin resistance and polycystic ovarian disease and was advised to follow lifestyle modification and Metformin.

DISCUSSION

Acanthosis nigricans (AN) is characterized by dark, coarse and thickened skin with a velvety texture, being symmetrically distributed on the neck, the axillae, antecubital and popliteal fossae, and groin folds, histopathologically characterized by papillomatosis and hyperkeratosis of the skin. AN is usually asymptomatic, but occasionally, it can be pruritic. Diagnosis is largely clinical with histopathology only for the confirmation. The lesions are symmetrically distributed and affect the back and sides of neck, axillae, groin, and antecubital and popliteal areas. The back of the neck is the most common site affected (99%).

Clinical recognition of AN is important because the disorder can occur in association with a variety of systemic abnormalities, many of which are characterized by insulin resistance. Obesity and diabetes mellitus are among the most frequently associated disorders. Rarely, AN develops as a sign of internal malignancy.

Acanthosis nigricans is associated with the following conditions:
1. *Obesity and diabetes mellitus*: Obesity and diabetes mellitus are the most common medical disorders linked with AN. Insulin resistance likely accounts for the development of acanthosis nigricans in individuals with these conditions.
2. *Polycystic ovarian syndrome*: Polycystic ovarian syndrome (PCOS) is associated with insulin resistance and hyperinsulinemia, and studies suggest 5–33 percent of women with PCOS have AN.[1]
3. *Syndromic acanthosis nigricans*: Multiple genetic disorders have been associated with acanthosis nigricans, many of which are characterized by insulin resistance that results either from defects in the insulin receptor or the production of antibodies against the insulin receptor.
   - Two disorders associated with insulin resistance are the type A and type B insulin resistance syndromes. The type A insulin resistance syndrome is also known as the HAIR-AN (hyperandrogenemia, insulin resistance and acanthosis nigricans) syndrome. These patients are usually women with normal BMI presenting with insulin resistance, acanthosis nigricans, oligomenorrhea, hirsutism and acne. Around 10–20% of such patients have identifiable insulin receptor mutations, with an autosomal-dominant inheritance. Patients in whom receptor defects cannot be detected are presumed to have as yet unidentified defects in post-receptor signaling.
   - Type B insulin resistance is acquired, resulting from autoantibodies against insulin receptors. This type of insulin resistance occurs in patients with less severe AN and may be associated with other autoimmune disorders.
   - Other genetic syndromes characterized by insulin resistance and acanthosis include Down syndrome, leprechaunism, Rabson-Mendenhall syndrome, congenital generalized lipodystrophy (Berardinelli-Seip syndrome), familial partial lipodystrophy, and Alstrom syndrome.
4. *Malignancy associated*: Rarely, acanthosis nigricans occurs as a paraneoplastic disorder. Abdominal adenocarcinomas, particularly gastric adenocarcinomas, represent the majority of acanthosis nigricans associated tumors. Features that suggest the possibility of an underlying malignancy in a patient with acanthosis

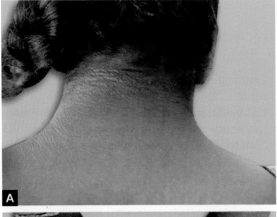

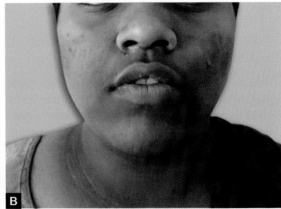

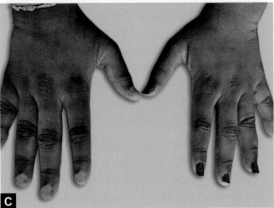

Figs. 1A to C: Velvety hyperpigmentation over the nape of the neck, over the face and the knuckles.

nigricans include a rapid onset of skin lesions, additional paraneoplastic findings, extensive involvement, lesions at atypical sites and older age.

5. *Drug related*: Rarely, acanthosis nigricans develops as a side effect of drug exposure. Drugs associated with this disorder include glucocorticoids , injected insulin, oral contraceptives, niacin, protease inhibitors, testosterone, and aripiprazole.

Pathogenesis—Hyperinsulinemia has a key role in the development of acanthosis nigricans. Elevated insulin levels stimulate the IGF 1 receptor, resulting in increased keratinocyte and dermal fibroblast proliferation. Transforming growth factor (TGF)-α, may contribute to the development of malignancy-associated acanthosis nigricans. Skin friction may play a role in the distribution of these lesions.[1]

CLINICAL FEATURES

A scale for grading of acanthosis nigricans was proposed by Burke et al. Severity was classified into four grades as follows.[2]

- *0—Absent*: not detectable on close inspection.
- *1—Present*: clearly present on close visual inspection, not visible to the casual observer, extent not measurable.
- *2—Mild*: limited to the base of the skull, does not extend to the lateral margins of the neck.
- *3—Moderate*: extending to the lateral margins of the neck (posterior border of the sternocleidomastoid, should not be visible when the participant is viewed from the front).
- *4—Severe*: extending anteriorly, visible when the patient is viewed from the front.

Cosmetic concerns are typically the primary indications for treatment. Weight loss has been linked to improvements in acanthosis nigricans in obese patients. Agents that improve insulin sensitivity, such as metformin and Pioglitazone may have some benefit for AN related to insulin resistance. Topical retinoids and vitamin D analogues have been found to be effective in several case series.

REFERENCES

1. Flier JS, Eastman RC, Minaker KL, et al. Acanthosis nigricans in obese women with hyperandrogenism. Characterization of an insulin-resistant state distinct from the type A and B syndromes. Diabetes. 1985;34(2):101–7.
2. Burke JP, Hale DE, Hazuda HP, et al. A quantitative scale of acanthosis nigricans. Diabetes Care. 1999;22(10):1655–9.

CASE 2

A 51-year-old gentleman presented with 2 year history of increased urinary urgency and precipitancy without any other associated urinary symptoms. He had past history of having been treated conservatively for renal calculi 16 years back. He had history of persistent lower back pain with dark-staining of underclothes and blackish discoloration of urine after prolonged stagnation. The clinical image of the patient is shown in Figures 1 and 2. The plain X-ray of the pelvis is shown in Figure 3.

WHAT IS THE RADIOLOGICAL ABNORMALITY SEEN AND WHAT IS THE DIAGNOSIS?

The pigmentation of the sclera and ear cartilage (Figs. 1 and 2) is suggestive of Alkaptonuria. On questioning, he recollected that his underclothes tended to have dark stains from his young age. A subsequent urine for Homogentisic acid was positive thereby confirming the diagnosis of alkaptonuria.

DISCUSSION

The conditions associated with extensive prostatic calcification are Tuberculosis, granulomatous diseases, malignant and Alkaptonuria or ochronosis.

Ochronosis usually results in blackish pigmentation of the joints, ocular sclera, skin over the ear cartilages, gentourinary and cardiovascular system. The deficiency of the enzyme homogentisate 1,2-dioxygenase leads to the accumulation of homogentisic acid in the cartilages, tendons and also scleral tissues. The arthritis does not affect the small joints and unlike ankylosing spondylitis the sacroiliac joints are usually spared which is the main differentiating feature.

The connective tissues where the homogentisic acid gets precipitated especially the intervertebral disk shows a dystrophic calcification. Apart from the darkening of urine, prostatic and urethral stones also can occur.

Regular physiotherapy spinal flexion extension exercises and static neck exercises help these patients to lead

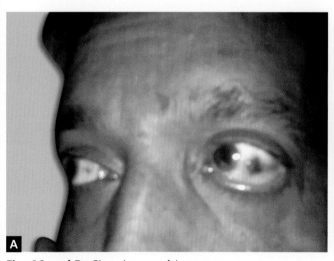
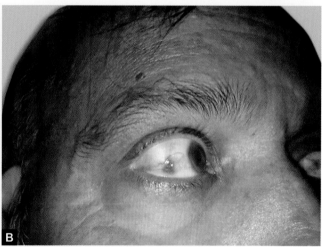

Figs.1A and B: Clinical image of the patient.

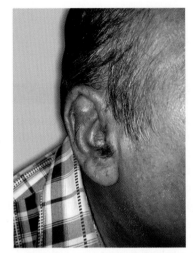

Fig. 2: Clinical image of the patient's hyperpigmented ear lobule.

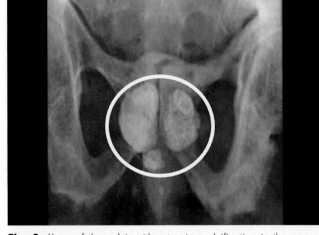

Fig. 3: X-ray of the pelvis with extensive calcification in the area of the prostate (shown with a circle).

a life without much disability. A large dose of vitamin C has been tried with an unproven value. Nitisinone, a tyrosine hydroxylase inhibitor can be theoretically tried, however the tendency for tyrosinemia while on these drugs and consequent adverse effects pose a major problem.[1,2]

REFERENCES

1. Phornphutkull C, Introne WJ, Perry MB, et al. Natural History of Alkaptonuria. N Engl J Med 2002;347:2111-21.
2. Sener RN. Prostatic and renal stones and unilateral obstruction of the urinary tract caused by Ochronosis. Am J Roentgenol 1992;158:214-5.

CASE 3

A 27-year-old, unmarried lady presented to endocrinology OPD with history of primary amenorrhea. She had noted deepening of voice and pubarche around age 11. However, she had noticed clitoromegaly much later. She did not notice any other features of virilization symptoms such as hirsutism, temporal balding or masculinization of body habitus. She did not have spontaneous breast development and had not attained menarche which had brought her to the hospital.

An initial evaluation elsewhere one year before presentation showed a hypoplastic uterus on a CT scan with a high total serum testosterone (146 ng/dL) and an elevated 17-OH progesterone (4.6 ng/mL). Subsequently she was diagnosed to have virilizing congenital adrenal hyperplasia (CAH) and a trial of oral dexamethasone for 3 months was given which failed to induce menstrual cycles. So she was prescribed cyclical estrogen-progesterone pills for the regularization of menstrual cycles. Normal breast development occurred following the estrogen only pills and regular withdrawal bleeding occurred only while she was on the combination (estrogen and progesterone) pill.

A clinical examination revealed that she was 159 cm tall with arm span of 170 cm and an upper segment to lower segment ratio of 0.89 confirming an eunuchoidism feature. She was normotensive.

Axillary hair was normal and pubic hair was Tanner stage 5 with male escutcheon. Breasts were Tanner stage 3. She had prominent clitoromegaly with a clitoral index of 600 mm² (Fig. 1). Labia were poorly developed but not fused. Urethral and vaginal orifices were seen separately. The gonads were not palpable and no inguinal masses or surgical scars were evident.

Follicle stimulating hormone level (FSH) was elevated at 80 mIU/mL. Other investigations revealed normal serum electrolytes, a serum total testosterone of 119 ng/dL (normal female range 50–100) and an elevated serum basal 17-hydroxyprogesterone of 10.6 ng/mL (0.11–1.2), in the range seen in congenital adrenal hyperplasia. Karyotyping revealed normal 46XX pattern with no detectable Y element on Fluorescent in situ hybridization.

WHAT COULD BE THE DIAGNOSIS?

Our patient was a virilized female and had a uterus with elevated basal 17 hydroxyprogesterone levels and a strikingly elevated serum testosterone levels. The history

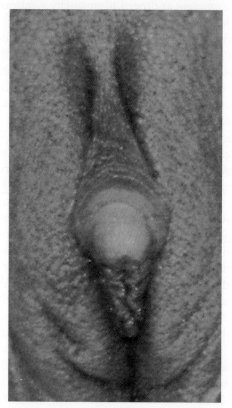

Fig. 1: Clinical image of clitoromegaly.

of parental consanguinity and neonatal sibling death raised the possibility of virilizing congenital adrenal hyperplasia. But the presence of eunuchoid body habitus with a tall rather than a short stature, failure of spontaneous breast development and a high serum FSH indicative of ovarian failure pointed towards the diagnosis of aromatase deficiency. The lack of response to glucocorticoid therapy also rules out the diagnosis of simple virilizing congenital adrenal hyperplasia. Our patient was started on estrogen-progesterone based contraceptive pills.

DISCUSSION

The causes of primary amenorrhea can be classified depending upon the stature of the patient comparing the mid parenteral height/expected target height. The differentials considered for short stature with primary amenorrhea are Turners syndrome, CGDP, hypothyroidism and hypopituitarism of any cause. In patients with normal stature the differentials include Mayer-Rokitansky-Kuster-Hauser syndrome, complete androgen insensitivity syndrome and aromatase deficiency. The differentials for tall stature and primary amenorrhea are hypogonadotropic hypogonadism, complete androgen insensitivity syndrome, Aromatase deficiency and Fragile X syndrome.

An ovotesticular type of disorder of sexual differentiation (True hermaphroditism) the other differential diagnosis to be considered, would have presented with palpable or visible gonads, variable karyotype (46XX/46XY/Mosaic), spontaneous breast development and menarche and histological demonstration of functioning ovarian and testicular tissues.

Estrogen resistance was not considered as a differential diagnosis as she had a developed secondary sexual characters and withdrawal bleeding with cyclical estrogen therapy. Further estrogen resistant females would not have shown an elevated serum testosterone or virilization.

Though most of the features fit in with aromatase deficiency in our patient, there were atypical features like absent infant deaths in the family, lack of maternal virilization during pregnancy, history of 'normal' genitalia at birth, raised 17 OHP and absence of demonstrable cystic ovaries. Maternal virilization during pregnancy may not be noted or may be absent if aromatase deficiency is partial.

Aromatase deficiency is an autosomal recessive condition presenting in girls as _disorder of sexual differentiation_ (46XX DSD) with ambiguous genitalia. Children with this disorder have a genital ambiguity at birth with 46XX karyotype. The failure of conversion of androgenic precursors to estrogen in the ovaries leads to the androgen/testosterone excess thereby an estrogen deficiency and the characteristic clinical features in this condition. The classic clinical features include virilization of the mother during the second half of pregnancy and clitoromegaly with posterior labioscrotal fusion of the neonate at birth; Infants are unlikely to have an adrenal crisis. They usually have an absence of growth spurt, absence of spontaneous breast development at the time of puberty and primary amenorrhea. The virilization worsens at puberty as ovarian androgens are produced in response to the normal pubertal gonadotropin surge and thereby the stimulated ovaries may become multicystic. The lack of estrogen leads to the tall stature and eunuchoid proportions if these patients present at a later age similar to our patient. These patients can have a delayed bone age and a high propensity for osteoporosis due to estrogen deficiency. However, the clinical picture may vary depending upon the severity of aromatase deficiency and may be modified by prior treatment with estrogen and progesterone.[1,2]

REFERENCES

1. Serdar E Bulun. Aromatase deficiency and oestrogen resistance: From molecular genetics to clinic: Semin Reprod Med 2000;18.
2. Nagasaki K, Horikawa R, Fujisawa K, et al. A Case of female pseudo-hermaphroditism caused by aromatase deficiency. Clin pediatr Endocrinol 2004;13:59–64.

CASE 4

A 17-year-old, boy presented to the endocrine out patient department, with complaints of progressive visual loss predominantly towards the evening and newly diagnosed diabetes mellitus. He was born of a second degree consanguineous marriage. Historically he had a developmental delay with poor scholastic performance. He was noticed to have night blindness by the age of 3 years. On examination he was obese with a BMI of 30kg/m² and had signs of insulin resistance in the form of grade 3 acanthosis nigricans (Fig. 1). He had polydactyly involving both the upper and lower limbs (Figs. 2A and B). Fundoscopy revealed pigmented retina that had the appearance of bony corpuscles with arteriolar attenuation and a pale optic disk. He had features of hypogonadism with poor development of secondary sexual characteristics.

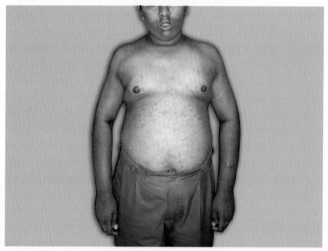

Fig. 1: Clinical image of the patient.

WHAT IS THE MOST PROBABLE DIAGNOSIS IN THIS PATIENT? WHAT ARE THE OTHER CONDITIONS THAT CAN PRESENT WITH SIMILAR FINDINGS?

This patient was diagnosed to have Bardet-Biedl syndrome. This syndrome can be diagnosed in the presence of at least 4 of 6 cardinal signs—mental retardation, obesity, hypogonadism in males, distal limb anomalies, renal involvement and progressive tapetoretinal degeneration.[1]

It is important to consider other syndromes with obesity, mental retardation and visual problems in the differential diagnosis. Genetic multisystem disorders with these features include the following.

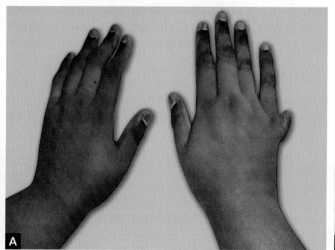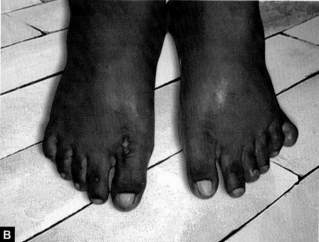

Figs. 2A and B: Images showing polydactyly of the upper and lower limbs.

Disorder	Clinical features
Prader-Willi syndrome	Obesity, neonatal hypotonia, mental retardation, short stature, hypogonadism and characteristic facial features
Laurence-Moon syndrome	Mental retardation, obesity, retinopathy, hypogonadism, spastic paraplegia and ataxia
Alstrom syndrome	Obesity, normal intelligence and height, retinopathy, hypogonadism, hearing disorders, diabetes mellitus, kidney disease
Cohen syndrome	Obesity, craniofacial anomalies including cleft lip, hypotonia, mild mental retardation, hypogonadotropic hypogonadism
Carpenter syndrome	Normal height, gynoid obesity, polydactyly or syndactyly, acrocephaly and mild mental retardation.

Other rare genetic obesity syndromes include Albright's hereditary osteodystrophy (pseudohypoparathyroidism), MOMO (Macrosomia, obesity, Macrocephaly, Ocular abnormality) syndrome, Rubinstein-Taybi syndrome and Börjeson-Forssman-Lehman syndrome.

DISCUSSION

Bardet-Biedl syndrome is a genetic autosomal recessive disease characterized by abdominal obesity, postaxial polydactyly, retinal dystrophy, mental retardation, hypodonadism and renal abnormalities. Other features, which are not always present, include hepatic fibrosis, Type 2 diabetes mellitus, reproductive tract abnormalities, short stature, developmental delay, and speech deficits. The typical facial features in this syndrome are a round moon face, premature frontal balding, enophthalmos and downward slanting palpebral fissures. Bardet-Biedl syndrome has been associated with mutations in different genetic loci. The most common mutation is the one found in chromosome 11q13.[2] Mental retardation is mild to moderate with a minority of patients having severe mental retardation. Central obesity of the android type is present in most of the patients. Obesity is associated with insulin resistance and type 2 diabetes mellitus, as well as other components of the metabolic syndrome including hypertension, hyperuricemia and a prothrombotic state. Limb anomalies are a common clinical finding in most series of patients with Bardet-Biedl syndrome and are seen in up to 70% of patients. Renal disease leading on to chronic kidney disease is seen in upto 60% of patients. Renal abnormalities reflect a defect in maturation of the kidneys. The various limb anomalies that can be seen are polydactyly, syndactyly, brachydactyly and clinodactyly. Other skeletal abnormalities include macrocephaly, hip dysplasia, skull deformities and tibia vara. Retinal dystrophy with structural or functional abnormalities or a typical retinitis pigmentosa is seen in almost all patients. Primary optic atrophy can be associated with retinitis pigmentosa. Visual deterioration in this syndrome is early in onset and prognosis is poor as the majority of patients have significant visual loss by the third decade. Hypogonadism is more frequently seen in male patients, as compared to female patients. A high incidence of various congenital heart defects have been reported. Neurological findings which have been observed are nystagmus, ataxia, dysdiadochokinesia and hypotonia. A higher risk for hypertension, prothrombotic state and renal anomalies have also been noted in heterozygous carriers of the mutation.

Bardet-Biedl syndrome differs from the much rarer Laurence-Moon syndrome, in which retinal pigmentary degeneration, mental retardation, and hypogonadism occur in conjunction with progressive spastic paraparesis and distal muscle weakness, but without polydactyly.

REFERENCES

1. Beales P, Elcioglu N, Woolf A, et al. New criteria for improved diagnosis of Bardet-Biedl syndrome: results of a population survey. J Med Genet. 1999;36(6):437–46.
2. Iannello S, Bosco P, Cavaleri A, et al. A review of the literature of Bardet-Biedl disease and report of three cases associated with metabolic syndrome and diagnosed after the age of fifty. Obes Rev Off J Int Assoc Study Obes. 2002; 3(2):123–35.

CASE 5

A 25-year-old gentleman was treated with phenytoin for ataxia since past 5 years. Clinically he had recurrent episodes of syncopal attack mainly in the early morning with seizure off and on. On routine biochemical evaluation, he had a random plasma glucose of 16 mg/dL in the casualty. He developed hypoglycemia within two hours of the initiation of 72 fast (glucose of 28 mg/dL)

with a corresponding non suppressed serum insulin level of 15.2 units/mL, characteristic of hyperinsulinemic hypoglycemia. His MRI brain is shown in Figures 1A and B. His CT abdomen revealed an exophytic mass in the inferior aspect of the tail of pancreas with endoscopic ultrasonography confirming the same (Figs. 2 and 3).

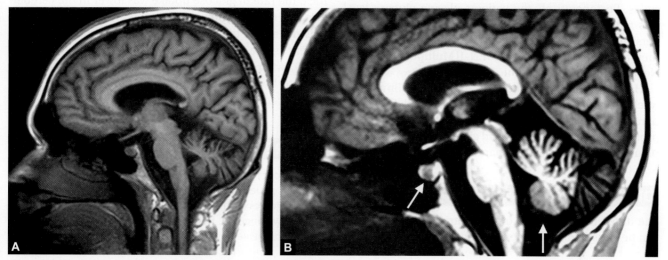

Figs. 1A and B: MRI of brain showing a pituitary microadenoma and gross cerebellar atrophy (shown with arrows).

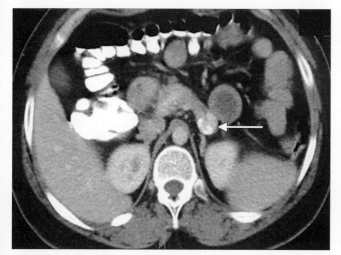

Fig. 2: CT abdomen showing a lesion in the tail of the pancreas (shown with arrow).

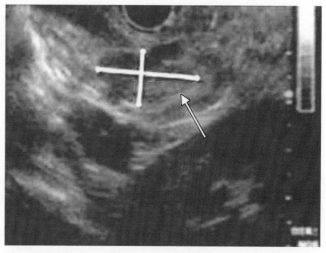

Fig. 3: Endoscopic ultrasonography (EUS) showing a hypodense space occupying lesion (shown with arrow).

WHAT IS THE DIAGNOSIS?

A further biochemical evaluation revealed an elevated serum prolactin of 161 ng/mL (Normal 2.5–17 ng/mL) indicating that he had a prolactinoma, hypercalcemia with albumin corrected calcium of 10.8 mg/dL (Normal 8.3–10.4 mg/dL) and also an elevated serum parathormone level of 185 pg/mL (Normal 8–50 pg/mL) suggestive of primary hyperparathyroidism.

Thus he was diagnosed to have Multiple Endocrine Neoplasia Type 1 (MEN1) with an insulinoma, primary hyperparathyroidism and a prolactinoma. The cerebellar atrophy was due to repeated untreated hypoglycemic episodes. Postoperatively the patients plasma glucose level was within normal limits. But his cerebellar symptoms persisted. Since the patient also had hypercalcemia he was thereby diagnosed to have MEN-1(Multiple Endocrine Neoplasia Type-1) syndrome.

He was given cabergoline in the dose of 0.5mg twice weekly for the treatment of prolactinoma. His Sestamibi parathyroid scintigraphy was negative for an adenoma probably due to all 4 parathyroid glands hyperplasia. He is planned for 3 and half gland parathyroid excision.

DISCUSSION

The differential diagnosis of symmetric cerebellar ataxia can be classified into acute, subacute, and chronic. Acute causes include cerebellar hematoma, viral cerebellitis, drug or alcohol ingestion, vertebrobasilar ischemic attacks, Wernicke's encephalopathy, and post-infectious syndrome, especially after varicella infection. Subacute presentations may also include chemotherapeutic agents, paraneoplastic syndromes, and nutritional deficiencies including thiamine and vitamin B-12.

The cerebellum is normally protected from hypoglycemia. In normal controls, glucose uptake is higher in the cerebellum relative to the cerebrum, but the rate of glucose metabolism is lower in the cerebellum. In case of the case patient (patient's with insulinoma) by contrast, the rate of glucose uptake was lower in the cerebellum and metabolism was similar to that of the cerebrum. This metabolic difference would seem to make the case patient more susceptible to hypoglycemic cerebellar injury, whereas in the controls, the cerebrum is more likely to be adversely affected by prolonged and severe hypoglycemia.[1,2]

REFERENCES

1. Kapoor N, Shetty S, Asha HS, et al. An unusual presentation of a patient with multiple endocrine neoplasia- 1. J Clin Diagn Res JCDR. 2014;8(12):MJ01–2.
2. Schwaninger M, Haehnel S, Hess K, et al. Cerebellar ataxia after repeated hypoglycemia. Eur J Neurol. 2002;9:544–5.

CASE 6

A 37-year-old male born to a 2nd degree consanguineous marriage, presented with left heel pain for 1 month without any antecedent history of trauma. He had an episode of left elbow pain 1 year back. He is on metformin for type 2 diabetes mellitus. He also complained of decreased libido.

His height was 158 cm, weight is 35 kg, BMI is 14 kg/m². He had a high-pitched voice. Physical examination revealed a pinched nose, dry wrinkled skin, loss and greying of hair, dystrophied nails and diffuse muscle wasting (Figs. 1 to 4). He had an ainhum of right 4th and 5th toes that resulted in auto-amputation. He had cataract in both the eyes that was corrected surgically 3 years ago. Callosities were present on the posterior aspect of calcaneum. He had a stretched penile length of 5 cm, testicular volume of 2 mL bilaterally and Tanner stage 2 pubic hair. X-ray of the elbow joint showed calcification of triceps near its insertion on the olecranon process.

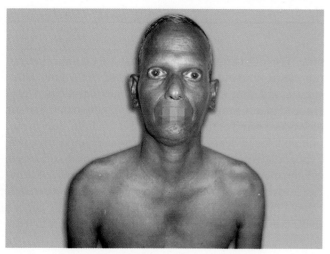

Fig. 1: Characteristic facial appearance with prominent eyes and a pinched or beaked nose.

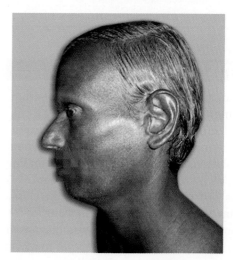

Fig. 2: Premature graying and loss of scalp hair.

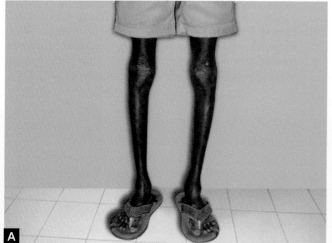

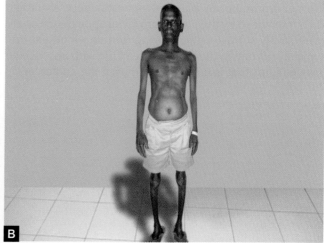

Figs. 3A and B: Severe muscle atrophy and loss of subcutaneous adipose tissue.

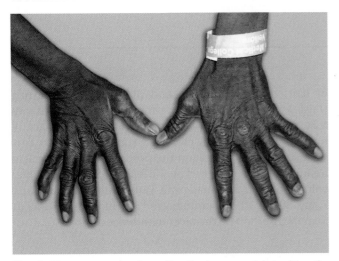

Fig. 4: Characteristic scleroderma-like skin changes and dystrophic nails.

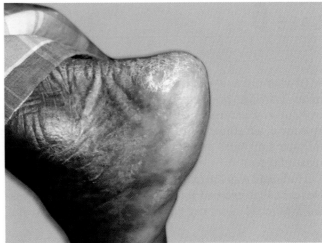

Fig. 5: Soft tissue calcification on the Achilles tendon region.

WHAT IS THE DIAGNOSIS?

Investigations revealed a HbA1C of 5.9%. Serum uric acid was 3.8 mg% (3–6) and CRP was 2.97 mg/L (<6). FSH was 57.8 mIU/mL (0.7-11.1) and testosterone was 197 ng/dL (270–1030) indicating hypergonadotropic hypogonadism. LDL cholesterol was 148 mg%, 8 am serum cortisol was 27.85 ug/dL (7–25), prolactin was 9.26 ng/mL (2.5–17) and TSH was 6.54 µIU/mL (0.3–4.5). With the classical facial appearance and the genetic study showing loss of function mutations of the WRN gene, he was diagnosed to have Werners syndrome. He is at present on metformin along with testosterone and on regular follow-up.

DISCUSSION

Werner syndrome, an inherited autosomal recessive trait, is characterized by the premature facial appearance associated with normal aging. Growth and development are typically normal in the first decade of life with absence of growth spurt that is usually seen during the adolescence time. The four cardinal signs are bilateral ocular cataracts, premature greying and/or thinning of scalp hair, short stature and characteristic dermatologic pathology. Deep, chronic ulcers around the ankle are highly characteristic of Werner syndrome. Other features include thin limbs, pinched facial features, osteoporosis, change in voice, hypogonadism, type 2 diabetes mellitus and soft tissue calcification (Fig. 5). There is an increased risk of atherosclerosis and cancers in such patients. The disease is caused by loss of function mutations of the WRN gene, a RecQ family member with both helicase and exonuclease activities.[1,2]

REFERENCES

1. Agrelo R, Cheng WH, Setien F, et al. Epigenetic inactivation of the premature aging Werner syndrome gene in human cancer. Proc Natl Acad Sci 2006;103(23):8822-7.
2. Epstein CJ, Martin GM, Schultz AL, et al. Werner's syndrome, a review of its symptomatology, natural history, pathologic features, genetics and relationship to the natural aging process. Medicine (Baltimore). 1966;45(3):177-221.

CASE 7

A 14-year-old boy presented to the OPD with the complaints of swelling in the region of his right breast for the past 3 months (Fig. 1). Examination revealed the presence of a disc of glandular tissue measuring 4 × 4 cm in the right retroareolar region. The swelling was tender. General physical examination showed a testicular volume of 10 mL bilaterally, with a pubic hair Tanner staging 4. He did not have any testicular mass.

WHAT IS THE DIAGNOSIS IN THIS PATIENT?

Our patient was diagnosed to have pubertal gynecomastia. A transient imbalance in the estrogen to androgen ratio during puberty is responsible for this condition. It usually resolves spontaneously within 6 months to two years of onset of the puberty and therefore the patients may be reassured regarding the same.However surgical correction may be required if the gynecomastia does not regress spontaneously.

DISCUSSION

Gynecomastia is a benign proliferation of the glandular tissue in males. It is common in adolescence and in middle aged or older men (Fig. 2). Clinically gynecomastia has to be differentiated from pseudogynecomastia/lipomastia, which is an accumulation of adipose tissue seen in obese men. Pseudogynecomastia is characterized by increased subareolar fat without enlargement of the breast glandular component. Carcinoma of the male breast has to be ruled out in older men if it occurs at that age. Gynecomastia can be physiological or pathological. Causes for gynecomastia include the following.[1]

1. *Pubertal Gynecomastia*: Usually resolves spontaneously.
2. *Drug induced Gynecomastia*: Drugs commonly associated with Gynecomastia are ketoconazole, spironolactone, cimetidine, anti androgens and 5 alpha eductase inhibitors.[2] Drug abuse, especially with anabolic steroids, alcohol, marijuana, or opioids, also should be considered in patients of adolescent age.
3. *Hypogonadism*: Both hypergonadotropic hypogonadism and hypogonadotropic hypogonadism.
4. *Testicular tumors*: Germ cell tumors which secrete hCG.
5. *Other causes*: Hyperthyroidism, chronic liver disease, chronic renal failure.
6. Familial or sporadic excessive aromatase activity, incomplete androgen insensitivity, feminizing testicular or adrenal tumors.

Pubertal gynecomastia usually regresses spontaneously. Gynecomastia, which has been present for less than 6 months often regresses after correction of the primary cause. However glandular tissue is gradually replaced

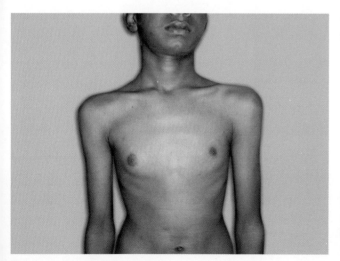

Fig. 1: Unilateral gynecomastia.

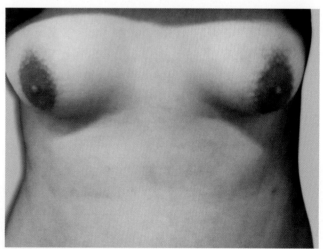

Fig. 2: Bilateral gynecomastia.

by fibrous tissue in patients with long standing Gynecomastia. In adults who present with the acute onset of painful Gynecomastia without an obvious cause, hormonal evaluation, including measurements of serum hCG, testosterone, luteinizing hormone, and estradiol levels, should be performed in order to rule out other causes of Gynecomastia. Pharmacological management is unlikely to be successful once this change has taken place and surgical correction may become necessary. Although not approved, the selective estrogen-receptor modulator tamoxifen, administered orally at a dose of 20 mg daily for 3 months, has been shown to be effective in the regression of the Gynecomastia. However, there are no definitive guidelines in the treatment of the Gynecomastia.

REFERENCES

1. Braunstein GD. Clinical practice. Gynacomastia. N Engl J Med. 2007;357(12):1229–37.
2. Deepinder F, Braunstein GD. Drug-induced Gynacomastia: an evidence-based review. Expert Opin Drug Saf. 2012; (5):779–95.

CASE 8

A 14-year-old boy presented with history of multiple bony swellings involving almost all the long bones, since the early childhood (Fig. 1). He had undergone surgery four times, for excision of these exostoses. He was the first child, born of a non consanguineous marriage. His parents had also noticed that he was short compared to his peers, from 3–4 years of age. He had history of two hospital admissions for lower respiratory tract infections. He also had history suggestive of developmental delay.

On examination he had loose skin folds on the back of his neck. He had multiple exostoses, short metacarpals and clinodactyly (Fig. 2). He had characteristic facial features in the form of a prominent nose, wide prominent philtrum, thin upper lip, small mandible and

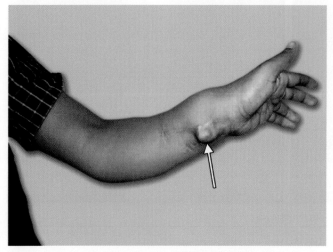

Fig. 1: Bony swelling/Exostosis at the wrist (shown with arrow).

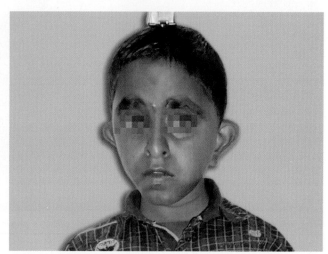

Fig. 2: Clinical image with characteristic facial features.

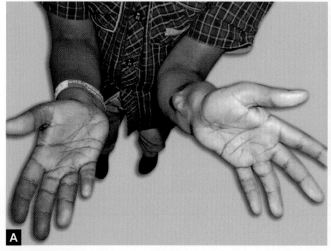

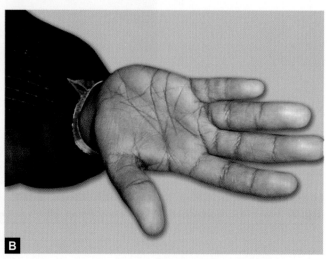

Figs. 3A and B: Small hands with short metacarpals and clinodactyly.

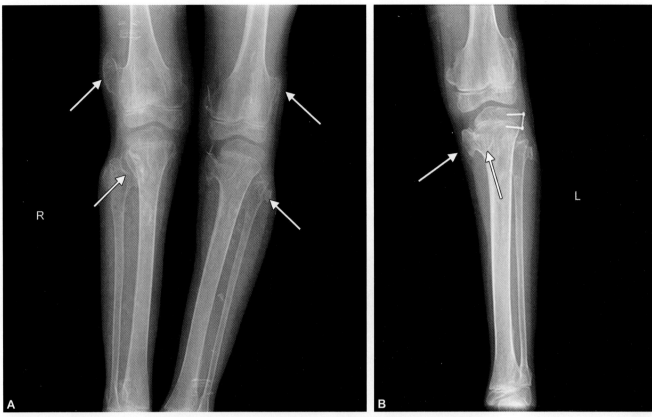

Figs. 4A and B: X-ray of the knee joint with multiple exostosis (shown with the arrows).

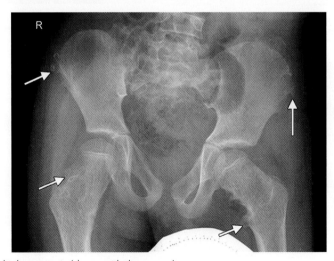

Fig. 5: X-ray of the pelvis with multiple exostosis (shown with the arrows).

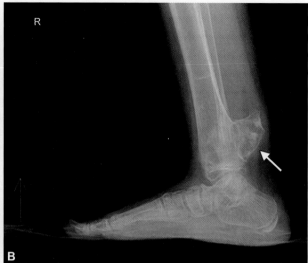

Figs. 6A and B: X-ray of the ankle joint showing an exophytic growth in the ankle joint (shown with arrow).

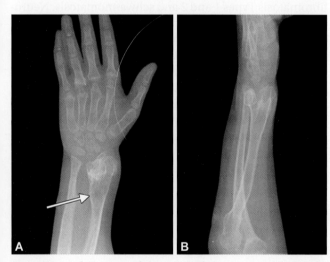

Figs. 7A and B: X-ray of the wrist with an exostosis (shown with arrow) and a bone age of around 11 years.

large ears (Figs. 3A and B). His X-rays are displayed in Figures 4 to 7.

WHAT IS THE DIAGNOSIS?

A diagnosis of Langer Giedion syndrome was made in this patient based on the presence of multiple exostosis, epiphyseal changes and the characteristic facial features.

DISCUSSION

Langer-Giedion syndrome or trichorhinophalangeal syndrome type 2 is a genetic disorder with characteristic face with fine sparse scalp hair, broad eyebrows, deep-set eyes, bulbous nose, elongated philtrum, thin upper lip, hypoplastic mandible, irregular teeth, small head and large laterally protruding ears (Fig. 2). In addition to the aforementioned features, other symptoms like hearing loss, submucous cleft palate, skin and joint laxity, melanocytic nevi, myopia, growth delay, mental deficiency, epilepsy, psychological disturbances, sarcomatous changes in exostoses, ureterohydronephrosis, hematometra, endocrine problems such as diabetes mellitus can occur.

It is usually inherited in an autosomal dominant manner. The disease is caused by a microdeletion in chromosome 8q23.3-q24.13 leading to the loss of at least two genes: *TRPS1* and *EXT1*.[1] Respiratory infections are frequent in these patients. As these patients grow older morbidity is mainly related to joint problems, manifesting as increased or decreased mobility, and in some patients an increased fracture rate. The multiple exostoses seen in these patients, usually do not progress after puberty. However, there is an increased risk of malignant change (0.5%) over 21 years of age. Exostoses may also cause neurovascular compression. Other orthopedic problems reported are clubfoot, joint laxity with increased risk of trauma and avascular necrosis of the hip joint. Ectodermal dysplasia with involvement of hair, teeth and nails may be present.[2]

REFERENCES

1. Schinzel A, Riegel M, Baumer A, et al. Long-term follow-up of four patients with Langer-Giedion syndrome: clinical course and complications. Am J Med Genet A. 2013; (9):2216–25.
2. Maas SM, Shaw AC, Bikker H, et al. Phenotype and genotype in 103 patients with trichorhino-phalangeal syndrome. Eur J Med Genet. 2015 May;58(5):279-92.

CASE 9

Mr A is a 23-year-old gentleman, who presented to the out patient department (OPD) for the evaluation of decreased muscle mass and multiple subcutaneous swellings all over the body which had progressively increased in size and number over the past 10 years. The clinical images are displayed in Figures 1 to 6.

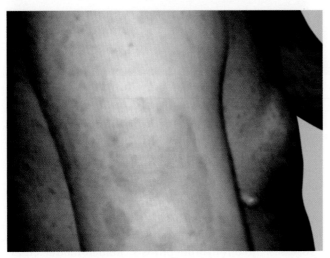

Fig. 1: Clinical image showing coffee colored macules on the right upper arm.

WHAT IS THE DIAGNOSIS?

On examination, the patient had several café au lait macules (Fig. 1) and multiple firm, painless, mobile subcutaneous swellings (Figs. 2 and 3). The café au lait spots were more than 6 in number with each measuring >1.5 cms in size. He had bony deformity in the form of pectus excavatum (Figs. 2A and B). He also had Lisch Nodules in the eyes (Figs. 5A and B). All these features are suggestive of neurofibromatosis Type 1.

DISCUSSION

There are three major forms of neurofibromatosis: neurofibromatosis Types 1 and 2 and schwannomatosis. Neurofibromatosis Type 1, also known as von Recklinghausen disease or NF1, is the most common type. NF1 is an autosomal dominant genetic disorder, that results from a mutation in the NF1 tumor suppressor gene found on chromosome 17. The hallmarks of NF1 are multiple café-au-lait macules and neurofibromas. Patients can develop characteristic bony deformities including osteopenia, scoliosis, sphenoid wing dysplasia, congenital tibial dysplasia, and pseudarthrosis.[1] Formal diagnostic criteria for NF1 were established by the NIH.[2]

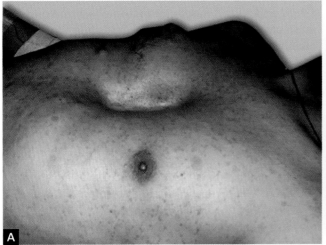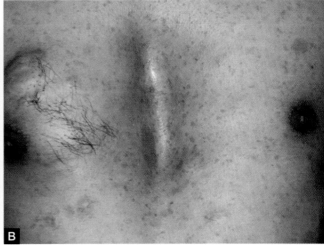

Figs. 2A and B: Image showing pectus excavatum and multiple mobile subcutaneous swelling on the anterior chest wall.

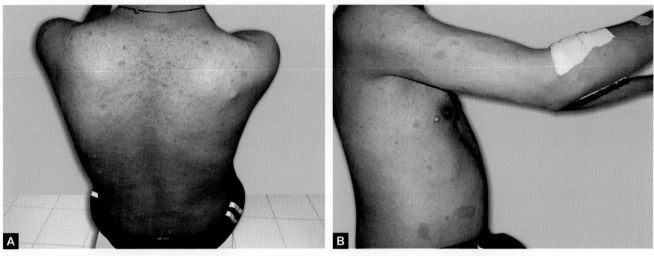

Figs. 3A and B: Multiple fleshy and boggy skin lesions in the back and the chest wall with multiple coffee colored skin lesions.

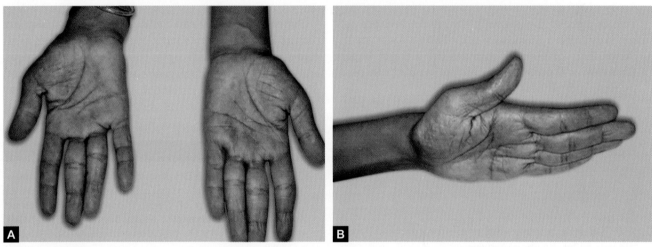

Figs. 4A and B: Patrick Yesudian sign: Palmar freckling.

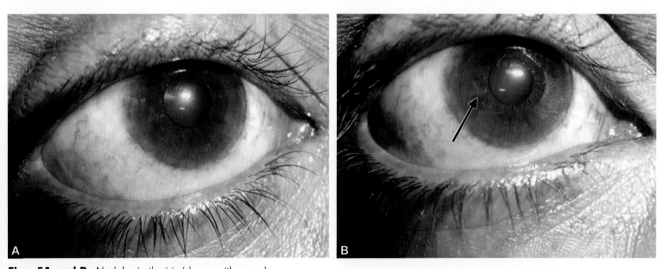

Figs. 5A and B: Nodules in the iris (shown with arrow).

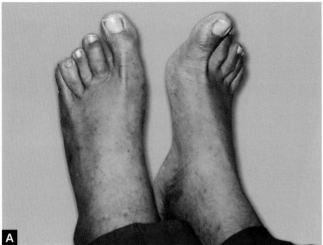 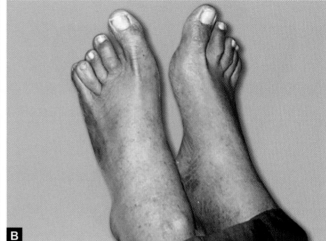

Figs. 6A and B: Bony changes in neurofibromatosis.

Two or more of the following clinical features are sufficient to establish a diagnosis of neurofibromatosis type 1:

1. Six or more café-au-lait macules (>0·5 cm at largest diameter in a prepubertal child or >1·5 cm in postpubertal individuals).
2. Axillary freckling or freckling in inguinal regions – Crowe's sign.
3. Two or more neurofibromas of any type or one or more plexiform neurofibromas.
4. Two or more Lisch nodules (iris hamartomas).
5. A distinctive osseous lesion (sphenoid wing dysplasia, long-bone dysplasia).
6. An optic pathway glioma.
7. A first-degree relative with neurofibromatosis Type 1 diagnosed by the above criteria.

Patients with NF1 can develop benign or malignant tumors affecting various parts of the body. Tumors associated with NF1 include optic glioma, malignant peripheral nerve sheath tumors, gastrointestinal stromal tumor, pheochromocytoma, carcinoid tumor, rhabdomyosarcoma, carcinoma breast and leukemia.

REFERENCES

1. Hirbe AC, Gutmann DH. Neurofibromatosis type 1: a multidisciplinary approach to care. Lancet Neurol. 2014;(8):834-43.
2. National Institutes of Health Consensus Development Conference Statement: neurofibromatosis. Bethesda, Md., USA, July 13-15, 1987. Neurofibromatosis. 1988;1(3): 172–8.

CASE **10**

A 23-year-old man presented for the evaluation of short stature and small penile size. He had a male gender identity with heterosexual orientation and normal libido. He was born at full term via normal vaginal delivery. There were no history of any maternal drug ingestion during pregnancy or recurrent hospital admissions during childhood. His parents noted ambiguous genitalia during the infancy but did not seek any medical intervention. He also reported accelerated linear growth during childhood. There is no evidence of pituitary insufficiency. Two of his siblings had died at the age less than 4 months.

His height was 143 cms (with mid parenteral height of 156 cm), weight was 61.6 kg, body mass index of (BMI) of 30.1 kg/m² (Fig. 1). Physical examination revealed clitoromegaly, phallus like structure of 4 cm with chordee and perineal hypospadias (Fig. 2). Labioscrotal folds were not fused and testes were not palpable. Urethral orifice and vaginal openings were visualized separately. There was no palpable breast tissue. He had male pattern hair distribution with temporal balding. He was normotensive.

WHAT IS THE DIAGNOSIS?

Vagina, uterus and fallopian tubes were visualized on genitogram. The USG pelvis showed a hypoplastic uterus but did not show any evidence of gonadal tissue. CT abdomen/pelvis showed bilaterally enlarged adrenal glands and streaked ovaries, and confirmed the absence of testes. The serum level of 17-hydoxyprogesterone level was 46.9 ng/mL, testosterone 732 ng/dL (50–120), Adrenocorticotropic hormone (ACTH) 1210 pg/mL (0-46) and 8 am cortisol 8.04 mcg/dL (7–25) with an insufficient post synacthen serum cortisol response. However, the serum electrolytes and plasma renin activity were within the normal range. The clinical, biochemical and radiological features were suggestive of classic congenital adrenal hyperplasia – simple virilizing form. He was referred to the Department of Urology for the corrective genitoplasty surgery. He was started on oral dexamethasone 0.5 mg once daily in the evening with hydrocortisone protocol during stress.

DISCUSSION

Congenital adrenal hyperplasias (CAH) are autosomal recessive disorders. 90% of cases are caused by 21-hydroxylase deficiency due to mutations in the *CYP 21A2* gene, resulting in an inadequate production of glucocorticoids and mineralocorticoids, and excess production of androgens. There are two major subtypes—the classic and the nonclassic (late-onet) types. The classic 21-hydroxylase deficiency can present in 2 forms: a salt-losing form and a simple virilizing form. CAH presents during the neonatal period and early infancy with adrenal insufficiency, or in toddlers with virilization. Female children have ambiguous genitalia at birth. The "nonclassic" form presents

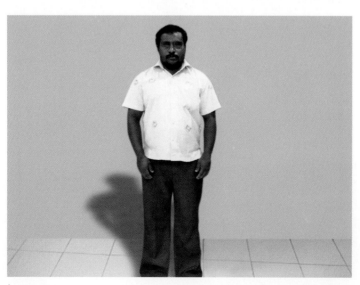

Fig. 1: Clinical image showing short stature.

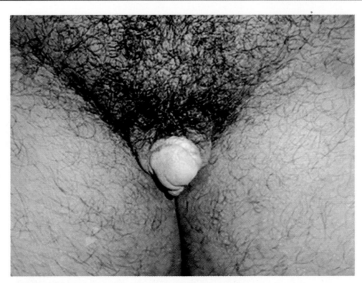

Fig. 2: Clinical image showing a phallus like structure with chordae and hypospadias.

later in life with signs of androgen excess, and without genital ambiguity. It presents as hirsuitism and menstrual irregularity in young women, early pubarche or sexual precocity in school age children, or may remain asymptomatic throughout life with problems in fertility. The main aim of treatment is to prevent hypocortisolemic crisis and to suppress the excess testosterone levels. Though the patients have suppressed androgen levels with dexamethasone or prednisolone, most of the female patients have fertility issues due to poor development of the uterine and fallopian tubes as well as due to fertilization related problems.[1,2]

REFERENCES

1. Speiser PW, Azziz R, Baskin LS, et al; Endocrine Society. Congenital adrenal hyperplasia due to steroid 21-hydroxylase deficiency: an Endocrine Society clinical practice guideline. J Clin Endocrinol Metab. 2010;95(9):4133-60.
2. Merke DP, Bornstein SR. Congenital adrenal hyperplasia. Lancet. 2005;365(9477):2125-36.

CASE **11**

A 17-year-old boy presented to the out patient department (OPD) for the evaluation of progressive spinal deformity. He was the first child of a non consanguineous marriage. On examination he was 165 cm tall with an arm span of 175 cm (Figs. 1A and B). He had an upper segment to lower segment ratio of 0.8. He had long slender fingers with hyper extensible joints (Figs. 2 and 3). The thumb sign and wrist sign were positive. Bony deformities in the form of pectus excavatum and kyphoscoliosis were also present. He had a divergent squint (Figs. 4A and B). He also had a high arched palate (Fig. 5). An echocardiogram was done as part of evaluation which showed a mitral valve prolapse.

WHAT IS THE DIAGNOSIS IN THIS PATIENT AND WHAT ARE THE OTHER DISORDERS WITH SIMILAR CLINICAL FEATURES?

A diagnosis of Marfans syndrome was made in our patient. Serial echocardiograms were planned annually as part of follow-up to look for aortic root dilatation. Conditions related to Marfans syndrome, presenting with similar clinical features include Ehlers-Danlos syndrome, Homocystinuria, mitral valve prolapse syndrome, Ectopia lentis

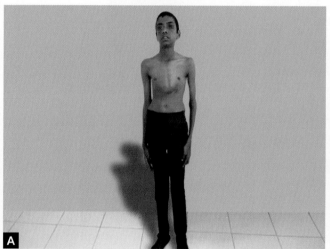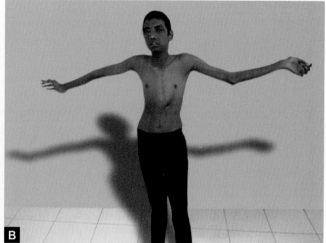

Figs. 1A and B: Patient's clinical image.

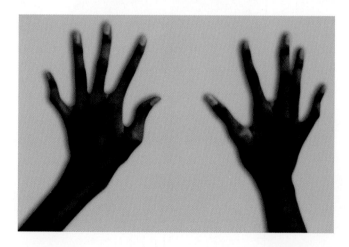

Fig. 2: Arachnodactyly.

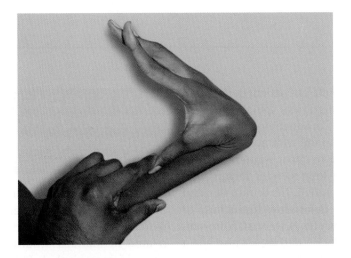

Fig. 3: Hyperextensible joints.

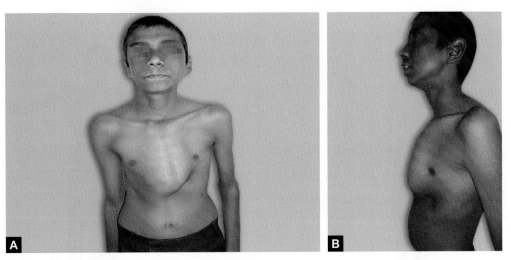

Figs. 4A and B: Pectus Carinatum.

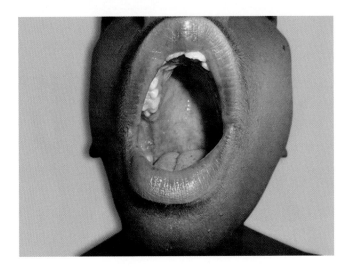

Fig. 5: High arched palate.

syndrome, and MASS phenotype (mitral valve prolapse, borderline but no progressive aortic dilatation, striae atrophica and at least one skeletal deformity).

DISCUSSION

Marfan syndrome is an inherited disorder of connective tissue whose cardinal features affect the cardiovascular system, eyes and skeleton. It is inherited in an autosomal dominant manner in majority of cases, but about 25% of patients may have de novo mutations. Most patients harbor mutations involving the gene (*FBN1*) encoding the connective tissue protein fibrillin-1. Fibrillin 1 is a main constituent protein of extracellular microfibrils that contribute to the formation of elastic fibers. Mutations in the transforming growth factor beta receptor are seen in patients with atypical Marfan syndrome.[1]

Cardiovascular complications of Marfan syndrome include aortic root dilatation, mitral valve prolapse and regurgitation, left ventricular dilatation and cardiac failure and pulmonary artery dilatation. Aortic root disease, leading to aneurysmal dilatation, aortic regurgitation, and dissection, is the main cause of morbidity and mortality in the Marfan syndrome.[2] Dilatation of the aorta is found in approximately 50 percent of children with Marfan syndrome and progresses with time. The risk of aortic dissection increases when the diameter of the aortic root exceeds 5 cm or when the rate of dilatation exceeds 1.5 mm per year.

Individuals affected by Marfan syndrome are tall for their genetic background. They have excess linear growth of their long bones. They have joint laxity and hypermobility which predisposes them to injuries. They typically have arachnodactyly with positive thumb and wrist signs. Deformities of the spine in the form of kyphoscoliosis are common and are seen in around 60% of the patients. A higher prevalence of osteoporosis and low bone mass has also been reported.

The eyes are commonly affected in Marfan syndrome in the form of Ectopic lentis in 50–80% of patients. Other ocular features include high myopia predisposing to retinal detachment, a flat cornea, hypoplastic iris or ciliary muscle, glaucoma and cataract.

Pectus excavatum occurs in approximately two-thirds of patients with Marfan's syndrome, can be associated with a restrictive ventilatory defect. Bullae in the lungs and spontaneous occurance of pneumothorax is common and should be looked for. Dural ectasia is another common problem and usually affects the lumbar spine. Patients with Marfans syndrome may have facial deformities including dolichocephaly, enophthalmos, downslanting palpebral fissures, malar hypoplasia, and retrognathia.

Early diagnosis and appropriate surgical and medical management of various conditions associated with Marfan syndrome can improve life expectancy significantly in these patients.

REFERENCES

1. Dean JCS. Marfan syndrome: clinical diagnosis and management. Eur J Hum Genet EJHG. 2007;15(7):724–33.
2. Adams JN, Trent RJ. Aortic complications of Marfan's syndrome. Lancet. 1998;352(9142):1722–3.

CASE **12**

A 17-year-old lady presented with history of delay in onset of puberty. She had short stature and report a normal height gain during the early childhood. Her mother and father were significantly taller than her. She was born at term of a normal vaginal delivery to a non-consanguineous marriage. She achieved all the developmental milestones at an appropriate age. At the age of 12 years, she was diagnosed to have primary hypothyroidism and was started on thyroxine replacement therapy. However, she was poorly compliant to the medications. There were no history of headache, galactorrhea, visual defects, anosmia or radiation/chemotherapy in the past.

Her height was 130 cms (< 5th centile) (Figs. 1A and B). Vital signs were within normal limits. Physical examination revealed dry skin, short 4th metacarpal (Figs. 2 and 3), wide carrying angle and widely spaced nipples. Bilateral lymphedema was present. She had normal axillary hair growth. Pubic hair and breast development were Tanner stage 1 and 2 respectively. Thyroid gland was not enlarged.

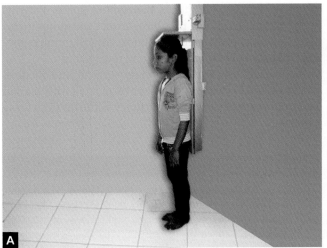
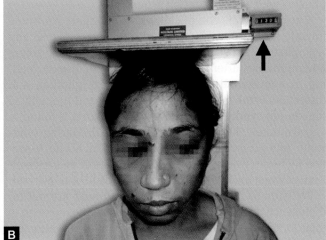

Figs. 1A and B: Patient's height of 130 cm with multiple lentinges on the face.

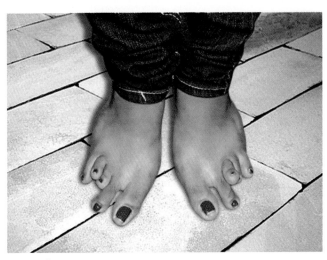

Fig. 2: Bilateral short 3rd and 4th metatarsals.

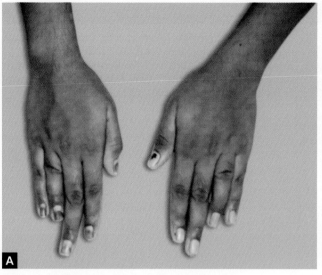
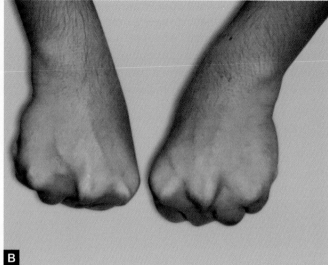

Figs. 3A and B: Bilateral short 4th metacarpals.

WHAT IS THE DIAGNOSIS?

The biochemical investigations revealed TSH of 142.46 uIU/mL (0.3–4.5) and FSH of 48.3 mIU/mL.

Laboratory tests were confirmed of the diagnosis of primary hypothyroidism. Inadequate dosage and poor compliance were responsible for the high Thyroid Stimulating Hormone (TSH) despite being on thyroxine replacement therapy. Follicular Stimulating Hormone (FSH) was in the postmenopausal range and was suggestive of primary ovarian failure. Karyotyping revealed 45XO phenotype confirming the diagnosis of turners syndrome. Thus, this patient's clinical and biochemical features were in favour of Turner's syndrome.

DISCUSSION

Turner's syndrome is the leading cause of primary amenorrhea and short stature in females. Turner's syndrome is the most common chromosomal abnormality in females, affecting 1:2500 live female births. It is a result of absence of an X chromosome or the presence of a structurally abnormal X chromosome.

1. Pure 45X monosomy is the most common karyotype seen in TS and is associated with the most abnormal phenotypic features. In about two thirds of the women with TS, the normal X chromosome is of maternal in origin. Monosomy X results from the nondisjunction as a result of failure of the sex chromatids to separate during meiosis in the parental gamete or in the early embryonic divisions.

2. Isochromosome Xq is the most common structural abnormality and is associated with autoimmune disorders and deafness, but congenital abnormalities are conspicuously absent.

3. Women with 45X/46,XY mosaicism have an increased risk of developing gonadoblastoma, and a minority of these women are also masculinized.

4. Women with the ring X chromosome are more likely to have psychological sequelae but are less likely to have structural congenital abnormalities, and the spontaneous menses occur in about a third of TS patients.

The gene, known as SHOX (short stature homeobox-containing gene), or PHOG (pseudoautosomal homeobox containing osteogenic gene), is expressed on both the inactive and active X and Y chromosomes. SHOX/PHOG point mutations have been shown to be associated with short stature.[1,2]

In treating patients with TS, estrogen is usually started at one tenth to one eighth of the adult replacement dose and then increased gradually over a period of 2–4 years. Low-dose estradiol therapy can be initiated as early as 12-years of age. The following are equivalent doses that achieve estradiol levels in the normal range for young adult women: oral estradiol, 2 mg/d; transdermal estradiol, 0.1 mg/d; and injectable estradiol cypionate, 2.5 mg/month. The main aim of the treatment is to allow for normal breast and uterine development; it is advisable to delay the addition of progestin for at least 2 years after starting estrogen or until breakthrough bleeding occurs. The use of oral contraceptive pills to achieve the pubertal development is best avoided, in view of the fact that the synthetic estrogen preparations in most fixed dose formulations are too high and the typical synthetic progestin may interfere with optimal breast and uterine development. It is important to educate the patients about continuing the estrogen replacement until the time of normal menopause to maintain feminization and importantly to prevent osteoporosis.[1]

REFERENCES

1. Elsheikh M, Dunger DB, Conway, et al. Turner's Syndrome in Adulthood. Endocr Rev. 2002;23(1):120–40.
2. Bondy CA. Care of Girls and Women with Turner Syndrome: A Guideline of the Turner Syndrome Study Group. J Clin Endocrinol Metab. 2007;92(1):10–25.

CASE 13

An 18-year-old girl was brought by her parents to our Endocrine out patient department (OPD) with complaints of their daughter being short than her younger sibling and delay in her menarche. The clinical images are displayed in Figures 1 to 3.

WHAT IS THE DIAGNOSIS?

On clinical examination she was found to be short with height of 135 cm (midparenteral height of 156 cms)

(Fig. 1). She had multiple lentigines on her face (Figs. 2A and B). She had pubic hair tanner stage 2 and breast Tanner stage 3. She also had Madelung deformity of the hand (Figs. 3A and B). The karyotyping showed 45XO suggestive of Turners syndrome.The patient was started on 0.005 mg of ethinyl estradiol and the dose was increased to 0.01 mg till her breast had developed to Tanner stage 3. Subsequently she was started on levonorgestrel 0.1 mg and ethinyl estradiol 0.02 mg for 21 days/cycles.

DISCUSSION

Madelung's deformity is usually characterized by malformed wrists and wrist bones, accompanied by short stature. Madelung deformity, a spontaneous forward subluxation of the hand was first described by Malgaigne and Madelung in the later part of the 19th century. Madelung deformity is an ulnar and dorsal curvature of the distal radius due to deficient growth of the volar and ulnar aspect of distal radial physis, increased inclination of the distal radial joint surface, triangulation of the corpus with proximal and volar migration of and a prominent dorsal subluxation of ulnar head. Madelung deformity, besides Turner's syndrome is also found in pseudohypoparathyroidism, mucopolysaccharidosis and achondroplasia of distal radial epiphysis. It has also been reported following trauma to the wrist, infection and neoplasia.

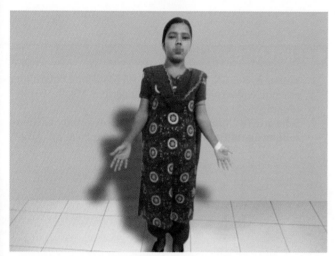

Fig. 1: Clinical image of the patient.

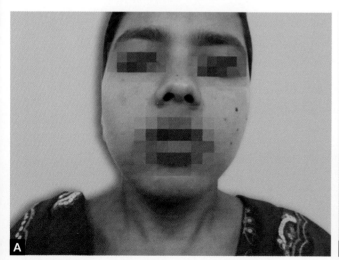
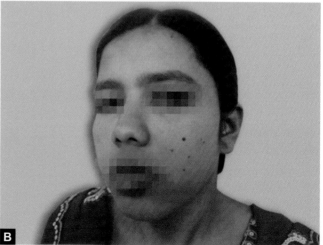

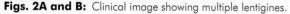

Figs. 2A and B: Clinical image showing multiple lentigines.

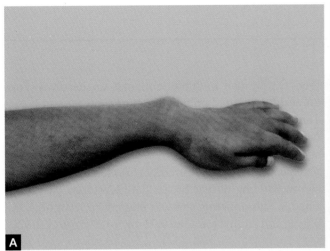
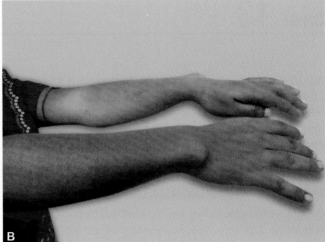

Figs. 3A and B: Clinical image of the patient's hands.

Leri-Weill's dyschondrosteosis (LWD) is an autosomal dominant condition characterized by mesomelic short stature and with Madelung deformity which is due to the deletion or mutation in Short Stature homeobox (SHOX) gene. Madelung deformity is also explained in Langers mesomelic dysplasia.[1,2]

REFERENCES

1. Kumar A, Rai GK, Akhtar J,et al. All Madelung deformities are not endocrine. Indian J Endocrinol Metab. 2013;17 (Suppl1):S231–3.
2. Schwartz RP, Sumner TE. Madelung's deformity as a presenting sign of Turner's syndrome. J Pediatr. 2000;136(4):563.

CASE 14

A 12-year-old girl presented with the history of progressive weight gain, breathlessness on exertion and nocturnal symptoms suggestive of Obstructive Sleep Apnoea, which had recently worsened over a period of 1–2 months. Born to consanguineous parents, she weighed 1.7 kg at birth, had a poor cry and required oxygen for respiratory distress. She had required nasogastric feeding in hospital for the first two weeks after birth. Her developmental milestones had been delayed. Although the subject had feeding difficulties initially, after one year of age, this was replaced by increasing weight and a voracious appetite. Genital examination was unremarkable.

WHAT IS THE DIAGNOSIS?

Clinically our patient had short stature, obesity, small hands and feet and history of hyperphagia suggestive of Prader-willi syndrome (Figs. 1 and 2). She also had almond shaped eyes, small appearing mouth with thin upper lip (Fig. 3). Her body composition revealed a fat percentage of 55.6% (Normally 20–30%) (Fig. 4). She did not have any metabolic complications of obesity. She was advised to follow strict diet and increase the physical activity.

DISCUSSION

Prader-willi syndrome (PWS) is traditionally characterized by hypotonia, short stature, hyperphagia, obesity, behavioral issues (specifically OCD-like behavior), small hands and feet, hypogonadism, and mild mental retardation. Prader-willi syndrome (PWS) is the most common syndromic cause of childhood obesity. In addition to the hyperphagia seen by one year of age, patients with PWS suffer from hypotonia and poor motor coordination. This combination of symptoms predisposes these children to choking and aspiration of food. In addition, patients with PWS have breathing disorders related to obstructive sleep apnoea (OSA) and central alveolar hypoventilation.

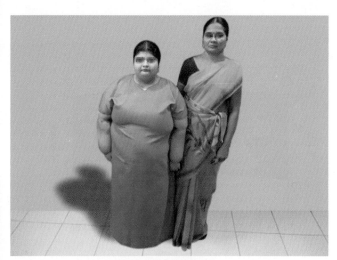

Fig. 1: Patients clinical image showing short stature with obesity.

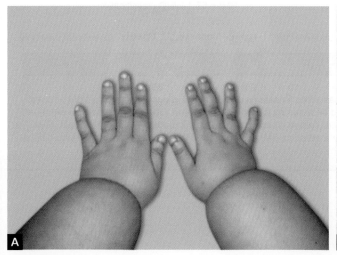
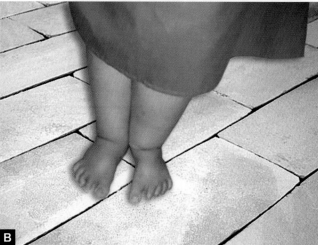

Figs. 2A and B: Clinical image showing small hands (Acromicria) and feet.

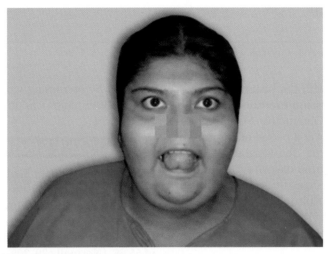

Fig. 3: Image with almond shaped eyes and small mouth with a thin upper lip.

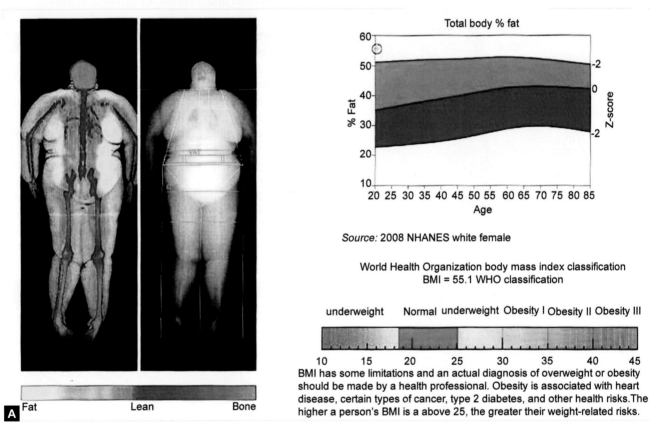

A | Fat   Lean   Bone

Total body % fat

Source: 2008 NHANES white female

World Health Organization body mass index classification
BMI = 55.1 WHO classification

underweight   Normal   underweight   Obesity I   Obesity II   Obesity III

BMI has some limitations and an actual diagnosis of overweight or obesity should be made by a health professional. Obesity is associated with heart disease, certain types of cancer, type 2 diabetes, and other health risks. The higher a person's BMI is a above 25, the greater their weight-related risks.

Fig. 4A

Body composition results

Region	Fat Mass (g)	Leanth BMC (g)	Total Mass (g)	% Fat	% Fat percentile YN	AM
L Arm	5110	2521	7631	67.0	99	99
R Arm	5712	2864	8576	66.6	99	99
Trunk	31422	23077	54498	57.7	99	99
L Leg	10230	9760	19990	51.2	94	94
R Leg	9091	8329	17420	52.2	95	95
Sbutotal	61565	46550	108115	56.9	99	99
Head	1271	3719	4990	25.5		
Total	**62836**	50269	113105	55.6	99	99
ANdroid (A)	5505	4545	10250	53.7		
Gynoid (G)	7156	8244	15400	46.5		

Adipose indices

Measure	Result	Percentile YN	AM
Total body % Fat	55.6	99	99
Fat mass/t	30.1	99	99
Android/gynoid ratio	1.16		
% Fat trunk% fat legs	1.12	97	98
Trunk/Limb fat mass ratio	1.04	86	91
Est. Vat mass (g)	744		
Est. Vat volume (cm^3)	804		
Est Vat area (cm^2)	154		

Lean indices

Measure	Result	Percentile YN	AM
Lean/height^2 (kg/m^2)	23.1	99	99
Appen lean height^2 (kg/m^2)	10.8	99	99

Est. VAT = Estimated viscreal adipose tissue
YN = Young normal
AM = Age matched

B

Figs. 4A and B: Body composition showing increased fat mass (shown with a circle).

PWS is characterized by an insatiable hunger starting from childhood, mental retardation, hypogonadism and growth deficiency; hypotonia, feeding problems and failure to thrive are the predominant features in the neonatal period.[1]

The clinical diagnosis of PWS is based on the criteria proposed by Holm et al in 1993 (1) Revised criteria published in 2001 proposed a lower clinical threshold to prompt DNA testing and a more definitive diagnosis.

Children with PWS suffer from a variety of breathing abnormalities. As these children are at high risk for developing apnoea and sudden deaths, they should undergo sleep study and therapy for the underlying problem. Appropriate therapy includes weight control, adenotonsillectomy and nocturnal ventilation.[2]

REFERENCES

1. Holm VA, Cassidy SB, Butler MG, et al. Prader-willi syndrome: consensus diagnostic criteria. Pediatrics 1993; 91:398-402.
2. Gunay-Aygun M, Schwartz S, Heeger S, et al. The changing purpose of Prader-willi syndrome clinical diagnostic criteria and proposed revised criteria. Pediatrics 2001;108:E92.

CASE 15

A 25-year-old gentleman born of a second degree consanguineous marriage presented with complaints of swelling over the joints for the past few years which was not resolving even after extensive removal. His brother also had a similar illness. His maternal uncle had premature coronary artery disease.

WHAT IS THE DIAGNOSIS?

His investigations revealed Total cholesterol –505 mg/dL (Normal <200), Triglycerides-160 mg/dL (Normal-<150 mg), Low Density Lipoprotein (LDL)-350 mg/dL (Normal <100 mg) and High Density Lipoprotein (HDL)-46 mg/dL. All other hormonal axes were within normal limits. There were no clinical and radiological features to suggest atherosclerotic change in the large vessels. He was diagnosed to have Familial Type 2a Hypercholesterolemia. He was started on Atorvastatin 40 mg and Ezetimibe 10 mg and advised for regular follow up.

DISCUSSION

Xanthoma tuberosum (also known as tuberous xanthoma) is characterized by xanthomas located over the joints (Figs. 1A, 1B, 1D, 1F, 2A, 2D, 2E and 4). Xanthoma tendinosum (also tendon xanthoma or tendinous xanthoma) is clinically characterized by papules and nodules in the tendons of the hands, feet, and heels (Figs. 1C, 1E, 2B, 2C and 2F). Xanthoma planum (also known as plane xanthoma), is clinically characterized by macules and plaques which diffusely spreads over large areas of the body (Figs. 3A to J). A xanthelasma is a sharply demarcated yellowish collection of cholesterol underneath the skin, usually on or around the eyelids (Fig. 5). Eruptive xanthoma which is associated with elevated triglyceride, is clinically characterized by small, yellowish-orange to reddish-brown papules that appear all over the body. Palmar xanthoma is clinically characterized by yellowish plaques that involve the palms and flexural surfaces of the fingers (Fig. 6).

Simon Broome Register Group has proposed a definition of familial hypercholesterolemia.

According to this group the definitive diagnosis of familial hypercholesterolaemia requires presence of (a) plus (b) below, Possible familial hypercholesterolaemia requires presence of (a) plus one of (c) or (d).

(a) At least two confirmed measurements of total cholesterol >7.5 m mol/L (285 mg%) and LDL cholesterol >4.9 mmol/L (185 mg%) in adults (total >6.7 mmol/L (255 mg%) and LDL >4.0 mmol/L (150 mg%) in children aged <16 years)

(b) Tendon xanthoma in patient or DNA based diagnosis of familial hypercholesterolemia in first or second degree relative

(c) Family history of myocardial infarction in second degree relative aged <50 years or in first degree relative aged <60 years

(d) Family history of high cholesterol in first degree relative or concentration >7.5 mmol/L (285 mg%) in second degree relative.

Fredrickson had classified familial hypercholesterolemia into five types which is shown in Table 1. In children aged 10–14 years, an LDL level of <160 mg/dL or >30% reduction from baseline levels is targeted. A rigorous target lipid level of <130 mg/dL is recommended in children between the ages of 14 and 18 years. In patients older than 18 years, a lipid target of <100 mg/dL is deemed appropriate. Mipomirsen, an antisense oligonucleotide that targets apoB-100 mRNA in the liver, and Lomitapide, a new lipid-lowering agent with a novel mechanism of action of inhibiting the microsomal triglyceride transfer protein is presently under investigation in the therapy of FH. The role of MTP in the production of LDL involves assisting in the transfer of triglycerides to apolipoprotein B.[1,2]

Table 1: Fredrickson classification of hyperlipoproteinemias.

Type	Lipoprotein Elevated	Lipid Elevation Major	Lipid Elevation Minor
I (rare)	Chylomicrons	TG	↑↔g
IIa	LDL	C	-
IIb	LDL, VLDL	C	TG
III (rare)	IDL	C,TG	-
IV	VLDL	TG	↑↔g
V (rare)	Chylomicrons, VLDL	TG	↑↔

(C : Cholesterol; TG : Triglycerides; LDL : Low density lipoprotein; VLDL: Very low density lipoprotein; IDL : Intermediate density lipoprotein).

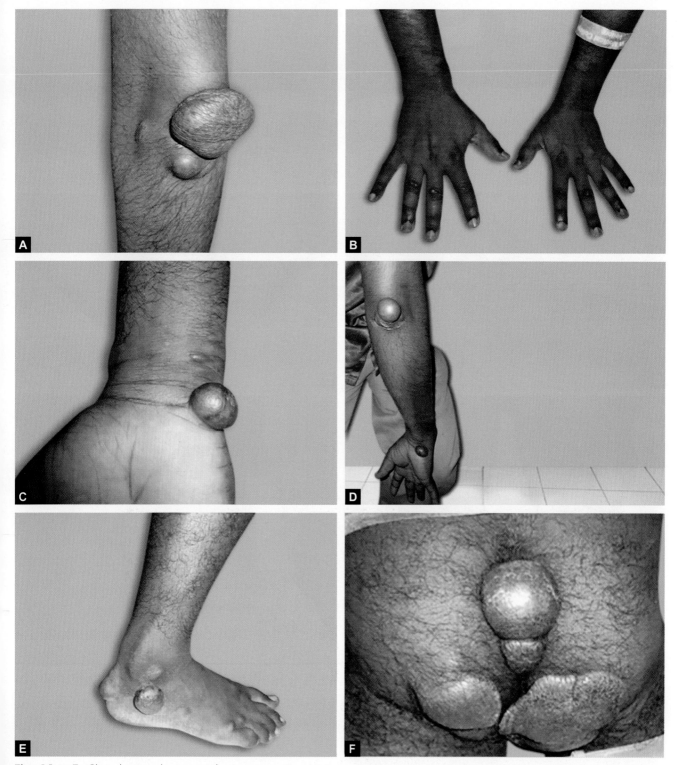

Figs.1A to F: Clinical image showing xanthomas over various joints.

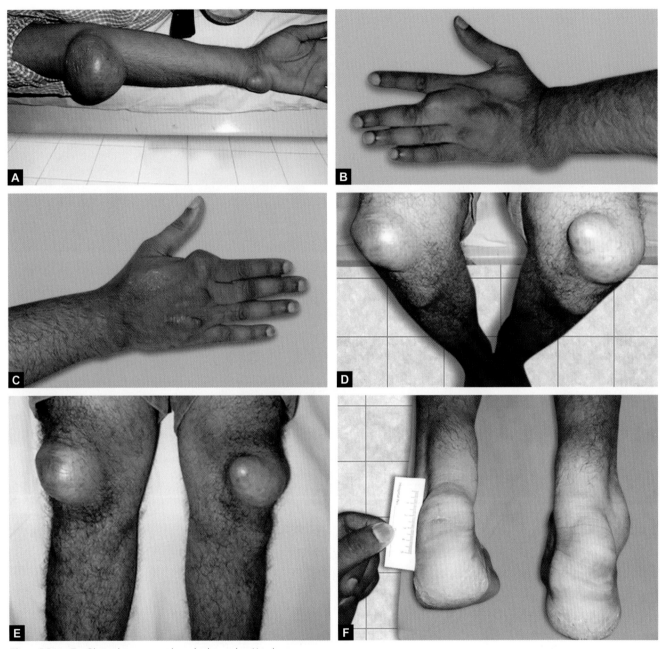

Figs. 2A to F: Clinical images with multiple tendon Xanthomas.

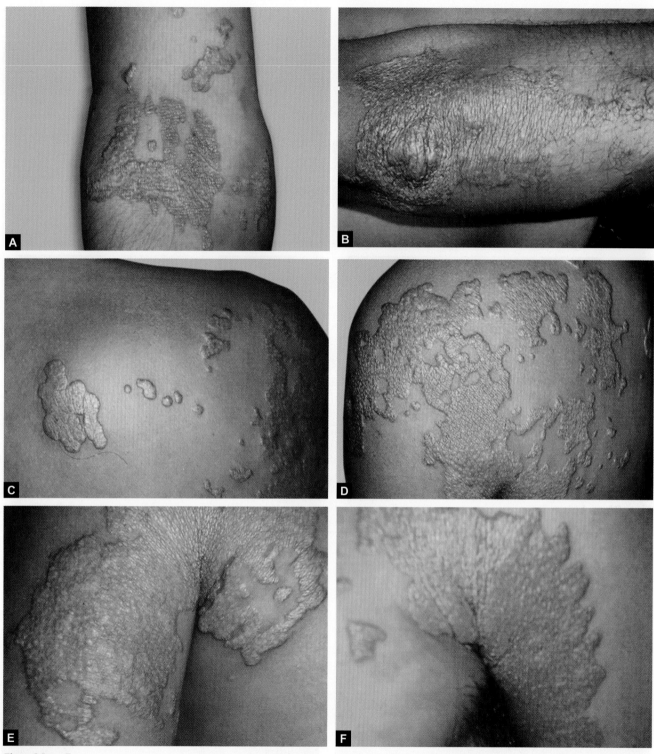

Figs. 3A to F

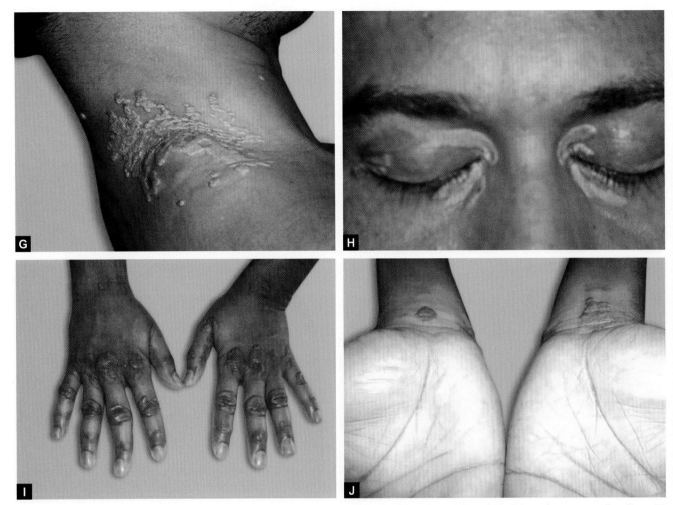

Figs. 3A to J: Extensive xanthomas over the elbows (Figs. 3A and B), both shoulders (Figs. 3C and D), bilateral anterior axillas (Figs. 3E and F), right side neck (Fig. 3G), Bilateral xanthomas (Fig. 3H) and tendon Xanthomas in the hands (Figs. 3I and J).

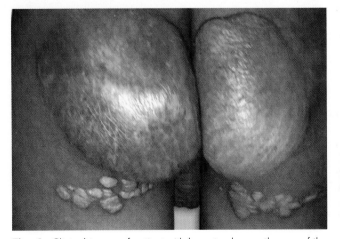

Fig. 4: Clinical image of patient with large tendon xanthomas of the Gluteal cleft.

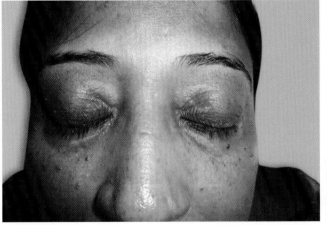

Fig. 5: Bilateral xanthelasmas are seen commonly in clinical practice which warrants a lipid profile in such patients.

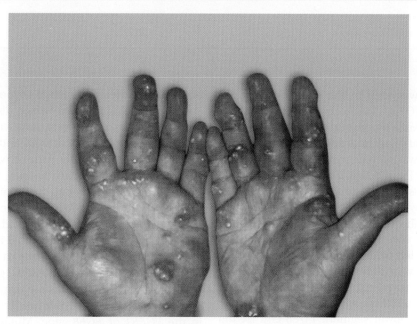

Fig. 6: Palmar Xanthomas.

REFERENCES

1. *National Institute for Health and Clinical Excellence.* Identification and management of familial hypercholesterolaemia. Clinical guideline 71. *NICE, August* 2008

2. Raal FJ, Santos RD, Blom DJ, et al. Mipomersen, an apolipoprotein B synthesis inhibitor, for lowering of LDL cholesterol concentrations in patients with homozygous familial hypercholesterolaemia: A randomised, double-blind, placebo-controlled trial. Lancet. 2010;375(9717):998–1006.

CASE 16

A 20-year-old Mr P was seen in the endocrinology out patient department (OPD) for the evaluation of symptoms of small sized penile length and testicular size (Figs. 1A and B). His parents had noticed this anomaly since his childhood. There was no hair growth over his body or beard area(Fig. 1C). He did not have any hair growth over the body or his growth of facial hair (Fig. 1C). The child was born with a cleft lip and cleft palate, had surgery for cleft lip at the age of 4 years and asymptomatic at present (Figs. 1D and E). His clinical examination showed that he had cleft palate which was not operated. He also had difficulty in differentiating various odors. His testicular volume was 2 mL with pubic hair Tanner stage 3. His height was 162 cm with arm span of 178 cm and upper segment to lower segment 74/88 cm. He did not have nystagmus or bimanual synkinesis. Retinal examination did not reveal any features of optic dysplasia.

WHAT IS THE DIAGNOSIS?

His investigations revealed a serum Luteinizing Hormone (LH) < 0.10 mIU/mL and Follicular Stimulating Hormone (FSH)-0.325 mIU/mL with serum testosterone of < 20.0 ng/dL with other hormonal axes being normal. MRI Brain revealed an absent olfactory bulb bilaterally (Figs. 2A and B & Fig. 3) suggestive of Kallmann's syndrome. He was started on injection testosterone 100 mg once in 3 weeks and was advised to escalate the dose to 250 mg once in 3 weeks after 3 months of initiation of testosterone.

DISCUSSION

Kallmann syndrome (KS) is a form of hypogonadotropic hypogonadism (HH) characterized by delayed or absent puberty and an impaired sense of smell. This disorder affects the production of hormones that direct sexual development. In Kallmann syndrome, the sense of smell is either diminished (hyposmia) or completely absent (anosmia) a feature which distinguishes Kallmann syndrome from most other forms of hypogonadotropic hypogonadism. Additional signs and symptoms of KS are renal agenesis, a cleft lip with or without a cleft palate, abnormal eye movements, hearing loss, and abnormalities of tooth development. Some affected patients have bimanual synkinesis, in which the movements of one hand are mirrored by the other hand. There are four forms of Kallmann syndrome, designated as 1 through 4, which are distinguished by their genetic cause. Mutations in the *KAL1*, *FGFR1*, *PROKR2*, and *PROK2* genes cause Kallmann syndrome. KAL1 mutations are responsible for Kallmann syndrome 1. Kallmann syndrome 2 results from mutations in the *FGFR1* or *FGF8* gene. Mutations in the *PROKR2* and *PROK2* (prokineticin receptor-2 and prokineticin-2) genes causes Kallmann syndrome types 3 and 4, respectively. Additional features, such as the cleft palate occur only in types 1 and 2. Mutations in the *KAL1*, *FGFR1*, *PROKR2*, or *PROK2* genes disrupt the migration of olfactory nerve cells and GnRH-producing nerve cells in the brain and therefore these patients have anosmia or hyposmia. Kallmann syndrome 1 (caused by KAL1 mutations) has an X-linked recessive pattern of inheritance and the gene is located on the X chromosome. Other forms of Kallmann syndrome are inherited in an autosomal dominant pattern. The goal of therapy in these patients is to restore sexual function, libido, well-being and behavior, and to optimize bone density and to prevent osteoporosis. Various forms of testosterone is available for replacement and the main aim is to keep the serum testosterone levels above the lower limit of normal, in the range of 250 to 300 ng/dL, just before the next injection. Fertility treatments in KS involves the administration of the gonadotropins LH and FSH in order to stimulate the production and release of eggs and sperms. Women with KS have an advantage over men as their ovaries usually contain a normal number of eggs.[1,2]

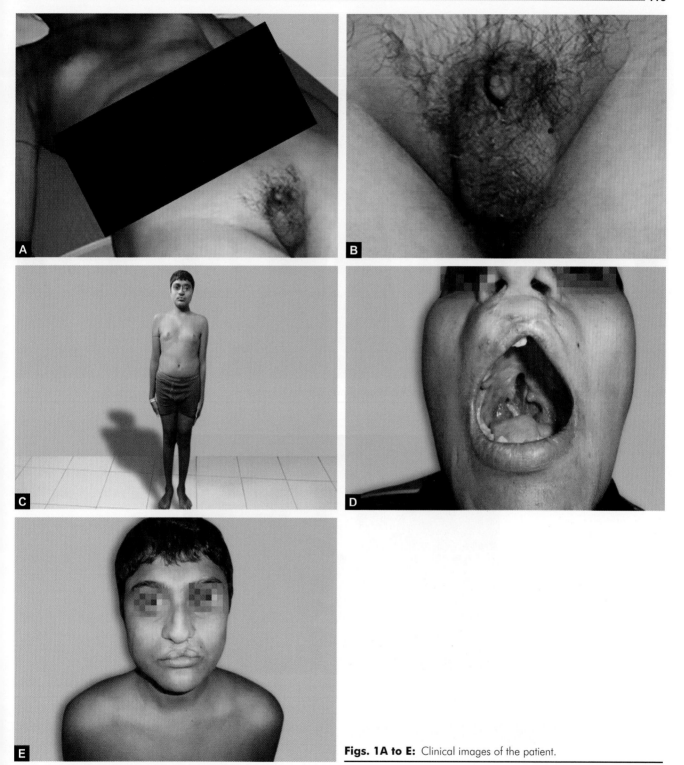

Figs. 1A to E: Clinical images of the patient.

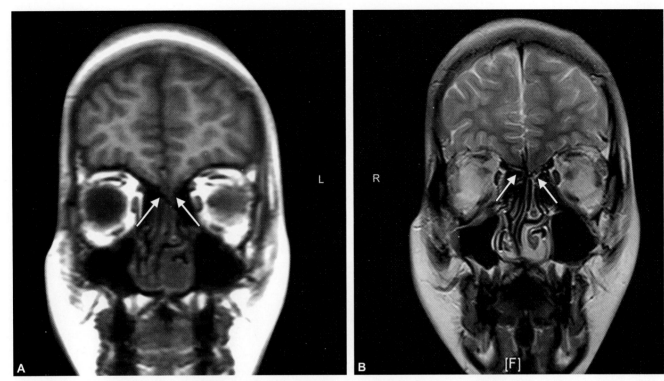

Figs. 2A and B: MRI of the brain showing absent olfactory bulbs (shown with the arrows).

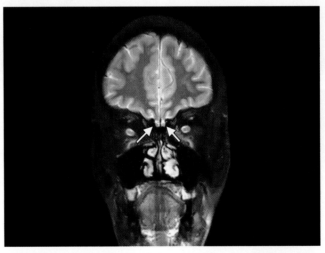

Fig. 3: Normal MRI of the brain showing olfactory bulbs (shown with the arrows).

REFERENCES

1. Fechner A, Fong S, McGovern P. A review of Kallmann syndrome: genetics, pathophysiology, and clinical management. Obstet Gynacol Surv. 2008;63(3):189–94.

2. Dodé C, Hardelin J-P. Kallmann syndrome. Eur J Hum Genet. 2008;17(2):139–46.

CASE 17

A 16-year-old boy born of a second degree consanguineous marriage was brought by his father with the complaints of small phallus as compared to his younger brother who was 14 years of age. A detailed clinical examination revealed only a small penis (Fig. 1). His height was 145 cm with mid parenteral height of 168 cm. His sexual maturity scoring was Tanner-1 with testes size of 1 mL bilaterally and poorly developed scrotum (Fig. 1).

WHAT ARE THE DIFFERENTIAL DIAGNOSIS?

His investigation revealed a suppressed testosterone level of < 20.0 ng/dL with follicular stimulating hormone (FSH) of 3.3/mL and leutinising hormone (LH) of 0.731. Other hormonal axes were within normal limits. His MRI brain revealed an absent Olfactory bulb and he was diagnosed to have Kallmann syndrome and was started on parenteral testosterone therapy.

DISCUSSION

A stretched penile length below minus 2.5 standard deviation of the mean in a patient with normal internal and external male genitalia warrant a diagnosis of micropenis. Traditional methods utilize a ruler or caliper to measure penile length. A modified syringe method also is used for the penile length measurement. The penile length should be measured when the penis is fully stretched, not flaccid; the measurement should be taken from the pubic ramus to the distal tip of the glans penis over the dorsal side. A different approach involves the use of a 10 mL disposable syringe wherein the needle-side of the syringe is cut off, and the piston is inserted into the syringe on the cut side. The piston is pulled back while pressing the fat pads inwards, which causes the penis to be pulled inside the syringe as a result of suction. This technique helps in the elimination of measurement differences caused by the suprapubic fat pad. Most patients referred to the endocrine out patient department (OPD) with a suspicion of micropenis are prepubertal and obese, and the small size of their penis is most often due to "buried penis", because of the suprapubic fat.

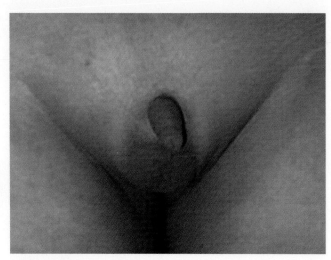

Fig. 1: Clinical image of the patient.

The differential diagnosis for the micropenis are:

Impaired testosterone production-Hypogonadotrophic hypogonadism- Kallmann syndrome, Prader-Willi syndrome, Laurence-Moon syndrome, Bardet-Biedl syndrome, Rud's syndrome or Primary hypogonadism- Anorchia, Klinefelter and poly-X syndromes, Gonadal dysgenesis (incomplete form), Luteinizing hormone receptor defect (incomplete form), Testosterone steroidogenesis (incomplete form), Noonan syndrome, Trisomy 21, Robinow syndrome.

Testosterone activation defects -Growth hormone/IGF-1 deficiency, androgen receptor defects (incomplete form), 5-α reductase deficiency (incomplete form) and fetal hydantoin syndrome.

The primary goals of the treatment for micropenis are to provide an acceptable body image and to enable the patient to have a normal sexual function.[1,2]

REFERENCES

1. Hatipoğlu N, Kurtoğlu S. Micropenis: Etiology, Diagnosis and Treatment Approaches. J Clin Res Pediatr Endocrinol. 2013 Dec;5(4):217–23.
2. Nerli R, Guntaka A, Patne P,et al. Penile growth in response to hormone treatment in children with micropenis. Indian J Urol. 2013;29(4):288.

CASE 18

A 32-year-old lady, not known to have diabetes mellitus presented with the chief complaints of recurrent loss of consciousness mainly during the fasting state for the last 4 years with symptoms being relieved by food intake. She had a gradual weight gain of 16 kg over the same duration. She had documented recurrent hypoglycemic episodes (glucose levels as low as up to 25 mg %) in the past two years.

WHAT IS THE PROBABLE DIAGNOSIS AND THE LINE OF MANAGEMENT?

Her investigations revealed a normal liver function test and a normal 8 am serum cortisol levels. She was subjected to a 72-hour fast test and within 2 hours of the start of the test she had developed hypoglycemia with a corresponding blood glucose level of 35 mg %. Her simultaneous serum insulin and C-Peptide levels were 10.8 (>3mIU/l) and 2.8 (>0.6 ng/mL) respectively, which were inappropriately high for the low glucose levels. Her CT abdomen with MRI cuts revealed a single intensely enhancing focal lesion in the uncinate process- (Figs. 1A and B) which was confirmed by an Endoscopic ultrasonogram.

She was told to take complex carbohydrate meals at frequent intervals to prevent hypoglycemia and started on diazoxide, preoperatively for the control of neuroglycopenic and neurogenic symptoms of hypoglycemia.

Subsequently she underwent excision of the lesion following which she was relieved of her symptoms. Her histopathological reports showed a polygonal tumour cells which were positive for synaptophysin and chromogranin and a MIB1 proliferation index of approximately 1–2%, all suggestive of a neuroendocrine tumour. She had a prediabetic range plasma glucose levels at three months follow up and was advised to follow life style modification.

DISCUSSION

Hypoglycemia can result from deficient glucose production, excessive glucose use, excessive external glucose loss, or a combination of these. Hypoglycemia is further classified as fasting and postprandial hypoglycemia. Fasting hypoglycemia implies the presence of disease and requires further evaluation.

Hypoglycemia due to excessive endogenous insulin secretion can be caused by a primary pancreatic β-cell disorder including an insulinoma, β-cell hyperplasia or nesidioblastosis. Patients with an insulinoma usually present with the symptoms of fasting hypoglycemia secondary to excessive and uncontrolled secretion of insulin.

Hypoglycemic symptoms can be divided into two categories: neuroglycopenic and neurogenic symptoms. Neuroglycopenic symptoms are due to central nervous

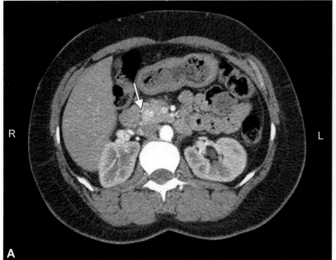
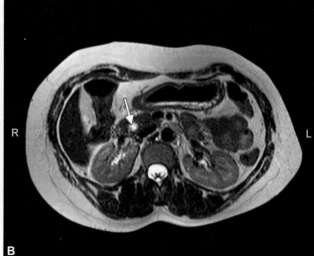

Figs. 1A and B: CT and MRI of the abdomen showing a discrete lesion in the uncinate process (shown with arrow).

system neuronal glucose deprivation which includes behavioral changes, confusion, visual changes, fatigue, seizures and loss of consciousness. The neurogenic symptoms are due to autonomic nervous system discharges caused by hypoglycemia. There are cholinergic symptoms which include hunger, sweating and parasthesias, and adrenergic symptoms which include anxiety, tremor and palpitations.

The presence of hypoglycemic symptoms with fulfilment of the following criteria is diagnostic for insulinoma: plasma glucose level of 2.5 mmol/L or lower (less than 45 mg%), insulin level of 6 μunits/mL (3 units) or higher, C-peptide level 0·2 nmol/L (0.6 ng/mL) or higher, and a negative sulphonylurea screen. A rise in peak plasma glucose concentration by 1·4 mmol/L (25 mg %) or more within 30 minutes in response to 1 mg of intravenous glucagon at the end of a prolonged fast indicates hyperinsulinemia. A number of techniques are available to localize a suspected insulinoma. An arterography was considered the "gold standard" for insulinoma localization. Surgical resection is the treatment of choice and offers the only chance of cure. With advances in the laparoscopic techniques, both laparoscopic enucleation and resection of pancreatic insulinomas have been performed successfully without any complications.[1,2]

REFERENCES

1. Service FJ, Natt N. The prolonged fast. J Clin Endocrinol Metab 2000;85:3973-4.
2. Gouya H, Vignaux O, Augui J, et al. CT, endoscopic sonography, and a combined protocol for preoperative evaluation of pancreatic insulinomas. AJR Am J Roentgenol 2003;181: 987-92.

CASE 19

An 18-year-old girl was referred to the endocrinology OPD with complaints of short stature, compared to her peer group. She was born to a consanguineous marriage of a normal non assisted delivery with no perinatal illnesses. She was found to be short since her early school days. She attained menarche at the age of 14 years. However, she did not have any pubertal growth spurt.

WHAT IS THE PROBABLE DIAGNOSIS? HOW WILL YOU MANAGE THIS PATIENT?

The clinical examination revealed a doll-like, cherubic face with a height of 115 cm (Mid parenteral height-155 cm) and a height standard deviation of less than the 5th centile. All her hormonal axes were normal except for a low level of Insulin like Growth factor (IFG-1) for her age and sex. With the clinical and biochemical finding growth hormone deficiency was diagnosed. However, due to her financial background the family forgoes the treatment with growth hormone replacement at present.

DISCUSSION

There is a higher frequency of breech presentation and perinatal asphyxia in patients with growth hormone deficiency. Neonatal morbidity may include hypoglycemia and prolonged jaundice. Children with acquired Growth Hormone Deficiency (GHD) present with severe growth failure, delayed bone age, increased weight/height ratios, fat distribution often "infantile", "doll-like", or "angel-like" (cherubic) in pattern, and immature face with under-developed nasal bridge and frontal bossing (Fig. 1). The voice is infantile, and hair growth is sparse and thin. The penis may be small, and puberty is usually delayed.

The Consensus Statement Criteria to Initiate Evaluation for GHD are

1. "Severe" short stature (height < –3 SD below mean)
2. Height < –1.5 SD below mid-parental height
3. Height < –2 SD below mean and either height velocity < –1 SD below mean over past year or decrease in height SD of more than 0.5 SD over the past year

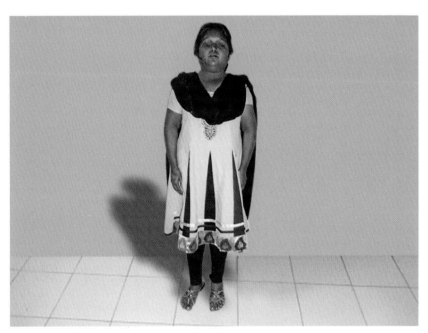

Fig. 1: Clinical image showing a cherubic face.

4. In the absence of short stature, height velocity < -2 SD below mean over 1 year or < -1.5 SD below mean over 2 years
5. Signs of an intracranial lesion
6. Signs of multiple pituitary hormone deficiency
7. Neonatal signs and symptoms of GHD, including hypoglycemia, prolonged jaundice, microphallus, or craniofacial midline abnormalities

Tools for the diagnosis of GHD include auxology, radiographic assessment of bone age, measurement of insulin-like growth factor 1 (IGF-I) and IGF binding protein 3 (IGFBP-3), provocative Growth Hormone (GH) testing, cranial magnetic resonance imaging (MRI), and, in certain cases, genetic testing. The most common provocative agents include insulin induced hypoglycemia, glucagon, clonidine, propranolol, arginine, GnRH or L-dopa. A peak stimulated Growth Hormone (GH) of less than 10 mcg/L is the usual cut-off for GH deficiency in children in the western countries, however we employ the cut-offs of 5 mcg/L . The exercise and sleep test, is not used very often in clinical practice for GHD. The dose of GH has traditionally been expressed as unit/kg/day. Recently there is a trend of using mg/kg/day or mg/m^2/week for calculation of dose of GH.

As per WHO standards 1 mg of recombinant GH has a bioactivity equivalent to 3 IU. Dose of 0.18–0.35 mg/kg/week (0.1–0.15 IU/kg/day, 25–50 mcg/kg/day, 4.5–9.5 mg/m^2/week, 15–30 IU/m^2/week) therefore represents physiological replacement dose for GHD. It is appropriate to give 2–4 units/m^2/day which is almost 1 mg/day GH therapy is associated with significant improvement in growth velocity, which increases from 3–4 cm/year before therapy to 10–12 cm/year during the first two years of treatment. This sustained growth is usually not maintained and the growth velocity declines to 7–8 cm/year after a period of two years. Inappropriate response to GH therapy should prompt evaluation of compliance, injection technique, hypothyroidism or reconsideration of the diagnosis of GHD.[1,2]

REFERENCES

1. Stanley T. Diagnosis of growth hormone deficiency in childhood. Curr Opin Endocrinol Diabetes Obes. 2012;19(1): 47–52.
2. Shalet SM, Toogood A, Rahim A,et al . The Diagnosis of Growth Hormone Deficiency in Children and Adults. Endocr Rev. 1998;19(2):203–23.

CASE **20**

A 21-year-old lady was brought by her mother for being shortest in the family. His brother was investigated and was on treatment for the same. She was born of a second degree consanguineous marriage. Her height was 110 cm with mid parenteral height of 155 cm. She had a small face with prominent forehead, depressed nasal bridge and small mandible (Fig. 1). She also had a high pitched voice. Otherwise her intelligence was normal.

WHAT IS THE CLINICAL DIAGNOSIS?

Her investigations revealed normal hormonal axes with high serum Growth Hormone and low Insulin like Growth factor (IGF-1) levels. With the clinical findings she was diagnosed to have growth hormone insensitivity syndrome-Larons dwarfism. Her X-ray of the wrist and hand showed fusion of all the long bones. So she was planned to be kept on follow-up.

DISCUSSION

Laron syndrome, or Laron-type dwarfism, is an autosomal recessive disorder characterized by an insensitivity to growth hormone (GH). The principal feature of Laron syndrome is abnormally short stature (dwarfism) with physical symptoms that include prominent forehead, depressed nasal bridge, underdevelopment of mandible, truncal obesity and a very small penis. Seizures are frequently seen secondary to hypoglycemia and prolonged jaundice and occur in neonates. Administration of GH has no effect on IGF-1 production, therefore treatment is mainly by biosynthetic IGF-1. IGF-1 must be offered before puberty to be effective. IPLEX (Mecasermin rinfabate) is composed of recombinant human IGF-1 (rhIGF-1) and its binding protein IGFBP-3 and was approved for the treatment of primary IGF-1 deficiency or GH gene deletion.[1,2]

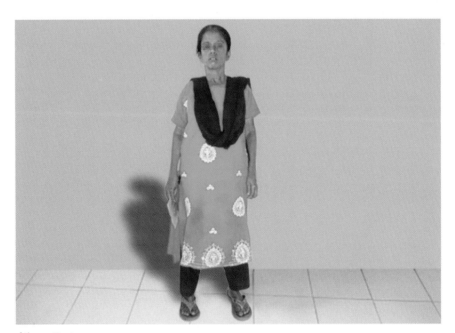

Fig. 1: Clinical image of the patient.

REFERENCES

1. Hardin D. Treatment of short stature and growth hormone deficiency in children with somatotropin (rDNA origin). Biol Targets Ther. 2008;655.

2. Berg MA, Argente J, Chernausek S, et al. Diverse growth hormone receptor gene mutations in Laron syndrome. Am J Hum Genet. 1993;52(5):998–1005.

CASE 21

A 45-year-old lady, Mrs. S presented with chief complaints of abdominal pain for the past 3 years, loose stools since the past 2 and 1/2 years and abnormal pulsations in the right side of the neck for the past 1 year. Her clinical examination showed a massive hepatosplenomegaly (Fig. 1). Her neck examination revealed a prominent V wave with a rapid Y descent (Figs. 2A to C). Her colonoscopy showed a thickened ileocecal junction. The Computed Tomography (CT) scan of the abdomen is shown in Figures 3A and B. The biopsy from the ileoceacal junction showed a tumor of neuroendocrine origin. So, a DOTATATE PET scan done to rule out metastasis is shown in Figures 3A to F.

WHAT IS THE DIAGNOSIS?

Echocardiography showed a severe Tricuspid Regurgitation (TR) with normal LV function. Based on the clinical and biochemical features she was diagnosed to have Carcinoid syndrome of the terminal ileum with metastasis and severe Tricuspid Regurgitation due to Carcinoid heart syndrome. She was referred to nuclear medicine department for the Lutetium-177 DOTATATE therapy. Her diarrhoea was managed with loperamide.

DISCUSSION

Tricuspid and pulmonary valve regurgitation occur usually as a secondary phenomena caused by dilatation of the valve ring consequent to right ventricular failure or pulmonary hypertension. Primary diseases of the tricuspid or pulmonary valves are uncommon. Carcinoid heart disease is a rare cause of intrinsic tricuspid and pulmonary valve disease leading to significant morbidity and mortality caused by right heart failure. Carcinoid tumours are a rare neuroendocrine malignancies arising from the neural crest amine precursor uptake decarboxylation

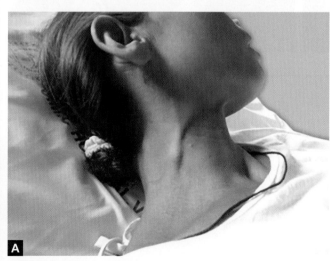

Fig. 1: Showing massive heapatosplenomegaly.

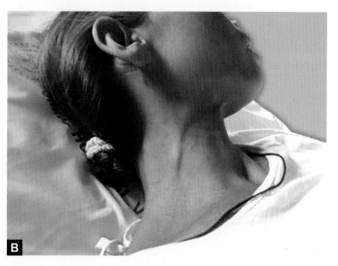

Figs. 2A and B

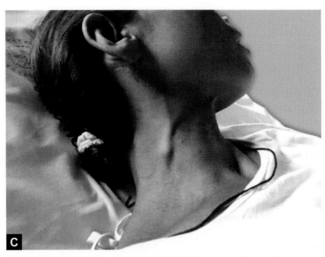

Figs. 2A to C: Sequential images showing prominent V waves and rapid y descents in the jugular venous pulse.

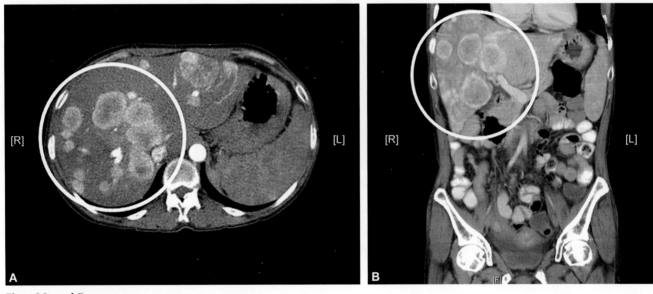

Figs. 3A and B

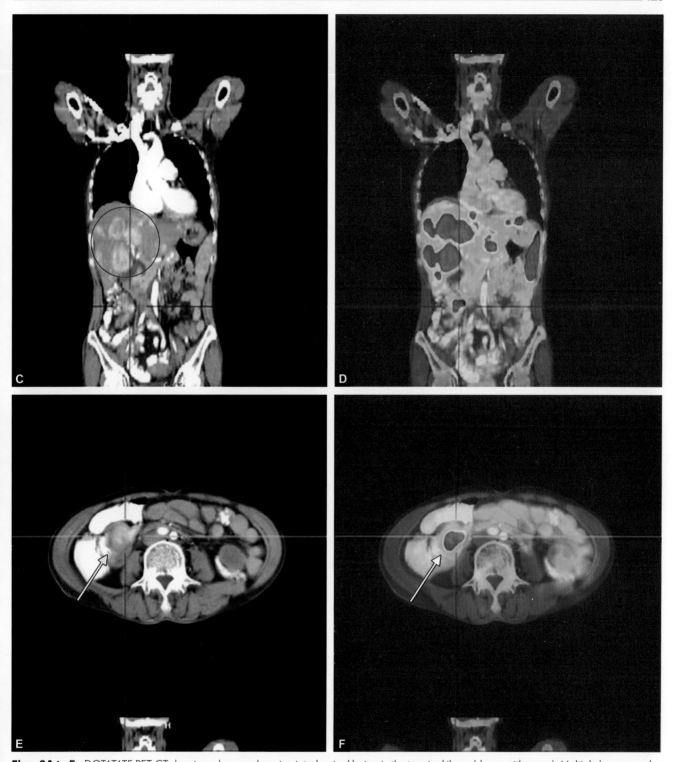

Figs. 3A to F: DOTATATE PET-CT showing a hyper enhancing intraluminal lesion in the terminal ileum (shown with arrow). Multiple hypervascular lesions of varying sizes in both lobes of the liver-hypervascular metastases (shown with a circle).

cells. Over 90% of all carcinoid tumors are located in the gastrointestinal system and the appendix and terminal ileum are the most common sites. The most malignant of the carcinoid tumors are characterized by facial flushing, intractable secretory diarrhea, and bronchoconstriction. Only the carcinoid tumors that invade the liver cause the pathological changes to the heart. The cardiac manifestations are caused by the paraneoplastic effects of vasoactive substances such as 5-hydroxytryptamine (5-HT or serotonin), histamine, tachykinins, and prostaglandins that are released by the malignant cells. Medical management consists of relieving symptoms of right heart failure with a combination of loop and thiazide diuretic therapy.[1,2]

REFERENCES

1. Fox DJ, Khattar RS. Carcinoid heart disease: presentation, diagnosis, and management. Heart. 2004;90(10):1224-8.
2. Bhattacharyya S, Davar J, Dreyfus G, et al. Carcinoid Heart Disease. Circulation. 2007;116(24):2860-5.

CASE **22**

A 45-year-old Bank officer was referred to the endocrine OPD from the dermatology department with history of skin hyperpigmentation and to rule out Addison's disease. He was normotensive on examination. He had palmar crease hyperpigmentation with no mucosal involvement (Fig. 1A). His central nervous system examination revealed a decreased vibration sense up to both the ankle joints with depressed ankle jerks and exaggerated knee joints reflexes. He had mild swaying while closing the eyes with negative cerebellar signs.

WHAT IS THE DIAGNOSIS?

Investigations revealed normal serum 8 AM cortisol levels and normal thyroid stimulating hormone (TSH) levels. He was a vegan since birth. His serum vitamin B12 levels were undetectable. He was started on parenteral vitamin B12 (1000 mcg daily for a week followed by once a week for 1 month and once a month). Within 3 months of the replacements, his palmar hyperpigmentation disappeared (Fig. 1B). Thus, he was diagnosed to have vitamin B12 deficiency causing skin hyperpigmentation.

DISCUSSION

The endocrine causes of hyperpigmentation are Addison's disease, Adrenocorticotropic Hormone (ACTH) dependent cushing's syndrome, acromegaly, Nelson's syndrome, vitamin B12 deficiency, thyrotoxicosis, primary hemochromatosis, porphyria and mercury poisoning.

Vitamin B12 deficiency was first described by Cook in 1944 and later by Baker et al., in 1963. Currently, vitamin B12 deficiency is defined as a plasma concentration of < 148 pmol/L (200 pg/mL) and marginal status defined as a concentration of 148–221 pmol/L. The main source of vitamin B12 (cobalamin) in humans is the consumption of meat, poultry and dairy products. The common systemic features reported are fatigue, glossitis, weight loss and anorexia with hyper pigmentation of skin being a rare symptom.

The histology from the hyper pigmented area show an irregular epidermal atrophy, absence of basal orientation of epidermal cells, patchy pigmentation of the lower epidermis, and numerous pigment-laden macrophages in the upper dermis and increase of melanin in the basal

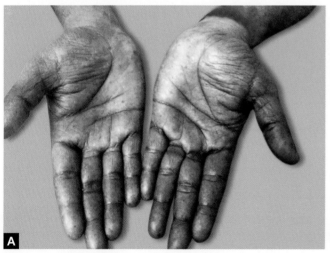
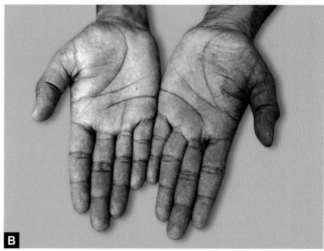

Figs. 1A and B: Patient's palms before and after treatment.

layer. It was suggested that deficiency of vitamin B12 causes a decrease in the intracellular reduction potential and thereby an oxidation of the reduced glutathione and decrease in Reduced Glutathione/Oxidised Glutathione GSH/GSSG ratio. Thus the epidermal melanocytes are stimulated to produce melanin as the tyrosinase inhibiting effect of GSH has been diminished. So, the predominant mechanism of hyperpigmentation in vitamin B12 is hypothesized as 1). Deficiency of vitamin B12 decreases the level of reduced glutathione, which activates tyrosinase and thus leads to transfer to melanosomes. 2) Defect in the melanin transfer between melanocytes and keratinocytes, resulting in pigmentary incontinence.[1,2]

REFERENCES

1. Mori K, Ando I, Kukita A. Generalized hyperpigmentation of the skin due to vitamin B12 deficiency. J Dermatol. 2001;28:282–5.
2. Aaron S, Kumar S, Vijayan J, et al . Clinical and laboratory features and response to treatment in patients presenting with vitamin B12 deficiency-related neurological syndromes. Neurol India. 2005;53:55–8.

CASE 23

A 45-year-old gentleman was referred to the endocrine OPD for the evaluation of recent onset weight gain of 26 kg over the past 6 months. He gave history of intake of unnamed medications which he was prescribed for his aches and pains by a traditional practitioner (Fig. 1). He did not have any addictions in the past. His clinical images are displayed in Figures 2A and B.

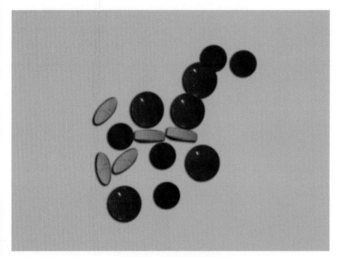

Fig. 1: Images of the unnamed medications the patient was on.

WHAT IS THE CLINICAL DIAGNOSIS?

His clinical evaluation revealed a round Cushingoid face (Fig. 2A) with purplish striae over the anterior abdominal wall (Fig. 2B). He was found to have normal liver and renal functions. However, his serum 8 am cortisol was undetectable. Thus, he was diagnosed to have exogenous cushings syndrome with hypothalamic pituitary and adrenal axis suppression. He was started on oral steroids and planned for tapering of the same over a period of 6 months. He was instructed to follow stress hydrocortisone protocol during any acute illness or stress. He was also found to have impaired glucose tolerance and was advised lifestyle modification.

DISCUSSION

Glucocorticoid misuse is an important problem which has been inadequately addressed in the rural and semi-urban communities in most part of the Indian subcontinent. With the easy availability of the steroids over the counter has been one of the most misused drugs. The patients are prescribed steroids by uncertified doctors due to their potential effect as analgesics. Thus, it is used mainly by the people who are engaged in heavy works. Patients continued to take without the knowledge of

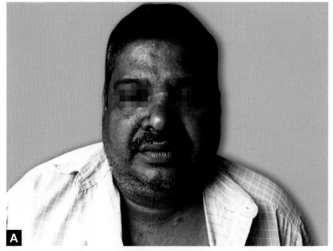

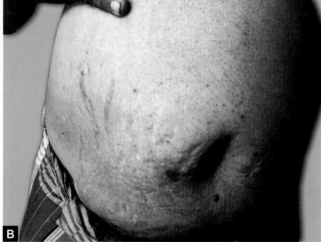

Figs. 2A and B: (A) Clinical image showing a cushingoid face, (B) purplish striae over the abdomen.

the side effects caused by the steroids and most often report to the higher centers with features of cushings syndrome or hypoadrenal crisis. Hypoadrenal crisis is a medical emergency and has to be treated with parenteral hydrocortisone or dexamethasone. Subsequently with oral steroids once the patient recovers. Some patients need to be on oral steroids, which are gradually tapered over a period of 6 to 12 months allowing for the complete recovery of the Hypothalamic-Pituitary-Adrenal axis.[1,2]

REFERENCES

1. Nalli C, Armstrong L, Finny P, et al. Glucocorticoid misuse in a rural and semi-urban community of North Bihar: a pilot study. Trop Doct. 2012;42(3):168–70.
2. Tempark T, Phatarakijnirund V, Chatproedprai S, et al. Exogenous Cushing's syndrome due to topical corticosteroid application: case report and review literature. Endocrine. 2010;38(3):328–34.

CASE **24**

A 24-year-old gentleman presented to the diabetes clinic for the evaluation of his glycemic status. Detailed history revealed that he also planning for the treatment of his primary infertility. He explained that he had never shaved in his life time as he had absent facial hair growth with absent axillary and pubic hair too. (Fig. 1). He had slate like hyperpigmentation of the skin involving the whole body (Fig. 2).

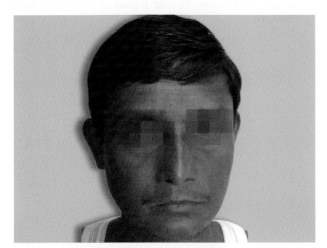

Fig. 1: Clinical image of the patient.

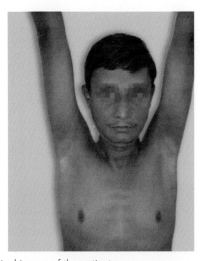

Fig. 2: Clinical image of the patient.

WHAT IS THE CLINICAL DIAGNOSIS?

He had testicular volume of 5 mL bilaterally and he explained that he had erectile dysfunction. He did not have signs of hypocalcaemia. He had poor Glycaemic control with fasting and post prandial plasma glucose being high with a HbA1c level of 12%. His investigations revealed low FSH, LH and a suppressed testosterone levels. He also had low serum 8 am cortisol with biochemical features of central hypothyroidism. His serum calcium and phosphate levels were within normal limits. He was found to have a high ferritin level of 2236 ng/mL (10–290) with serum iron of 262 mcg/dL (40–145). The MRI brain showed a small pituitary gland (Fig. 3).

Hence, he was diagnosed to have primary hemochromatosis with panhypopituitarism with Bronze diabetes. He was initiated on hormonal supplements and was initiated on insulin for his insulinopenic status. He was referred to the Department of Hematology for repeated venesection as a treatment for hemochromatosis.

DISCUSSION

Classic hereditary hemochromatosis (HH) is an autosomal recessive iron-overload disorder associated with the

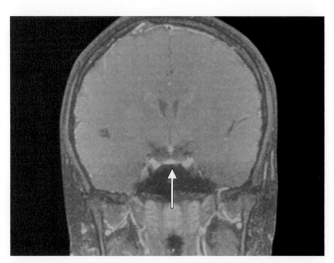

Fig. 3: MRI of the brain showing a small pituitary gland (shown with arrow).

mutation of the *HFE* gene located on chromosome 6. Symptomatic organ involvement often begins in the mid-life. Liver disease (ranging from a slightly elevated aminotransferase levels, with or without hepatomegaly, to cirrhosis and even hepatocellular carcinoma) usually predominates, but endocrine disorders (diabetes, hypogonadotropic hypogonadism, impotence, and hypothyroidism), cardiac problems (arrhythmias and heart failure), and joint disease (destructive arthritis) are also found in patients with HH. These patients have inappropriately high duodenal transfer of iron to the plasma. Once the diagnosis of hereditary hemochromatosis (adult- or juvenile-onset) has been established, further clinical workup is necessary to define its possible visceral or metabolic consequences. In young adults with signs of juvenile-onset disease (with hypogonadotropic hypogonadism or unexplained heart failure), the biochemical workup of HH is warranted. Phlebotomy is the safest, most effective, and most economical therapeutic approach which is done weekly until the serum ferritin level is less than 50 ng per milliliter and the transferrin saturation drops to a value below 30 percent of the baseline.[1,2]

REFERENCES

1. Whittington CA, Kowdley KV. Review article: haemochromatosis. Aliment Pharmacol Ther. 2002 Dec;16(12):1963–75.
2. Pietrangelo A. Hereditary Hemochromatosis — A New Look at an Old Disease. N Engl J Med. 2004 Jun 3;350(23): 2383–97.

CASE 25

An 18-year-old lady presented to the endocrine OPD for evaluation of short stature and primary amenorrhea. She had been diagnosed with diabetes mellitus and hypothyroidism at the age of 10 years and was on treatment. On examination she had excessive body hair with a Ferriman gallwey score of 12. She had icthyotic hyperpigmented patches on her legs and lower abdomen. She had short stature and widely spaced eyes. She had bilateral sensory neural hearing loss. She had poor development of secondary sexual characteristics. She was also found to have clinodactyly (Figs. 1 to 5).

WHAT IS THE DIAGNOSIS?

Further biochemical evaluation revealed hypogonadotropic hypogonadism. She was found to have a normal female karyotype. Echocardiogram showed a bicuspid aortic valve. Genetic analysis was done and next generation

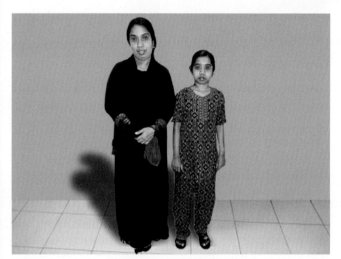

Fig. 1: Short stature.

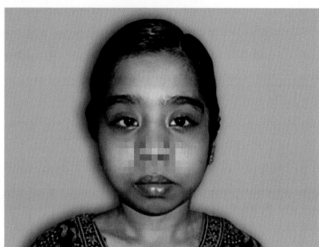

Fig. 2: Hypertelorism.

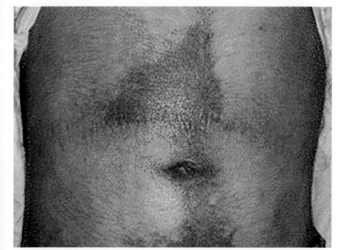

Fig. 3: Hyperpigmented patches over the abdomen.

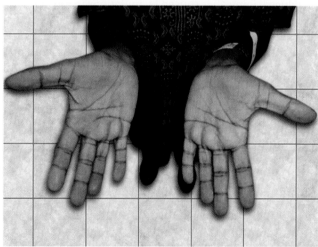

Fig. 4: Clinodactyly.

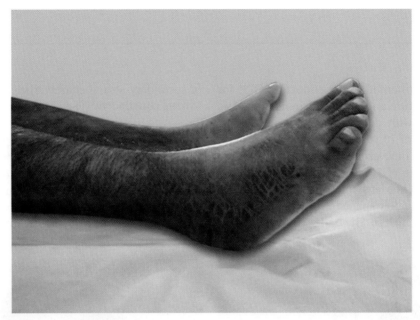

Fig. 5: Hypertrichosis, fixed ankle contracture.

sequencing revealed a mutation in the *SLC29 A3* gene, which encodes the equilibrative nucleoside transporter hENT3.

DISCUSSION

The H syndrome is an autosomal-recessive disorder characterized by cutaneous hyperpigmentation, hypertrichosis, hepatosplenomegaly, heart anomalies, hearing loss, hypogonadism, short stature, hallux valgus, and fixed flexion contractures of the toe joints and the proximal interphalangeal joints. It is caused by mutations in the *SLC29A3* gene, which encodes the equilibrative nucleoside transporter hENT3.[1] The term H syndrome refers to the major clinical and laboratory findings of *h*yperpigmentation and *h*ypertrichosis, *h*epatosplenomegaly, *h*eart anomalies, *h*earing loss, *h*ypogonadism, low *h*eight, and occasionally,

*h*yperglycemia.[2] These patients have characteristic hyperpigmented, hypertrichotic, and indurated cutaneous patches involving the middle and lower parts of the body. Histopathological examination of involved skin shows hyperpigmentation of the basal layer with seborrheic keratosis-like acanthosis and infiltration of CD68-positive histiocytes. Awareness of this disorder helps in early diagnosis when patients present with this distinctive constellation of clinical features.

REFERENCES

1. Molho-Pessach V, Lerer I, Abeliovich D, et al. The H Syndrome Is Caused by Mutations in the Nucleoside Transporter hENT3. Am J Hum Genet. 2008 Oct 10;83(4):529–34.
2. Priya TP, Philip N, Molho-Pessach V, et al. H syndrome: novel and recurrent mutations in SLC29A3. Br J Dermatol. 2010 May 1;162(5):1132–4.

MULTIPLE CHOICE QUESTIONS

1. In humans, the androgen receptor is encoded by the *AR*-gene located on the X chromosome at Xq11-12. The *AR* gene contains a variable tract of CAG/CAA triplets that encode a polyglutamate repeat. Diseases associated with shortened variations in the androgen receptor glutamine repeat include all *EXCEPT:*
   A. Coronary artery disease
   B. Kennedy's disease
   C. Prostate cancer
   D. Androgenic alopecia

2. A 28-year-old married lady presented with history of primary infertility. Her menstrual cycle was normal. No significant hormonal abnormality was detected. Hysterosalpingogram (HSG) followed by laparoscopy finding was suggestive of tubal block. Evaluation of her male partner was not significant. What is the best treatment option of her infertility?
   A. Clomiphene citrate (*see* below) with or without intrauterine insemination (IUI),
   B. Gonadotropins with or without IUI
   C. In vitro fertilization (IVF)
   D. Expectant management

3. Which of the following is true regarding neuroendocrine tumor?
   A. Somatostatinoma is associated with characteristic skin lesion necrolytic migratory erythema
   B. Gastrinoma is characterized by triad of diabetes mellitus ,steatorrhoea and cholelithiasis
   C. Gastrinoma is the most common enteropancreatic tumor associated with MEN
   D. Endoscopic ultrasonography is very sensitive for the detection of insulinomas located at pancreatic tail

4. All the following can cause an increase in serum sodium *EXCEPT:*
   A. Tolvaptan
   B. Demeclocycline
   C. Carbamazepine
   D. Lithium

5. A 30-year-old gentleman, a long distance runner presents with chest pain on exertion. Historically, he is a nonsmoker and teetotaler. On examination he is 178 cm tall and has an arm-span of 190 cm. An ECG shows evidence of an anterior wall myocardial infarction. What other clinical anomaly would you find in this patient?
   A. Mitral regurgitation
   B. Aortic aneurysm
   C. Dislocated lens
   D. Aortic regurgitation

6. Following his recovery, he has a fall while climbing down the staircase and fractured his tibia on trivial trauma. A DXA scan of the spine is done, the most likely finding in this patient is:
   A. T score +1.0, Z score +1
   B. T Score -2.5, Z score -3.5
   C. T score +1.0, Z score +0.0
   D. T score-3.0, Z score -.2.0

7. One therapeutic agent that has been tried in this condition is:
   A. Hematin
   B. Betaine
   C. Ascorbic acid
   D. Xanthine

8. A 25-year-old gentleman presents with a sudden onset of loss of consciousness. He is found to have serum sodium of 106 mmol/L (Normal 135–144 mmol/L). He does not have any previous history of illness and is not on any medications. He has not had vomiting or been on diuretics. His urine spot sodium is 60 mmol/L.

   Which of the following are not relevant in this situation to establish a conclusive diagnosis:
   A. 8.00 am Cortisol
   B. Urinary delta ALA levels
   C. TSH/T4
   D. Serum electrophoresis

9. He is an occasional social drinker, but claims he had a binge the previous night with a large ingestion of alcohol. He is started on 3% saline and thiamine as well. He recovers. The next day, he passes very dark colored urine. The urinary microscopy is negative. What other symptom would you expect him to have:
   A. Renal stones
   B. Peripheral neuropathy
   C. Angina
   D. Emphysema

10. This condition is commonly:
    A. Autosomal dominant
    B. Autosomal recessive
    C. X-linked Dominant
    D. X-linked recessive

    Match the following (Applicable for 11 to 15)

    Options –
    A. Sertoli cell only syndrome

B. 11-Deoxycorticosterone

C. 17- hydroxyprogesterone

D. Complete androgen Insensitivity Syndrome

E. 17 alpha hydroxylase deficiency

F. MRK syndrome

G. Partial androgen insensitivity syndrome with non scrotal gonads

H. 3 beta-hydroxysteroid type 2 deficiency

I. 17 beta HSD deficiency

J. Ovotesticular testicular DSD

11. One-month-old new born child presented with history of ambiguous external genitalia with small penis and hypospadias. The baby was apparently asymptomatic for initial 3 weeks current admitted with nausea, vomiting, low blood pressure with signs of dehydration. On examination, bilateral gonads were palpable in labioscortal fold. Biochemical investigations showed elevation of 17 hydroxypregnenolone to cortisol ratio. What is the likely diagnosis in this case?

12. A 15-year-old female attended endocrine OPD for the evaluation of primary amenorrhea. Clinical evaluation revealed poor development of secondary sexual features (SMR- B2P1). She had history of taken medication for a period of 1 year however, she failed to menstruate. Her BP was 150/100 mm Hg, and pulse was – 87/min. An ultrasound of abdomen showed hypoplastic uterus and presence of fallopian tube and ovary. What is the likely diagnosis?

13. What is most likely cause of hypertension in the previous case?

14. A 17-year-old female attended endocrine OPD for evaluation of primary amenorrhea. She was tallest of all her siblings. On examination she had appropriate breast development (Tanner stage of B3) along with scanty axillary and pubic hair. External genitalia showed a blind vaginal pouch, bilateral inguinal hernia resemblance like that of gonads on palpation. Ultrasound of the abdomen showed no mullerian structure. Hormonal evaluation showed marked elevation of testosterone, Leutinising Hormone (LH) with mild elevation of Follicular Stimulating Hormone (FSH).

15. Higher risk for germ cell malignancy is seen in patients of which disorder of sex development.

Match the following (Applicable for 16 to 19)

Options:

A. Noonan syndrome

B. Turner syndrome

C. Father height + mother height /2 ± 6.5

D. SDS equal the child height – mean height for age and sex/SD of height of normal child for age and sex

E. Russell Silver syndrome

F. Pseudohypoparathyroidism

G. Elevated FSH and LH level

H. Low calcium, high PTH

I. Mauriac syndrome

J. Double diabetes

16. Growth failure can occur in diabetic children with long-standing type -1 diabetes with poor glycemic control. This is characterized by severe growth failure, and hepatosplenomegaly due to excess hepatic glycogen deposition. This type of growth retardation has become increasingly rare with modern diabetes care. What is the name of this clinical condition?

17. Height Standard Deviation Score (SDS) for age is calculated by:

18. A 10-year-old girl was evaluated for short stature. On examination she her height was below < 3rd centile. She had rounded face, shortened fourth and other metacarpals and obesity. Her MRI brain showed basal ganglia calcification. What is the likely diagnosis?

19. A 10-year-old girl attended Endocrine Outpatient Department for evaluation of short stature. Her birth weight of 2100 gm, length at birth was 43 cm. She had failure to thrive and had history post natal growth failure. On examination she had triangular facies and side hemi hypertrophy. What is the likely diagnosis?

20. State whether the following statements are true or false in patients with lipodystrophy

A. Patients with lipodystrophy are severely insulin resistant

B. Pioglitazone can be used in patients with Human Immunodeficiency Virus (HIV) lipodystrophy

C. Koeberling Dunnigan syndrome is a partial lipodystrophy

D. The Koberling syndrome can have a Lamin gene mutation

ANSWERS FOR THE MULTIPLE CHOICE QUESTIONS

Chapter 1: The Terrific Thyroid

| 1. C | 2. D | 3. D | 4. D | 5. D | 6. D | 7. D | 8. C | 9. B | 10. D |

| 11. D | 12. D | 13. D | 14. D | 15. B | 16. D | 17. C | 18. C |

19. A. *True* B. *True* C. *False* D. *True*   20. A. *False* B. *False* C. *False* D. *True*

Chapter 2: Diabolical Diabetes

| 1. B | 2. D | 3. A | 4. D | 5. C | 6. C | 7. D | 8. B | 9. A | 10. C |

| 11. D | 12. A | 13. A | 14. C | 15. A | 16. C | 17. B | 18. C | 19. A | 20. A |

| 21. D | 22. C | 23. B | 24. D | 25. B | 26. B | 27. A | 28. B | 29. A |

30. A. *False* B. *False* C. *True* D. *True*

Chapter 3: Aggressive Adrenal

| 1. D | 2. A | 3. C | 4. B | 5. D | 6. A | 7. B | 8. C | 9. C | 10. B |

Chapter 4: Pituitary Passions

| 1. C | 2. A | 3. D | 4. B | 5. B | 6. A | 7. A | 8. D | 9. B | 10. D |

| 11. B | 12. C | 13. B | 14. B |

15. A. *True* B. *True* C. *True* D. *True*

Chapter 5: Bountiful Bone

| 1. C | 2. B | 3. A | 4. B | 5. B | 6. D | 7. B | 8. a. D b. A c. B |

9. a. I b. D c. G   10. a. D b. I c. B d. G e. F

Chapter 6: Endocrine Miscellany

| 1. B | 2. C | 3. C | 4. C | 5. C | 6. B | 7. B | 8. D | 9. B | 10. A |

| 11. H | 12. E | 13. B | 14. D | 15. G | 16. I | 17. D | 18. F | 19. E |

20. A. *True* B. *True* C. *True* D. *True*

Index